HANDBOOK

....

OF DIFFICULT AIRWAY

....

MANAGEMENT

....

Carin A. Hagberg, MD

Associate Professor of Anesthesiology and Director of
*   Residency Education*
University of Texas Medical School at Houston
Staff Anesthesiologist
Hermann Hospital
Lyndon B. Johnson General Hospital
Houston, Texas

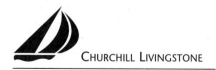

CHURCHILL LIVINGSTONE

A Division of Harcourt Brace & Company

Philadelphia   London   Toronto   Montreal   Sydney   Tokyo   Edinburgh

CHURCHILL LIVINGSTONE
A Division of Harcourt Brace & Company

The Curtis Center
Independence Square West
Philadelphia, Pennsylvania 19106

Library of Congress Cataloging-in-Publication Data

Handbook of difficult airway management / [edited by] Carin A. Hagberg. —1st ed.

p.   cm.

ISBN 0–443–07788–6

1. Respiratory organs—Obstructions—Treatment—Handbooks, manuals,
    etc.   2. Trachea—Intubation—Handbooks, manuals, etc.   I. Hagberg,
    Carin A.

RC776.03H36 2000   615.8′36—dc21

DNLM/DLC   98-31197

HANDBOOK OF DIFFICULT AIRWAY MANAGEMENT   ISBN 0–443–07788–6

Printed in the United States of America.

Last digit is the print number: 9   8   7   6   5   4   3   2   1

To my three wonderful daughters,
Alessandra, Ellie, and Catherine,
who constantly inspire me
and never cease to amaze me.
God bless.

Contributors

Ramiro Arellano, MD, MSc, FRCP(C)
Assistant Professor, Department of Anesthesia, Dalhousie University, Halifax, Nova Scotia, Canada

The Airway and Clinical Postoperative Conditions; Medical Conditions Affecting the Airway: A Synopsis

Jonathan L. Benumof, MD
Professor of Anesthesia, University of California, San Diego, School of Medicine; University of California, San Diego, Medical Center, La Jolla, California

ASA Difficult Airway Algorithm: New Thoughts and Considerations

Michelle Bowman-Howard, MD
Chief of Anesthesiology, Sugar Land Methodist Health Center, Sugar Land, Texas

Management of the Traumatized Airway; Effective Dissemination of Critical Airway Information

Jon P. Bradrick, DDS
Associate Professor and Director, Division of Oral and Maxillofacial Surgery, University of Texas Medical School at Houston; Associate Professor, Oral and Maxillofacial Surgery, Lyndon B. Johnson General Hospital, Houston, Texas

Surgical Approaches to Airway Management for Anesthesia Practitioners

D. John Doyle, MD, PhD

Associate Professor, Department of Anesthesia, University of Toronto Faculty of Medicine, Toronto, Ontario, Canada

The Airway and Clinical Postoperative Conditions; Medical Conditions Affecting the Airway: A Synopsis

Anita Giezentanner, MD

Assistant Professor of Anesthesiology, University of Texas Medical School at Houston; Staff Anesthesiologist, Hermann Hospital, Lyndon B. Johnson General Hospital, Houston, Texas

The Difficult Obstetric Airway

Carin A. Hagberg, MD

Associate Professor of Anesthesiology and Director of Residency Education, University of Texas Medical School at Houston; Staff Anesthesiologist, Hermann Hospital, Lyndon B. Johnson General Hospital, Houston, Texas

The Difficult Obstetric Airway; Extubation of the Difficult Airway

Harold S. Minkowitz, MD

Anesthesiologist, Memorial Hospital-Memorial City, Houston, Texas

Airway Gadgets; Laryngeal Mask Airway and Esophageal Tracheal Combitube

Debra E. Morrison, MD

Assistant Clinical Professor of Anesthesiology, University of California, Irvine, Irvine Medical Center, Orange, California

Preparation of the Patient for Awake Intubation; Retrograde Intubation

Andranik Ovassapian, MD

Professor of Clinical Anesthesia, Department of Anesthesia and Critical Care, University of Illinois College of Medicine; Director, Airway Study and Training Center, University of Illinois Hospital at Chicago Medical Center, Chicago, Illinois

Prediction and Evaluation of the Difficult Airway; Flexible Fiberoptic Tracheal Intubation

C. Lee Parmley, MD, JD

Associate Anesthesiologist and Associate Professor of Anesthesiology and Critical Care, Department of Critical Care, M. D. Anderson Cancer Center, Houston, Texas

Difficult Airway in the Intensive Care Unit

Ronald J. Redden, DDS

Clinical Assistant Professor of Anesthesiology, Oral and Maxillofacial Surgery, Oral Pharmacology, University of Texas Health Science Center—Dental Branch; Clinical Assistant Professor of Anesthesiology, Oral and Maxillofacial Surgery, Lyndon B. Johnson General Hospital, Houston, Texas

Anatomic Airway Considerations in Anesthesia

Tyce Regan, MD

Staff Anesthesiologist, Spring Branch Medical Center, Houston, Texas

Extubation of the Difficult Airway; Effective Dissemination of Critical Airway Information

Antonio F. Sanchez, MD

Associate Clinical Professor of Anesthesiology, University of California, Irvine, Irvine Medical Center, Orange, California

Preparation of the Patient for Awake Intubation; Retrograde Intubation

Melissa Wheeler, MD

Assistant Professor of Anesthesiology, Northwestern University Medical School; Attending Anesthesiologist, Department of Anesthesiology, Children's Memorial Hospital, Chicago, Illinois

Prediction and Evaluation of the Difficult Airway; Flexible Fiberoptic Tracheal Intubation; The Difficult Pediatric Airway

Mark E. K. Wong, MD

Associate Professor, Oral and Maxillofacial Surgery, University of Texas Health Science Center—Dental Branch; Chief of Service, Oral and Maxillofacial Surgery, Lyndon B. Johnson General Hospital, Houston, Texas

Surgical Approaches to Airway Management for Anesthesia Practitioners

Foreword

This volume is entitled "Handbook of Difficult Airway Management," but it is actually far more than that. In my opinion, it is the most comprehensive, well-planned, and useful compendium summarizing the vast amount of work relating to airway management that has appeared over the last 10 years.

It is generally known that management improvements have led to a documented decline in the incidence of airway-related perioperative morbidity. Both the dissemination of information and the development of new techniques and devices have contributed to this gratifying fact.

As a student of the difficult airway, I have kept abreast of publications relating to the topic and witnessed the valuable efforts of the ASA and the multidisciplinary, international *Society of Airway Management.* All of this activity, focused on a single but complex topic, has improved the quality of care.

Dr. Carin Hagberg has planned this text in a most pleasing and thorough manner. She has literally thought of everything. Moreover, the editorial attention has been superb. The result is easy to read and maximally informative. Overlap, when it inevitably occurs in the multi-authored text, is not confusing, nor does it feel particularly redundant. By starting at the beginning, as it were, with assessment, planning, and preparation, and continuing with execution and follow-up, the book presents the reader with a program of study. The chapters on extubation and on issues in the intensive care unit contain new material and make a serious contribution to the literature. The chapters on the pediatric and obstetrical airway are mini-handbooks in themselves. The chapter on medical conditions affecting the airway is a unique and very useful presentation. It is practical for quick reference, touching on essential airway aspects of a wide array of comorbidities.

The contributors have been recruited from both the traditionally acknowledged experts, such as Ovassapian and Benumof, and a newer, obviously experienced group, as well.

I predict this volume will achieve a high degree of acceptance by anesthesiologists, intensivists, and emergency medicine physicians.

My congratulations to the editor, authors, and publisher.

CHARLES BEATTIE, PHD, MD

Professor and Chair
Anesthesiologist-in-Chief
Department of Anesthesiology
Vanderbilt University Medical Center
Nashville, Tennessee

Preface

....

The *Handbook of Difficult Airway Management* is designed to serve as an easy guide to practical management of airway problems for physicians including anesthesiologists, surgeons, emergency medicine physicians, and critical care physicians, both in training and in practice, as well as other health care practitioners who are involved with airway management. The approach to airway management has changed considerably in the last decade. These years have seen many technological improvements, such as the introduction of new devices and techniques as well as the development of the ASA Difficult Airway Algorithm, which has provided a more systematic approach to airway management. Despite the considerable progress in medicine, adverse events surrounding airway management continue to remain an important cause for litigation. The intent of this book is not simply to add to the current literature on this subject, but rather to attempt to make all recent concepts available in a pocket-sized book that can be used in daily practice and can serve as a quick reference during an encounter with a difficult airway.

The contributors, who are respected experts in the field of airway management, provide succinct and comprehensive discussions of managing challenging airways in both pediatric and adult patients. This handbook also provides important information regarding routine airway evaluation and management, as well as practical approaches to the common problems encountered in managing an airway.

CARIN A. HAGBERG

Acknowledgments

I would like to sincerely acknowledge the scholarly efforts of all the contributors. I would also like to thank my colleague and mentor, Dr. Jacques Chelly, for his generous support, and to thank my secretary, Callye Bowie, for her devoted efforts on my behalf.

Contents

Chapter 1

Anatomic Airway

Considerations

in Anesthesia

Ronald J. Redden

One of the prime considerations when providing anesthesia at any level is the appreciation and management of the patient's airway. Armed with a fundamental recognition of airway anatomy, the anesthesia practitioner can successfully anticipate potential life-threatening problems and can better use the full spectrum of anesthetic techniques needed to provide safe and effective care of patients. The upper airway involved with normal respiration consists of the nasal cavity, mouth, pharynx, larynx, and trachea. An understanding of structures, innervation, and function is important before mastering the techniques of maintaining or reestablishing a patent airway.

NOSE

The surface anatomy of the nose is formed by nasal bones, upper and lower lateral cartilages, cartilage of the nasal septum, and skin. Nasal bones are located superior to the cartilage and are not movable, whereas the tip and lower portion of the nose are cartilaginous and more flexible. The bony framework comprises two nasal bones (in the upper portion), the vomer (located inferiorly), and the perpendicular plate of the ethmoid (located superiorly). The anterior and lower portions of the nose are mainly supported by cartilage, forming a vault or vestibule bounded by the medial and lateral crura (Fig. 1–1). This U-shaped dome of the nasal vestibule keeps the nostril patent. External deformity of the nose may indicate internal nasal obstruction of one or both sides, which may influence which side a nasal intubation should be performed on—if at all. The external openings to the nose are called the *nares* and are formed by the alae laterally, the columella centrally, and the nasal tip superiorly.

The *nasal septum* divides the cavity into two passages, or fossae, that open anteriorly at the nares and continue posteriorly, having an axis at right angles to the face. Posteriorly, the nasal passage opens into the nasopharynx at the *choanae*. The nasal septum, formed by the perpendicular plate of the *ethmoid*, the *vomer*, and the *septal cartilage*, is normally a midline structure but is frequently deviated to one side.[1] Naturally occurring deviations are often discovered during a preoperative anesthesia airway examination. By having the patient breathe through each nostril independently while occluding the contralateral nostril, airway patency can be established and may influence which naris is selected for nasotracheal intubation. The *fossa* is the internal part of the nose and is lined by mucous membrane that contains glandular structures. Within the walls in this area of the nasal passages are found four irregular ridges projecting medially (*supreme, superior, middle,* and *inferior turbinates,* or *conchae*) and covered by soft tissue and mucous membrane.[1, 2] The space beneath each turbinate is called a *meatus* and is

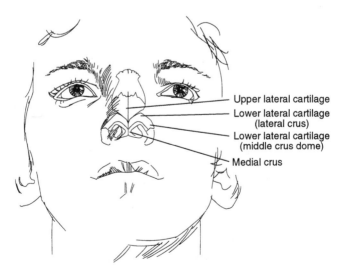

Upper lateral cartilage
Lower lateral cartilage (lateral crus)
Lower lateral cartilage (middle crus dome)
Medial crus

Figure 1–1   Upper and lower lateral cartilages forming a U-shaped dome that keeps the nostril patent.

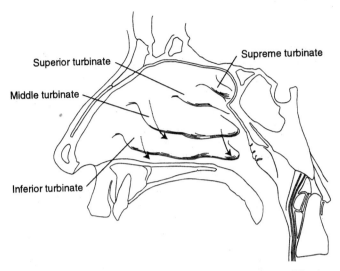

Figure 1–2   The space beneath each turbinate is called a *meatus* and is where the paranasal sinuses and the nasolacrimal duct drain into the nasal cavity.

where the *paranasal sinuses* and the *nasolacrimal duct* drain into the *nasal cavity* (Fig. 1–2). Prolonged intubation and subsequent obstruction of the paranasal sinuses can lead to sinusitis. The major nasal pathway for airway adjuncts is below the inferior turbinates (Fig. 1–3). During nasotracheal intubation, the endotracheal tube (ET) should be passed

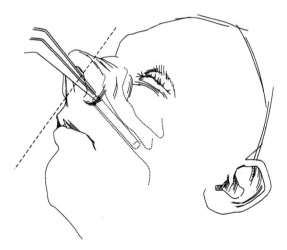

Figure 1–3   The major nasal pathway for airway adjuncts is below the inferior turbinates.

directly backward (perpendicular to the face) along the floor of the nose, preferably on the right side to avoid trauma from the beveled tip of the tube. Trauma to the mucosa may cause bleeding from the highly vascularized tissue (ethmoidal branches of the internal carotid artery via the ophthalmic artery, the sphenopalatine branch of the maxillary artery, and the superior labial branch of the facial artery) or perforation into the submucosal space with hematoma and abscess formation. At the posterior extent, the choana is oval and measures approximately 2.5 cm vertically and 1.5 cm horizontally.[2] The posterior choana is generally symmetric or consistent and does not usually deviate in this region. Occasionally, however, cases of congenital choanal atresia or posttraumatic bony septal deviation may occur, resulting in posterior obstruction of the septum. A history of either problem should be exposed during a routine medical history and airway examination before anesthesia. Common sensation to the nasal cavity arrives from the nasociliary branch of the ophthalmic division (V1) and the maxillary division (V2) of the trigeminal nerve.[1] Given the complexity of nerve supply to this area, nasal anesthesia can be accomplished only with multiple blocks and infiltration as well as topical anesthetic applied to the nasal mucosa (cocaine 4%, lidocaine 4%, and phenylephrine 1% in combination).

More than just a respiratory pathway, the nose humidifies and warms inspired air, and the mucosal vasculature raises the temperature of inspired air to near body temperature. Evaporation of water from the mucosa produces almost 100% relative humidity of inspired gases. Endotracheal intubation bypasses the warming and humidifying effects of the nose and delivers cool, dry gas to the lungs.

MOUTH

The oral cavity lies within the alveolar arches and the teeth (front and sides) and the hard and soft palates (above). The floor of the mouth is occupied largely by the anterior two thirds of the tongue; the posterior third of the tongue lies in the oropharynx. The tongue musculature is divided into intrinsic muscles that run freely in the body of the tongue and alter its shape, and extrinsic muscles that attach to fixed points and move the tongue as a whole. These muscles attach the tongue to the mandible (*genioglossus*), the hyoid (*hyoglossus*), the styloid process (*styloglossus*), and the soft palate (*palatoglossus*). Understanding the function and importance of these muscles relative to anesthesia is important. For example, in the supine unconscious patient, the tongue tends to move backward, potentially producing airway obstruction. A forward jaw thrust pulls the tongue forward because of the genioglossus attachment to the *symphysis menti* of the mandible, establishing airway patency.[1] In addition, the genioglossus muscle may become inactive when associated with jaw fractures, anesthesia, or paralysis. The result is airway obstruction as the tongue falls backward into the pharynx. The floor of the mouth is mainly supported by the paired *mylohyoid* muscles arising from the mandible and inserting into the hyoid bone. The mylohyoid muscle subdivides the area beneath the jaw and tongue into two potential spaces: the *submandibular space* (below the muscle) and the *sublingual space* (above the muscle).[3] Facial trauma or mandibular fractures may result in hematoma formation or tissue edema in either of these fascial spaces, causing posterior displacement of the tongue (Fig. 1–4). In addition, a cellulitis of the submandibular and submental spaces secondary to infection or tooth extraction may also involve the floor of the mouth superior to the mylohyoid muscle. Tongue muscles are soon involved and become edematous and displaced posteriorly. The result of this rapid progression of swelling is airway obstruction, often necessitating a tracheotomy. The tongue itself is a very vascular structure, supplied by the lingual artery through its dorsal, deep, and sublingual branches. A lingual artery hematoma from oral trauma or tongue laceration can cause bleeding into the sublingual and submaxillary spaces, resulting in elevation of the tongue and the floor of the mouth with subsequent upper airway obstruction.[4]

PHARYNX

The *pharynx* can be visualized as a musculofascial tube that connects the nasal and oral cavities with the lower larynx and esophagus. The tube is actually composed of a thin outer fascial layer that is inferiorly continuous with the adventitia of the esophagus and superiorly attached to the base of the skull.[2] The tube thickens posteriorly to become the *buccopharyngeal fascia* and is a common site of laceration

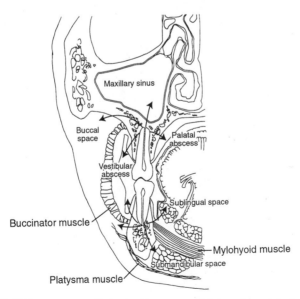

Figure 1–4   Trauma or mandibular fracture may result in hematoma, infection, or tissue edema in either the submandibular or the sublingual fascial space, causing posterior displacement of the tongue.

and retropharyngeal dissection during intubation attempts. In the event of an inadvertent posterior placement of an ET in this area, false passages are created within the mucosa, cervical fascia, and voluntary muscles of the neck (Fig. 1–5). As a result of a traumatic intubation attempt, bleeding and infection into the deep cervical layers could enlarge potential spaces, leading to swelling that may occlude the upper airway, or even involve fascial planes associated with the carotid sheath, pericardium, or diaphragm.

The pharynx can be divided into three segments: the nasopharynx, oropharynx, and hypopharynx (Fig. 1–6). The *nasopharynx* lies directly behind the nasal cavity with a roof formed by the sphenoid and occipital bones. Posteriorly, the nasopharynx is separated from the spinal column by prevertebral fascia and the longus capitis and deep prevertebral musculature. Communicating with the nasopharynx are five passages: two *nasal choanae*, two *eustachian tubes*, and the inferior continua-

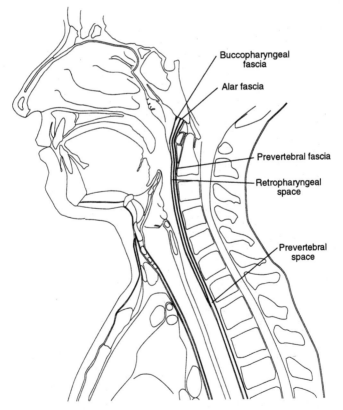

Buccopharyngeal fascia

Alar fascia

Prevertebral fascia

Retropharyngeal space

Prevertebral space

Figure 1–5 Inadvertent posterior placement of an endotracheal tube can cause false passages to be created within the mucosa and fascial spaces.

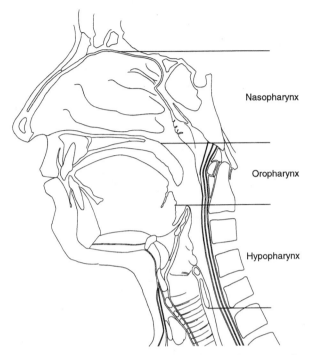

Figure 1–6 Pharynx divided into three segments: the nasopharynx, oropharynx, and hypopharynx.

tion with the oropharynx. In this area are found the *lymphoid* or *adenoid tonsil* tissues along the roof and posterior walls. Enlargement of these tissues may result in chronic nasal obstruction and difficulty in establishing a nasotracheal airway; it is certainly a factor contributing to sleep apnea. In patients with a history of sleep apnea, the minimal airway area in the retropalatal region was found to be significantly smaller than that in awake normal subjects.[5] The sensory nerve supply to the nasopharynx is via three divisions of the trigeminal nerve. Because of this broad distribution of afferents, topical application of local anesthetic is the only means to achieve effective anesthesia.

The *oropharynx* begins where the nasopharynx ends at the soft palate superiorly and extends inferiorly to the tip of the epiglottis. The lateral walls contain paired *tonsilar fossae* formed by the *palatoglossal* and *palatopharyngeal folds* (Fig. 1–7). Within these folds bilaterally are found the *palatine tonsils*, which may reach considerable size during childhood or recent upper respiratory infections and actually prohibit direct exposure of the larynx during direct laryngoscopy.

Because sensory innervation of the mouth and oropharynx comes from a variety of sources (maxillary nerve [VII] via the palatine and nasopharyngeal branches; lingual branch from mandibular division

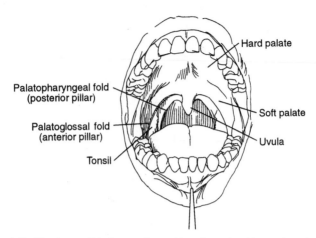

Figure 1–7   Structures within the mouth requiring direct visual inspection when one is preoperatively evaluating the airway.

[VIII] of the trigeminal nerve; glossopharyngeal nerve; and pharyngeal plexus), this area is amenable only to topically administered local anesthetic agents in preparation for awake intubation. However, it may be useful at times to anesthetize the posterior third of the tongue and anterior epiglottis by local anesthetics injected near the glossopharyngeal nerve medial to the base of the anterior tonsillar pillar.[6] This technique is used to attenuate the gag reflex and the patient's response to awake laryngoscopy.

The *hypopharynx* is the portion of the larynx that extends inferiorly from the superior edge of the *epiglottis* to the inferior edge of the *cricoid cartilage*. It is typically located at the level of the fourth through the sixth cervical vertebrae and is continuous with the oropharynx above and with both the esophagus and the laryngeal inlet below. The inlet of the larynx lies anteriorly and is defined by the epiglottis, the *aryepiglottic folds*, the *arytenoid cartilages,* and the *posterior commissure.*[1, 2] The larynx protrudes into the hypopharynx, forming funnel-shaped recesses on each side called *piriform fossae* or recesses (Fig. 1–8). The piriform recess diverts food boluses laterally and away from the larynx in transit to the esophagus. Each recess is bound laterally by aryepiglottic folds and the internal lining of the thyroid cartilage, and superiorly by the lateral *glossoepiglottic folds*. The paired lateral glossoepiglottic folds and single median fold bound two spaces called the *epiglottic valleculae* and attach the tongue with the epiglottis. The *valleculae* are where a curved laryngoscope blade is inserted in order to visualize the glottis during laryngoscopy. The *buccopharyngeal* and *prevertebral fascia* and deep prevertebral musculature cover the posterior border of the hypopharynx, which is also the sight of inadvertent posterior pharyngeal tears during traumatic endotracheal tube placement.

As in the oropharynx, the mucosa of the posterior pharynx is inner-

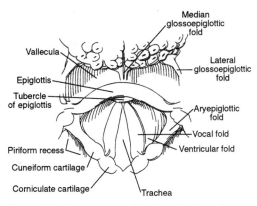

Figure 1–8 Larynx as visualized from the hypopharynx.

vated by the pharyngeal plexus (nerves X, XI, and IX), which supplies sensory innervation to the hypopharynx.[1, 2] Branches of the superior laryngeal nerve lie in the medial and lateral walls of the piriform sinuses and carry sensory innervation to the structures in the areas above the vocal cords. These sensory nerves can be blocked by diffusion of local anesthetic either by direct application or from soaked pledgets. The internal branch of the superior laryngeal nerve can also be blocked from an external approach before the nerve penetrates the thyrohyoid membrane inferior to the greater cornu of the hyoid bone.

LARYNX

The larynx begins at the base of the tongue and ends at the beginning of the trachea. It is anterior to the lower portion of the oropharynx and the larygopharynx. The larynx is a sophisticated structure composed of cartilages, fibroelastic membranes, muscles, and mucous membranes. It functions as an open valve in respiration, a partially closed valve (the orifice of which can be modulated in phonation), and a closed valve protecting the lower airway against aspiration during swallowing. Closure at this level also assists in the development of intrathoracic pressure associated with coughing, micturition, defecation, and heavy lifting.[7] The larynx is composed of nine cartilage structures, three single and three paired: the thyroid (the largest and most notable, also called the Adam's apple), cricoid, arytenoid (two), corniculate (two), and cuneiform (two) cartilages and the epiglottis.

The interior of the larynx is important anatomically because of two structures: the *epiglottis* and the *vocal cords*. The epiglottis acts as a valve protecting the conductive airway by closing during the act of swallowing. The vocal cords are primarily responsible for phonation. Skeletally, the larynx is formed by the *thyroid* and *cricoid cartilages*, the *arytenoid cartilages*, and the *epiglottis* and is suspended from the hyoid bone from above (Fig. 1–9). The thyroid cartilage at the level of C5

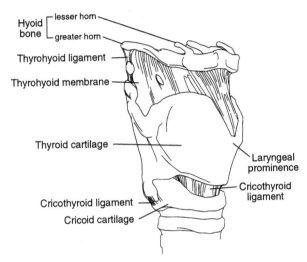

Figure 1–9 Cartilaginous and fibroelastic membranous components of the larynx.

comprises two broad laminae joined anteriorly at the midline. This angle forms a major anterior or visible prominence marking the level of the vocal cords. The two superior horns of the thyroid cartilage aid in the suspension from the hyoid bone (indicating the level of the epiglottis and the laryngeal entrance), and the two inferior horns articulate with the cricoid cartilage below.[2] The thyroid cartilage is attached to the hyoid bone above by the *thyrohyoid membrane* and below to the cricoid cartilage by the *cricothyroid membrane* (site of cricothyroidotomy because of its superficial location). The cricoid cartilage lies inferior to the thyroid cartilage at the level of C6[6] and aids in the support of the posterior laryngeal structures. It is the only complete ring in the entire airway. This signet-shaped ring is shorter in the anterior (5 to 7 mm) than in the taller posterior (2 to 3 cm) portion.[2] The paired *arytenoid cartilages* sit on the lateral superior surface of the broad posterior portion of the cricoid ring and are attached to the hyoid and thyroid cartilages by several ligaments. The intrinsic muscles of voice control are attached to the two arytenoid cartilages, and the vocal cords project anteriorly from the arytenoid cartilages to the thyroid cartilage.

On laryngoscopic inspection, the larynx begins at the base of the tongue with a leaflike projection called the *epiglottis*. The epiglottis is composed of cartilage and a covering mucous membrane. The epiglottic structure is connected with the base of the tongue anteriorly by a medial glossoepiglottic fold and lateral glossoepiglottic folds. The pair of depressions between the median fold and the lateral folds are the valleculae. From the lateral edges of the epiglottis there are two aryepiglottic folds that travel medially and posteriorly. Along this backward course, the folds pass over two paired small protuberances, the *cuneiform cartilages*, immediately before ending at two paramedian protuberances, the *corniculate cartilages*. These cartilages reinforce the walls of the aryepiglottic folds against the boluses of food deflected by the epiglottis during swallowing into the area lateral to the glottic opening between the aryepiglottic folds and the laminae of the thyroid cartilage (piriform recesses).

The epiglottis, aryepiglottic folds, and corniculate cartilages define the glottic opening, or the *aditus*.[6] Immediately within the aditus, the epiglottis is found projecting posteriorly into the glottis. Inferior to this appears the first set of lateral folds, the *vestibular folds* or *false vocal cords*. Inferior and parallel to the false cords lie the *true vocal cords*. The vocal cords extend from the arytenoid cartilages posteriorly to the thyroid cartilage anteriorly. The laryngeal recess between the false and true vocal cords is termed the *ventricle*, which at times can inadvertently catch the advancing ET while the tube approaches the *rima glottidis, the* opening between the true vocal cords.[2] Whereas the false cords point downward, the true cords are directed upward. This design facilitates the expiration of air but can passively resist up to 140 mm Hg of an incoming column of air and contributes to the ineffectiveness of positive-pressure ventilation through a closed glottis as occurs during laryngospasm.[6]

Innervation to the larynx can be divided into that in the area above and that in the area below the level of the vocal cords. At about the level of the hyoid bone, the vagus nerve gives off the *superior laryngeal nerve*, a branch of the vagus nerve, which further divides into both external and internal branches (Fig. 1–10). The larger internal branch pierces the thyrohyoid membrane and carries sensory input to the laryngeal mucosa down to the level of the vocal cords. The external

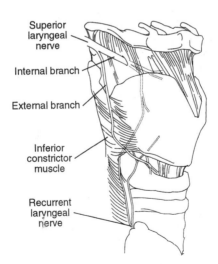

Superior
laryngeal
nerve

Internal branch

External branch

Inferior
constrictor
muscle

Recurrent
laryngeal
nerve

Figure 1–10   The superior laryngeal nerve, which supplies sensory innervation to the area above the vocal cords, may be accessed before entering the cricothyroid membrane.

branch courses through the cricoid cartilage and gives motor fibers to the cricothyroid muscle.[1, 2] Before an awake intubation, local anesthetics may be employed to attenuate sensation above the vocal cords by blocking the external branch, with the hyoid bone and the thyroid membrane used as palpable landmarks. The motor innervation of the intrinsic laryngeal muscles is by the *recurrent laryngeal nerve*, a branch of the vagus nerve. In addition, a branch of the recurrent laryngeal nerve penetrates the cricothyroid membrane and supplies sensory innervation to the subglottic larynx up through the level of the vocal cords. Because of the inaccessibility of the recurrent laryngeal nerves, the area below the cords requires topical application of anesthetic by either aerosolization from above or transtracheal injection through the cricothyroid membrane. The posterior pharynx and hypopharynx need separate topical applications of anesthetic to be rendered insensitive before an awake intubation.

PEDIATRIC AIRWAY

Many differences between adult and pediatric anatomy affect mask ventilation and intubation. For example, the neonate and the infant usually have a proportionately larger occiput that tends to place the head in a flexed position—one that can easily obstruct the premedicated child if unmonitored. Narrow nasal passages, a long epiglottis, and a short trachea and neck collectively contribute to making infants obligate nose breathers.[8] The tongue is typically larger in proportion to the oral cavity and often obstructs the airway or makes laryngoscopy more difficult. The narrow passages and large tongue, in combination with large tonsillar and adenoid tissues, can easily become obstructed by the copious secretions commonly seen in younger patients. The larynx is usually more anterior and cephalic, with the glottis located at C3 in premature babies and at C3 to C4 in newborns, compared with C5 in adults.[9] The cricoid cartilage is the narrowest point of the airway in children younger than 5 years, as opposed to the glottis in adults. In addition, the larynx and trachea are funnel-shaped in children. As a result of these factors, as little as 1 mm of edema has a proportionately greater effect in children than in adults, and this may contribute to postoperative croup. The vocal cords themselves slant anteriorly, making the insertion of an ET more difficult; thus, cricoid pressure may be required to visualize the glottis.

Anatomic differences like those described can influence anesthetic techniques and the management of the unconscious pediatric airway. A prominent occiput can interfere with a sniffing position for intubation but can be remedied by slightly elevating the shoulders with towels and placing the head on a doughnut-shaped pillow. Oral airways can sometimes contribute to displacement of an oversized tongue into the posterior pharynx, and nasal airways can traumatize small nares and prominent adenoids, resulting in bleeding. Compression of submandibular soft tissues should be avoided during mask ventilation in order to prevent the occurrence of upper airway obstruction. Because of the subglottic narrowing of the conducting airway, the patient younger than 10 years should be intubated with a cuffless ET demonstrating a leak of less than 10 to 25 cm H_2O.[8, 9] A leak is paramount in preventing excessive pressure on the mucosa, which may contribute to the development of postoperative croup. The approximate internal diameter of an ET is estimated by a formula based on age:

17 + odd age / 4 = tube diameter in millimeters

16 + even age / 4 = tube diameter in millimeters

Exceptions include premature (2.5- to 3-mm tubes) and full-term (3- to 3.5-mm tubes) neonates. When formulas are used as rough guidelines, endotracheal tubes 0.5 mm smaller and larger than predicted should always be readily available. The approximate length of the ET may be estimated by the following formula:

Age/2 + 12 = length of tube in centimeters (orally)

Age/2 + 15 = length of tube in centimeters (nasally)

Again, formulas provide only an estimation, and the actual position must be confirmed by auscultation and clinical judgment.

REFERENCES

1. Morris IR: Functional anatomy of the upper airway. Emerg Med Clin North Am 6:639, 1988.
2. Sykes JM, Isaacs RS: Applied anatomic considerations in airway management. *In* Hanowell LH, Waldron RJ (eds): Airway Management. Philadelphia, Lippincott-Raven, 1996, p 3.
3. Teichgraeber JF, Rappaport NH, Harris JH: The radiology of upper airway obstruction in maxillofacial trauma. Ann Plast Surg 27(2):103, 1991.
4. Kattan B, Snyder HS: Lingual artery hematoma resulting in upper airway obstruction. J Emerg Med 9:421, 1991.
5. Schwab RJ, Gupta KB, Gefter WB, et al: Upper airway and soft tissue anatomy. Am J Respir Crit Care Med 152:1673, 1995.
6. Fung DM, Devitt JH: The anatomy, physiology, and innervation of the larynx. Anesthesiol Clin North Am 13:259, 1995.
7. Graney DO: Basic science: Anatomy. *In* Cummings CW, Fredrickson JM, Hacker LA, et al (eds): Otolaryngology—Head and Neck Surgery. St Louis, CV Mosby, 1986.
8. Agarwal R: Pediatric anesthesia. *In* Duke J, Rosenberg SG (eds): Anesthesia Secrets. Philadelphia, Hanley & Belfus, 1996, p 369.
9. Barash PG, Cullen BF, Stoelting RK: Clinical Anesthesia. Philadelphia, JB Lippincott, 1992.

Chapter 2

Prediction and Evaluation

of the Difficult Airway

Melissa Wheeler and Andranik Ovassapian

Although the importance of the prediction and evaluation of the difficult airway may seem to be self-evident in the practice of anesthesia, it is helpful to review recent data from the Closed Claims Project of the American Society of Anesthesiologists (ASA), particularly those findings that are important to management of the difficult airway. First, adverse respiratory events constitute the largest source of injury. Three types of adverse respiratory events resulted in three quarters of the claims: inadequate ventilation (38%), esophageal intubation (18%), and difficult intubation (17%). Of these adverse respiratory events, three quarters were judged to be preventable, three quarters were judged to result from substandard care, three quarters resulted in award of damages, and approximately 85% resulted in death or brain damage.[1] It is arguable that better prediction of and anticipation of the difficult airway might lead to a reduction in these numbers. For example, consider a specific clinical scenario, the patient at risk for aspiration. The most common approach to these patients is the rapid sequence induction. This approach assumes the ability to intubate the patient's trachea. If we have a method to better predict the difficult airway before we are committed to rapid sequence induction, we can consider alternatives to securing the airway and thus provide a safer induction for our patients.

DEFINITION OF TERMS

Four concepts important to the prediction of the difficult airway are *failed intubation, difficult intubation, difficult laryngoscopy,* and *difficult mask ventilation.*

Failed intubation is the simplest and most straightforward to define because it has a clear-cut end point, the inability to place the endotracheal tube. Thus there is fairly uniform reporting of the incidence of failed intubation in the literature; it occurs in approximately 0.05%, or 1:2230, of surgical patients and in approximately 0.13% to 0.35%, or 1:750 to 1:280, of obstetric patients.[2, 3]

The definition of *difficult intubation* is less straightforward than that of failed intubation, primarily because there is a less clear-cut clinical end point, and therefore there is a greater variety in the reported incidence. However, in 1993 the ASA Committee on Practice Guidelines for Management of the Difficult Airway proposed that difficult intubation be defined as intubation when "the proper insertion of the endotracheal tube with conventional laryngoscopy requires more than three attempts and/or . . . more than 10 minutes."[4] Unfortunately, this definition has some obvious shortcomings because difficult intubation may be independent of both the number of attempts and the time. For example, an experienced laryngoscopist may determine on the first attempt and within 30 seconds that this will be a difficult intubation and that therefore difficult intubation algorithms should be followed. It has been proposed, then, that the definition should be based on a uniform understanding of the best attempt at intubation and should use the number of attempts and time as boundaries only.[5] Clearly, this is a gray area in terms of defining a clinical end point for scientific study. Therefore, Cormack and Lehane defined what could be a more universally applicable and uniform clinical end point by introducing the concept of *difficult laryngoscopy.*[6] They describe four grades of laryngoscopy based on the structures visualized. Grade I is visualization of the entire laryngeal aperture, grade II is visualization of the posterior portion of the laryngeal aperture, grade III is visualization of the tip of the epiglottis, and grade IV is visualization of the soft palate only (Fig. 2–1). Many investigators who evaluate methods of prediction of the difficult intubation have adopted this grading system, variously defining grades III and IV or grade IV alone as correlating with a potentially difficult intubation.

Difficult mask ventilation is less often discussed in the literature. It is clear from clinical experience that there are grades of difficulty, just as with difficult intubation. Proposals for classification have been made,[4] but none are universally accepted. The lack of uniformity in acceptable

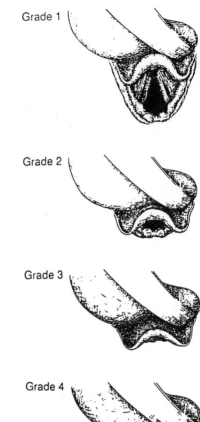

Grade 1

Grade 2

Grade 3

Grade 4

Figure 2–1 Four grades of laryngoscopic view (see text). (From Williams KN, Carli F, Cormack RS: Unexpected, difficult laryngoscopy: A prospective survey in routine general surgery. Br J Anaesth 66:38, 1991.)

definitions of airway-related terms limits the value and feasibility of comparisons between studies or meta-analysis of the predictors of difficult airway management.

PREDICTION OF THE DIFFICULT AIRWAY

Most investigations and reviews of prediction of the difficult airway have focused on prediction of the difficult rigid or conventional intubation. Thus the majority of this chapter reviews those studies. Most investigators rely primarily on physical signs, secondarily on historical clues, and lastly on diagnostic testing.

Physical Signs for Prediction of the Difficult Intubation

When considering physical signs as predictors of the difficult intubation, it is helpful to review the necessary steps or goals of laryngeal visualization during rigid laryngoscopy. Briefly, these involve the alignment of three anatomic axes—the laryngeal axis, the pharyngeal axis, and the oral axis—to allow successful exposure of the glottic opening. The pharyngeal and laryngeal axes are brought into alignment by flexion of the neck, and the oral axis is brought into alignment with the others by extension of the head (Fig. 2–2). Anatomic factors that interfere with this alignment have been reviewed in the literature.

Forty years ago, Cass and colleagues reported the first anecdotal review of physical factors that might interfere with alignment of the pharyngeal and laryngeal axes and thus with visualization of the larynx.[7] They described six factors: a short, muscular neck; a receding mandible; protruding maxillary incisors; poor temporomandibular joint mobility; a long, high-arched palate; and an increased alveolar–mental distance. Many of these factors are still considered potentially associated with a difficult intubation. Twenty years later, White and Kander reaffirmed the association of an increased depth of the mandible and decreased temporomandibular joint mobility with difficult intubation.[8] Additionally, they suggested that reduced cervical mobility is a sign of potentially difficult intubation (Table 2–1).

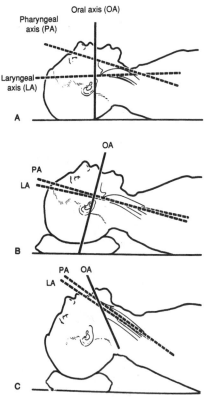

Figure 2–2 Optimal head position for rigid laryngoscopy. *A*, Patient supine with the head in neutral position. None of the anatomic axes are in alignment. *B*, Elevation of the head 10 cm results in alignment of the pharyngeal axis (PA) and laryngeal axis (LA). *C*, Head extension results in alignment of the oral axis (OA) with PA and LA. (*A–C*, From Stone DJ, Gal TJ: Airway management. *In* Miller RD [ed]: Anesthesia, 4th ed. New York, Churchill Livingstone, 1994, p 1408.)

Table 2–1   Traditional Physical Predictors of Difficult Intubation

Short, muscular neck
Receding mandible
Protruding maxillary incisors
Poor temporomandibular joint mobility
Long, high-arched palate
Increased alveolar–mental distance
Decreased cervical mobility

In 1983, Patil and associates described the concept of *thyromental distance*.[9] This is defined as the distance from the chin to the notch of the thyroid cartilage. They proposed this as a means of screening for patients with a potentially difficult airway. They noted that in the normal adult, this distance should be 6.5 cm, and that if this distance is less than 6 cm, it may be associated with difficult intubation.

In that same year, Mallampati suggested an entirely new approach to evaluation of the difficult intubation.[10] His theory was that a disproportionately large tongue base could hinder exposure of the larynx. Since the tongue base cannot easily be measured directly, the size of the tongue can be inferred by noting the relative visibility of pharyngeal structures when the patient is examined in a standard position with the mouth fully opened and the tongue fully extended.[10, 11] Although Mallampati originally proposed three oropharyngeal classes, Samsoon and Young[2] modified this to four classes, and most investigators have adopted this four-class system. Class I is exposure of the soft palate, uvula, and tonsillar pillars; class II is exposure of the soft palate and the base of the uvula with a portion of the posterior pharyngeal wall visible; class III is visualization of the soft palate only; and class IV is visualization of no pharyngeal structures except the hard palate (Fig. 2–3).[2] Most investigators would then consider class I and II airways to

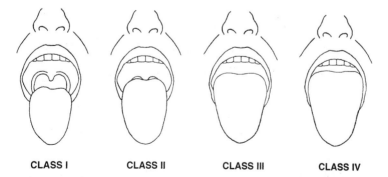

CLASS I   CLASS II   CLASS III   CLASS IV

Figure 2–3   Mallampati classification schematic (see text). (From Mallampati SR: Recognition of the difficult airway. *In* Benumof JL [ed]: Airway Management Principles and Practice. St Louis, Mosby–Year Book, 1996, p 126.)

be easy to manage and class III and IV airways to be more difficult, if not impossible, because more pharyngeal structures are obscured, thus leaving less space for exposure of the larynx. However, in prospective analyses the Mallampati test has achieved only moderate sensitivity and specificity. This may be related to the great deal of interobserver variability that many investigators report.[12–14] This variability may in turn arise because the structures evaluated are mobile and under voluntary control. One way to minimize these shortcomings is always to use the recommended technique when performing these tests. That technique is to have the patient sitting, head neutral, mouth fully opened, and tongue fully extended. Various authors have both advocated and condemned phonation during this test.[15–17] The best bet for consistency is always to perform the test in the same manner within the clinical practice and to conduct the test twice in each patient. For example, the test can be performed once at the beginning of a physical examination and again at the end of the examination.

In 1994, Savva proposed the concept of *sternomental distance*.[18] This is the distance from the tip of the chin to the sternal notch. In the normal adult, this distance should be greater than 12.5 cm, and if it is less than 12 cm it may be associated with difficult intubation. In his study, he found that this measurement was both more specific and more sensitive than the thyromental distance. He believed that this was because this measurement may better incorporate head extension. There has been no independent confirmation of these findings.

To evaluate the validity of any predictors, certain statistical parameters must be applied (Table 2–2). It would be reasonable to expect to predict at least 9 of 10 difficult intubations. This would correspond to a test with a sensitivity of 90%. In addition, a reasonable test would produce only one false alarm a week. In a hypothetical practice of 10,000 cases per year, this would correspond to a specificity of 99.5%. For example, for the Mallampati test, a class I oropharyngeal classification would always correlate with a grade I or II laryngoscopic view, and a class IV oropharyngeal classification would always correlate with

Table 2–2 Definitions of Statistical Terms

Sensitivity	The percentage of correctly predicted difficult intubations as a proportion of all intubations that were truly difficult
Specificity	The percentage of correctly predicted easy intubations as a proportion of all intubations that were truly easy
Positive predictive value	The percentage of correctly predicted difficult intubations as a proportion of all predicted difficult intubations
Negative predictive value	The percentage of correctly predicted easy intubations as a proportion of all predicted easy intubations

a grade IV laryngoscopic view, such that we would be able to predict all difficult intubations and never have a false alarm. However, multiple prospective analyses of single predictors have achieved, at best, only moderate sensitivity and moderate specificity. Perhaps the best way to improve the statistical accuracy of physical signs for prediction of the difficult intubation is to combine predictors. Combined predictors have been evaluated using various combinations of the physical signs that have been described over the past 40 years.

Physical Signs: Combined Predictors

The first category to consider is the "Mallampati plus." Three papers have explored the combination of Mallampati classification plus thyromental distance. Mathew and colleagues, in 1989, compared 22 patients with known difficult intubation and 22 matched controls.[19] All patients with difficult intubation had thyromental distances of less than 6 cm and had Mallampati classifications of III or IV. All the controls had thyromental distances greater than 6.5 cm and Mallampati classifications of I or II. Therefore, since there was no overlap between groups, the investigators described 100% specificity and sensitivity. However, this degree of accuracy has not been duplicated by other investigators. Frerk, in 1991, prospectively evaluated these same two factors in 244 patients and did not find 100% specificity and sensitivity.[20] Instead, he found 98% specificity, which in our hypothetical practice of 10,000 cases per year would correspond to approximately four false alarms per week (200 false alarms per 10,000 cases), and he found 80% sensitivity, which would miss 2 of 10 difficult intubations. Lewis and colleagues, in 1994, combined the thyromental distance and the Mallampati classification into a statistical formula called the Performance Index.[17] The value chosen for the Performance Index sets a cutoff that, depending on the incidence of difficult intubations in the clinical practice, can be used to predict the ratio of missed difficult intubations to false alarms.

Other investigators have examined combinations of more than two predictors. Wilson and colleagues examined a combination of five risk factors (Wilson Risk Sum): weight, head and neck movement, jaw movement, receding mandible, and buck teeth.[13] One of three levels is assigned per risk, with a level of zero representing no risk for difficult intubation and a level of 2 representing the greatest risk for difficult intubation (Table 2–3). Wilson's group suggested that a score of 2 would correspond to a test that was 85% specific and 75% sensitive. That is, there would be approximately 30 false alarms per week in a hypothetical practice (1500 false alarms per 10,000 cases), and 5 of 20 difficult intubations would be missed. Additionally, this test is not applicable to children or to pregnant women because of the weight classification. However, Oates and colleagues compared the Wilson Risk Sum with the Mallampati classification and found it to be slightly superior.[12] Although both tests predicted only 5 of 12 difficult intubations, the Wilson Risk Sum resulted in fewer false alarms (i.e., it was more specific) and displayed less interobserver variability.

Bellhouse and Doré examined radiographic measurements in 19

Table 2–3   Wilson Risk Sum

Risk Factor	Risk Level
Weight (kg)	
<90	0
90–110	1
>110	2
Head and neck movement (degrees)	
>90	0
~90	1
<90	2
Jaw movement	
Incisor gap >5 cm or subluxation >0	0
Incisor gap <5 cm and subluxation = 0	1
Incisor gap <5 cm and subluxation <0	2
Receding mandible	
Normal	0
Moderate	1
Severe	2
Buck teeth	
Normal	0
Moderate	1
Severe	2

patients with known difficult airways and compared these with measurements in 14 patients with known easy airways.[21] They then looked for clinical parameters that would correspond to the radiographic predictors that distinguished between these two patient groups. They found three suggestive clinical measures: Mallampati classification III or IV, limited atlantooccipital joint mobility, and receding chin. There has been no formal prospective evaluation of their findings, and thus the sensitivity and specificity of this combination of predictors are unknown.

In 1992, Rocke and colleagues studied 1500 obstetric patients to evaluate nine risk factors.[3] They found four of these factors to be predictive of a difficult intubation. These were the Mallampati classification, a short neck, a receding mandible, and protruding maxillary incisors. They then ranked combinations of these four factors in order of increasing probability of a difficult airway (Fig. 2–4).

In 1995, Tse and associates evaluated 471 patients and compared combinations of three variables: the Mallampati classification, head extension, and the thyromental distance. They found that the combination of tests improved the specificity of prediction, at a great cost in sensitivity, however.[22] They concluded that there would be too many false alarms with the routine application of these tests and therefore recommended that awake intubation be reserved for those patients in whom there was a high index of suspicion of difficult intubation and who were considered candidates for rapid sequence induction, had

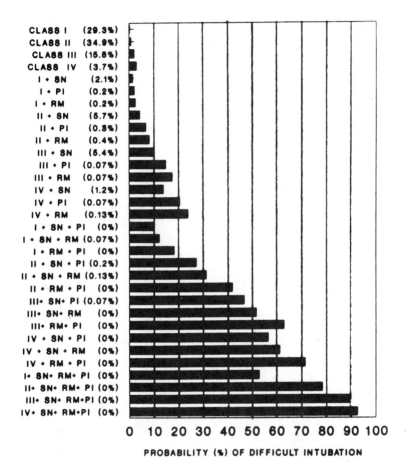

Figure 2–4 Combined physical predictors of difficult rigid intubation. The graph shows the incidence of these predictors and the probability of difficult intubation when various combinations of these predictors are observed according to the study of Rocke and associates. Class I–IV, Mallampati classification; SN, short neck; PI, protruding maxillary incisors; RM, receding mandible. (From Rocke DA, Murray WB, Rout CC, Gouws E: Relative risk analysis of factors associated with difficult intubation in obstetric anesthesia. Anesthesiology 77:67, 1992.)

known previous difficult intubations, or had clinical diseases that made the practitioner suspect difficult ventilation.

An algorithm proposed by Mallampati considers five risk factors: the Mallampati classification, the thyromental distance, head mobility, neck mobility, and the gross morphologic characteristics of the head and neck. He then combines these five factors to arrive at an index of likelihood of difficulty with airway management (Fig. 2–5).[23] Although

ALGORITHM FOR CLINICAL RECOGNITION OF DIFFICULT AIRWAY

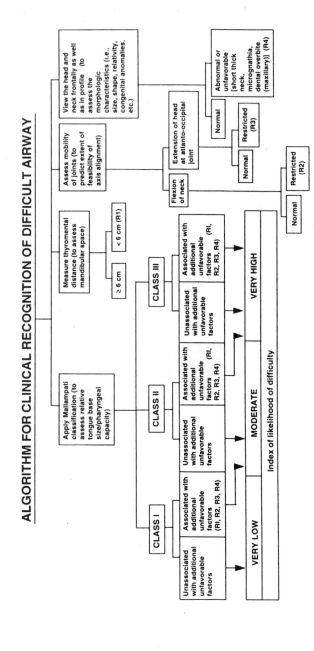

Figure 2–5 A reasonable approach to the prediction of the difficult airway. R1, thyromental distance <6 cm; R2, restricted neck flexion; R3, restricted extension of the head; R4, short, thick neck. (From Mallampati SR: Recognition of the difficult airway. *In* Benumof JL [ed]: Airway Management Principles and Practice. St Louis, Mosby–Year Book, 1996, p 126.)

this algorithm is reasonable, it has yet to be formally and prospectively evaluated.

In 1996, El-Ganzouri and colleagues reported a prospective analysis of 10,507 consecutive adult patients presenting for surgery under general anesthesia.[24] A multivariate model for stratifying the risk of difficult endotracheal intubation was developed from seven criteria evaluated for each patient: the mouth opening, the Mallampati classification, neck movement, ability to protrude the mandible, body weight, and a history of difficult intubation (Tables 2–4 and 2–5). Compared with Mallampati class I as a single predictor, a simplified airway risk index score of 3 demonstrated a similar positive predictive value (21.9% versus 21.0%) with greater sensitivity (59.5% versus 44.7%). For a score of 4, the sensitivity of the simplified airway risk index exceeded that of the Mallampati class III for the prediction of laryngoscopy grades of III or greater.

Historical Clues for Prediction of the Difficult Intubation

There are known congenital syndromes associated with difficult airway management, either difficult mask ventilation or difficult intubation, or both (Chapter 12). Enlarged lingual tonsils or epiglottic cysts can cause failed intubation when physical examination reveals no clues to increased risk for difficult intubation.[25, 26] To minimize airway-related morbidity and mortality, clinicians should be aware of this and proceed with caution in any patient who gives a history of difficult intubation. Also, certain disease states, such as sleep apnea, have been suggested to correlate with an increased risk of difficult intubation.[27]

Review of prior anesthetic records can be a valuable historical clue in determining the ease or difficulty of airway management.

The MedicAlert National Registry has added the category of difficult airway/intubation (Chapter 17). This registry provides a 24-hour emergency response center, and patients who are enrolled receive an identification bracelet and card. The information at the registry can be updated by any clinician. This registry may provide extremely useful information regarding previous encounters with a patient who has a difficult airway. The telephone number for this service is 800-432-5378.[28]

Diagnostic Evaluation of the Difficult Airway

Diagnostic evaluation is distinct from prediction of the difficult airway because it is usually limited to patients with a known or clinically suspicious difficult airway. Radiographic or endoscopic evaluation, or both, may be appropriate in some patients, and preoperative consultation with other specialists (otolaryngologist, thoracic surgeon, pulmonologist, oncologist) may be necessary.

Prediction of the Difficult Mask Ventilation

What is particularly interesting about the focus of the majority of the papers that evaluate methods of predicting the difficult airway is that

Table 2-4 Accuracy of Risk Factors in Predicting Difficulty with Tracheal Intubation

Risk Factor	Laryngoscopy Grade*	Sensitivity (%)	Specificity (%)	Positive Predictive Value (%)	Negative Predictive Value (%)
Mouth opening <4 cm	≥III/IV	26.3/46.7	94.8/93.9	25.0/7.4	95.2/99.4
Thyromental distance <6 cm	≥III/IV	7.0/16.8	99.2/99.0	38.5/15.4	94.3/99.1
Mallampati class III	≥III/IV	44.7/59.8	89.0/87.4	21.0/4.7	96.1/99.5
Neck movement <80°	≥III/IV	10.4/16.8	98.4/97.9	29.5/7.9	94.4/99.1
Inability to protrude the mandible	≥III/IV	16.5/26.2	95.8/95.3	20.6/5.4	94.6/99.2
Body weight >110 kg	≥III/IV	11.1/13.1	94.6/94.3	11.8/2.3	94.2/99.1
Positive history of difficult intubation	≥III/IV	4.5/9.3	99.8/99.7	69.0/23.8	94.1/99.1

*Laryngoscopy grade categorized as III and IV combined (≥III) or IV alone.
Data from El-Ganzouri AR, McCarthy RJ, Tuman KJ, et al: Preoperative airway assessment: Predictive value of a multivariate risk analysis. Anesth Analg 82:1197, 1996.

Table 2–5 Multivariate Predictors of Difficult Trachael Intubation

Variable	Classification	Incidence (%)	Simplified Airway Risk Index Weighting*
Mouth opening	≥4 cm	93.6	0
	<4 cm	6.4	1
Thyromental distance	>6.5 cm	89.0	0
	6.0–6.5 cm	9.9	1
	<6.0 cm	1.1	2
Mallampati class	I	46.2	0
	II	40.8	1
	III	13.0	2
Neck movement	>90°	91.4	0
	80°–90°	6.4	1
	<80°	2.2	2
Ability to protrude the mandible	Yes	95.1	0
	No	4.9	1
Body weight	<90 kg	77.6	0
	90–110 kg	16.6	1
	>110 kg	5.8	2
History of difficult intubation	None	98.2	0
	Questionable	1.4	1
	Definite	0.4	2

*The risk index score is the sum of the risk index–weighting factors.
Data from El-Ganzouri AR, McCarthy RJ, Tuman KJ, et al: Preoperative airway assessment: Predictive value of a multivariate risk analysis. Anesth Analg 82:1197, 1996.

the ease or difficulty of mask ventilation is virtually ignored. The Australian study of reported anesthetic complications indicated a 15% incidence of difficult mask ventilation in patients who had difficult or failed intubation.[29] This is extremely critical information to have, as the combination of a difficult intubation and a difficult mask ventilation is an emergency that necessitates urgent management.

One group of investigators reported the incidence of difficult face mask ventilation as part of their study predicting the difficult airway.[24] In this study, only 8 of 10,000 patients were reported to have a difficult mask ventilation. This incidence was too low to permit evaluation of predictors of difficult mask ventilation. Large prospective studies, probably requiring the cooperation of multiple centers, are needed to address this issue.

PREDICTING THE DIFFICULT AIRWAY: FUTURE DIRECTIONS
(Table 2–6)

Additional prospective evaluations of combined predictors that incorporate more sophisticated statistical analyses, such as the Performance Index, should be undertaken. Standardized definitions of terms and a standardized intubating position should be adopted so that results

Table 2–6   Predicting the Difficult Airway: Future Directions

Standardization of definitions of difficult airway terms
Further evaluation of historical predictors
Further evaluation of combined predictors
Evaluation of predictors for difficult mask ventilation
Evaluation of predictors for children
Technological advances

among studies may be more accurately compared. Further evaluation of historical clues such as sleep apnea should be pursued. Evaluation of predictors for difficult mask ventilation is needed. Predictors of the difficult airway in children also need to be explored.

New technology may lead to improved specificity and sensitivity of prediction. One example of this new technology is acoustic reflection analysis. This technique uses sound waves to measure pharyngeal volume. In the first paper to evaluate this technique, 14 patients with a history of failed intubation were compared with 14 matched controls who were known to have easy intubations. Those patients in the failed intubation group had pharyngeal volumes of 37.5 mL, and those patients in the control group had pharyngeal volumes of 43.4 mL. Since there was no overlap between groups, this test resulted in a specificity and sensitivity of 100%.[30] The test takes only 2 to 3 minutes; however, there needs to be prospective evaluation before it can be routinely recommended and applied.

A simpler technological device is the bubble inclinometer. This device measures the degree of laryngeal tilt. The theory is that a 40-degree tilt has good correlation with a grade III laryngeal view. In 50 patients studied, Roberts and colleagues found a positive predictive value of 78%, which corresponds to a reasonable sensitivity and specificity.[31] There has been no independent prospective confirmation of the value of a bubble inclinometer in detecting difficult intubation cases.

Indirect laryngoscopy as a method of difficult airway prediction has been reported.[32] This method involves the use of an otolaryngoscopic instrument that consists of a handle connected to a removable mirror that is illuminated by a halogen fiberoptic light source also incorporated into the handle. For the study, the patient was instructed to sit upright with the back straight and the head and trunk forward. The patient was asked to open the mouth fully, and then the tongue was pulled forward with a gauze. The mirror was placed in the patient's mouth until the back of the mirror touched the epiglottis and elevated the uvula. The laryngeal view was then graded: grade 1, vocal cords visible; grade 2, posterior commissure visible; grade 3, epiglottis visible; grade 4, no glottic structure visible. Grades 3 and 4 were considered to be predictive of a difficult intubation. The predictive value of this grading system was compared with the Mallampati test and the Wilson Risk Sum. The authors found a positive predictive value of 31% compared with 5.9% for the Wilson Risk Sum and 2.2% for the Mallampati test. Sensitivity was comparable to that of the Mallampati test (69.2% versus

67.9%) and slightly better than that of the Wilson Risk Sum. Specificity was improved for both tests. However, this method was attempted in 3572 patients but was successfully completed in only 2504. Patient refusal, patient intolerance because of gagging, poor physical status, and local infection were cited as reasons for unsuccessful examination. This low completion rate is a disadvantage of this technique.

CONCLUSIONS

Reviewing the *Index Medicus* to determine the number of airway-related articles published as a percentage of the total anesthesia-related articles published shows that since 1975 there has been a steady increase in academic discourse on this topic. Concurrently there has been a steady decline in adverse respiratory events, death, and brain damage as reported in the ASA Closed Claims Project. It is possible that improved information and increased discussion about difficult airway prediction and management have contributed to the decrease in catastrophic closed claims. Although current tests are less than ideal, a systematic and careful evaluation of the airway in each patient within the practitioner's own practice is still the best defense against the unexpected difficult intubation or difficult ventilation, or both. Additionally, when patients with a difficult airway or intubation are encountered, they should be registered with the MedicAlert system. Finally, the practitioner should always expect the unexpected: have a difficult airway cart ready and available, frequently review difficult airway drills such as the ASA Difficult Airway Algorithm, and practice special techniques that are helpful in the management of the patient with a difficult airway.

REFERENCES

1. Cheney FW, Posner KL, Caplan RA: Adverse respiratory events infrequently leading to malpractice suits. A closed claims analysis. Anesthesiology 75:932, 1991.
2. Samsoon GL, Young JR: Difficult tracheal intubation: A retrospective study. Anaesthesia 42:487, 1987.
3. Rocke DA, Murray WB, Rout CC, Gouws E: Relative risk analysis of factors associated with difficult intubation in obstetric anesthesia. Anesthesiology 77:67, 1992.
4. Practice guidelines for management of the difficult airway. A report by the ASA Task Force on Management of the Difficult Airway. Anesthesiology 78:597,1993.
5. Benumof JL: The difficult airway. *In* Benumof JL (ed): Airway Management Principles and Practice. St Louis, Mosby–Year Book, 1996, p 121.
6. Cormack RS, Lehane J: Difficult tracheal intubation in obstetrics. Anaesthesia 39:1105, 1984.
7. Cass NM, James NR, Lines V: Difficult direct laryngoscopy complicating intubation for anaesthesia. BMJ 1:488, 1956.
8. White A, Kander PL: Anatomical factors in difficult direct laryngoscopy. Br J Anaesth 47:468, 1975.
9. Patil VU, Stehling LC, Zauder HL: Predicting the difficulty of intubation utilizing an intubation guide. Anesthesiol Rev 10:32, 1983.
10. Mallampati SR: Clinical sign to predict difficult tracheal intubation (hypothesis). Can Anaesth Soc J 30:316, 1983.
11. Mallampati SR, Gatt SP, Gugino LD, et al: A clinical sign to predict difficult tracheal intubation: A prospective study. Can Anaesth Soc J 32:429, 1985.

12. Oates JD, Macleod AD, Oates PD, et al: Comparison of two methods for predicting difficult intubation. Br J Anaesth 66:305, 1991.
13. Wilson ME, Spiegelhalter D, Robertson JA, Lesser P: Predicting difficult intubation. Br J Anaesth 61:211, 1988.
14. Charters P, Perera S, Horton WA: Visibility of pharyngeal structures as a predictor of difficult intubation. Anaesthesia 42:1115, 1987.
15. Oates JD, Oates PD, Pearsall FJ, McLeod AD, Howie JC: Phonation affects Mallampati class. Anaesthesia 45:984, 1990.
16. Wilson ME, John R: Problems with the Mallampati sign. Anaesthesia 45:486, 1990.
17. Lewis M, Keramati S, Benumof JL, Berry CC: What is the best way to determine oropharyngeal classification and mandibular space length to predict difficult laryngoscopy? Anesthesiology 81:69, 1994.
18. Savva D: Prediction of difficult tracheal intubation. Br J Anaesth 73:149, 1994.
19. Mathew M, Hanna LS, Aldrete JA: Preoperative indices to anticipate the difficult tracheal intubation [abstract]. Anesth Analg 68:S187, 1989.
20. Frerk CM: Predicting difficult intubation. Anaesthesia 46:1005, 1991.
21. Bellhouse CP, Doré C: Criteria for estimating likelihood of difficulty of endotracheal intubation with the MacIntosh laryngoscope. Anaesth Intensive Care 16:329, 1988.
22. Tse JC, Rimm EB, Hussain A: Predicting difficult endotracheal intubation in surgical patients scheduled for general anesthesia: A prospective blind study. Anesth Analg 81:254, 1995.
23. Mallampati SR: Recognition of the difficult airway. *In* Benumof JL (ed): Airway Management Principles and Practice. St Louis, Mosby–Year Book, 1996, p 126.
24. El-Ganzouri AR, McCarthy RJ, Tuman KJ, et al: Preoperative airway assessment: Predictive value of a multivariate risk index. Anesth Analg 82:1197, 1996.
25. Mason DG, Wark KJ: Unexpected difficult intubation. Asymptomatic epiglottic cysts as a cause of upper airway obstruction during anaesthesia. Anaesthesia 42:407, 1987.
26. Cohle SD, Jones DH, Puri S: Lingual tonsillar hypertrophy causing failed intubation and cerebral anoxia. Am J Forensic Med Pathol 14:158, 1993.
27. Shapiro BA, Glassenberg R, Panchal S: The incidence of failed or difficult intubation in different surgical populations [abstract]. Anesthesiology 81:A1212, 1994.
28. Mark LJ, Beattie C, Ferrell CL, et al: The difficult airway: Mechanisms for effective dissemination of critical information. J Clin Anesth 4:247, 1992.
29. Williamson JA, Webb RK, Szekely S, et al: The Australian Incident Monitoring Study. Difficult intubation: An analysis of 2000 incident reports. Anaesth Intensive Care 21:602, 1993.
30. Eckmann DM, Glassenberg R, Gavriely N: Acoustic reflectometry and endotracheal intubation. Anesth Analg 83:1084, 1996.
31. Roberts JT, Ali HH, Shorten GD: Using the bubble inclinometer to measure laryngeal tilt and predict difficulty of laryngoscopy. J Clin Anesth 5:306, 1993.
32. Yanamoto K, Tsubokawa T, Shibata K, et al: Predicting difficult intubation with indirect laryngoscopy. Anesthesiology 86: 316, 1997.

Chapter 3

ASA Difficult Airway Algorithm: New Thoughts and Considerations

Jonathan L. Benumof

The American Society of Anesthesiologists (ASA) Difficult Airway Algorithm has been before the anesthesia community, in one form or form or another, since 1993. During this 6-year experience, a number of new issues have emerged that require modification of the ASA Difficult Airway Algorithm. These issues include the use of regional anesthesia (RA), the use of muscle relaxants, the role of the laryngeal mask airway (LMA), and appropriate options for the cannot-ventilate, cannot-intubate (CVCI) situation. This chapter first briefly reviews the algorithm in its present form and then discusses each of these issues. Additionally, definitions of *optimal or best attempt at conventional mask ventilation and laryngoscopy* and of *difficult endotracheal intubation* are reviewed.

BRIEF REVIEW OF THE ASA DIFFICULT AIRWAY ALGORITHM

The ASA Difficult Airway Algorithm is depicted in Figure 3–1. This is an all-inclusive algorithm that incorporates all previously approved concepts into one flow diagram.[1-2] The algorithm begins with preoperative evaluation and recognition of the difficult airway. Evaluation of the airway should include determination of the oropharyngeal classification, the mandibular space length, the range of motion of the head and neck (the ability to assume the sniffing position), the length and thickness (muscularity) of the neck, the length of the teeth, the degree of natural overriding of the maxillary on the mandibular teeth, the ability to bring the mandibular teeth anterior to the maxillary teeth, the configuration of the palate, and the presence of a beard, large breasts, or pathologic states (cancer, infection, bleeding, disruption, and so forth) (see Chapter 2 for further detail).

When management of the airway is expected to be difficult, it is logical to secure the airway while the patient is awake. In order for awake endotracheal intubation to succeed, it is essential to prepare the patient properly. The components of proper preparation for awake intubation consist of psychologic preparation (awake intubation proceeds more easily in the patient who knows and agrees with what is going to happen); appropriate monitoring (electrocardiogram, noninvasive blood pressure, pulse oximetry, and capnography); the administration of a drying agent; judicious sedation (keeping the patient in meaningful contact with the environment); the induction of vasoconstriction of the nasal mucous membranes; the topical application of local anesthetic; the performance of laryngeal nerve blocks; aspiration prevention; and the availability of appropriate airway equipment. Once the patient is properly prepared, any one of a number of intubation techniques can achieve endotracheal intubation (Table 3–1).[3] Oxygen supplementation during preparation and intubation is almost always desirable. The technique or techniques chosen depend on the anticipated surgery, the condition of the patient, and the skills and preferences of the anesthesia practitioner. Also, once the patient is prepared adequately, an "awake look" with a laryngoscope may be performed in order to further assess the degree of difficulty in securing the airway. If an adequate view is obtained, endotracheal intubation may be performed followed immediately by the administration of an intravenous induction agent.

Occasionally, awake intubation may fail owing to a lack of patient cooperation, equipment or operator limitations, or all of these. Depending on the precise cause of failure of awake intubation, (1) the surgery may be canceled (the patient needs further counseling, airway edema or trauma has resulted, or different equipment or personnel is necessary), (2) general anesthesia (GA) may be induced (the fundamental problem must be considered to be a lack of cooperation, and mask ventilation is considered to be nonproblematic), (3) RA may be induced (see the section Use of Regional Anesthesia and the Difficult Airway), or (4) a surgical airway may be created (the surgery is essential and GA is considered inappropriate until intubation is accomplished). Occa-

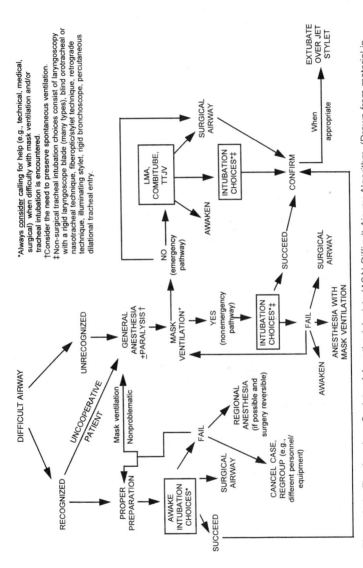

Figure 3–1 The American Society of Anesthesiologists (ASA) Difficult Airway Algorithm. (Drawn from material in ASA guidelines[1] and Benumof.[2]) LMA, laryngeal mask airway; TTJV, transtracheal jet ventilation.

Table 3–1   Techniques for Difficult Airway Management*

Techniques for difficult intubation
    Alternative laryngoscope blades
    Awake intubation
    Blind intubation (oral or nasal)
    Fiberoptic intubation
    Intubating stylet-tube changer
    Light wand
    Retrograde intubation
    Surgical airway access
Techniques for difficult ventilation
    Esophageal-tracheal Combitube
    Intratracheal jet stylet
    Laryngeal mask airway
    Oral and nasopharyngeal airways
    Rigid ventilating bronchoscope
    Surgical airway access
    Transtracheal jet ventilation
    Two-person mask ventilation

---

*These alphabetical lists of commonly cited techniques for difficult airway management are not comprehensive. No preferences are implied, and combinations of techniques may be employed.
From Benumof JL: The ASA management of the difficult airway algorithm and explanation—Analysis of the algorithm. *In* Benumof JL (ed): Airway Management Principles and Practice. St. Louis, Mosby–Year Book, 1996, p 147.

sionally, a surgical airway is the best choice for intubation (e.g., with laryngeal or tracheal fracture or disruption, upper airway abscess, combined mandibular-maxillary fractures).

It is appropriate to attempt endotracheal intubation after the induction of GA when a difficult airway is not recognized or when a difficult airway is recognized but the patient is extremely uncooperative and vigorously refuses an awake intubation. If GA is necessary, the clinician should consider the relative merits of the preservation of spontaneous ventilation versus the use of muscle relaxants (in an unrecognized difficult airway, the use of a muscle relaxant is ordinarily not an issue). Endotracheal intubation can be accomplished by any one of a number of intubation choices. If a given intubation choice should fail, gas exchange should be accomplished by mask ventilation. If the initial intubation choice is conventional laryngoscopy, the first laryngoscopic procedure should be optimal with respect to head and neck position and the use of external laryngeal manipulation (see the sections More Realistic Definition of Difficult Tracheal Intubation, and Definition of Optimal or Best Attempt at Conventional Laryngoscopy). If conventional laryngoscopy should fail, there are a number of acceptable alternative approaches that may facilitate endotracheal intubation. The repeated use of a conventional laryngoscope can cause laryngeal trauma (edema, bleeding), which may result in the loss of the ability to ventilate via mask. In fact, the most common scenario in the respiratory catastrophes in the ASA Closed Claims Project was the development of progressive difficulty in mask ventilation between persistent and prolonged failed intubation attempts, resulting in the inability to ventilate and provide adequate gas exchange. Consequently, if there does not appear to be anything different that can be atraumatically and quickly tried (a better sniffing position, an external laryngeal manipulation, a new blade, a new technique, reattempt at intubation by a much more experienced laryngoscopist, and so forth) after a few failed intubation attempts, and if ventilation by mask can still be maintained, it is prudent to cease attempting to intubate the trachea and to awaken the patient, continue anesthesia by mask ventilation, or create a surgical airway before the ability to ventilate by mask is lost.

If the ability to ventilate by mask is lost and the patient cannot be intubated (a CVCI situation), then a truly emergent imminent brain- and life-threatening situation exists and gas exchange must be restored immediately. There are now four acceptable responses to the CVCI situation: (1) the insertion of an LMA, (2) the insertion of an esophageal-tracheal Combitube (ETC), (3) the institution of transtracheal jet ventilation (TTJV), and (4) the creation of a surgical airway (if personnel, equipment, lighting, and positioning are appropriate) (see the section Appropriate Options for the Cannot-Ventilate, Cannot-Intubate Situation). One must remember that both the ETC and the LMA are supraglottic ventilatory devices and may not allow successful intubation when airway obstruction occurs at or below the glottic opening. Also, any of these rescue options should be pursued early and quickly to enhance the possibility of a positive patient outcome. Finally, those responsible for the patient must guarantee communication of this difficult airway experience to future caretakers so that the near-death experience is not repeated (see Chapter 17). There are four important messages in the ASA Difficult Airway Algorithm (Table 3–2).[3]

MORE REALISTIC DEFINITION OF DIFFICULT TRACHEAL INTUBATION

The ASA Difficult Airway Algorithm defines *difficult endotracheal intubation* as the proper insertion of an endotracheal tube (ET) with conventional laryngoscopy that requires more than three attempts, more than 10 minutes, or both.[1] In addition, *difficult laryngoscopy* is also defined according to the laryngoscopic view. This definition of a difficult endo-

Table 3–2 ASA Difficult Airway Algorithm Take-Home Messages

1. If suspicious of trouble → Secure the airway awake
2. If you get into trouble → Awaken the patient
3. Have plan B and C immediately available or in place → Think ahead
4. Intubation choices → Do what you do best

From Benumof JL: The ASA management of the difficult airway algorithm and explanation—Analysis of the algorithm. *In* Benumof JL (ed): Airway Management Principles and Practice. St. Louis, Mosby–Year Book, 1996, p 149.

tracheal intubation is illogical because an optimal attempt at laryngoscopy may be achieved on the first attempt (see Definition of Optimal or Best Attempt at Conventional Laryngoscopy) within 30 seconds and reveal a grade IV laryngoscopic view (whether due to inherent anatomy, a massive lesion, or both), and thus a difficult intubation may be readily apparent to a reasonably experienced intubationist on the first attempt and be *independent* of both the number of attempts and the time. Conversely, one may have a near-optimal grade II view (success close), and a slight improvement (optimal effort) may result in success. A more logical definition of a difficult endotracheal intubation would be based on the optimal view as well as periglottic abnormality and would retain the number and time of attempts as maximal boundary conditions.

DEFINITION OF OPTIMAL OR BEST ATTEMPT AT CONVENTIONAL MASK VENTILATION

If the patient cannot be intubated, gas exchange is dependent on mask ventilation, and if the patient cannot be ventilated by mask, a CVCI situation exists and immediate life-saving maneuvers must be instituted (see the section Appropriate Options for the Cannot-Ventilate, Cannot-Intubate Situation). Since each of the acceptable responses to a CVCI situation has its own risks, the decision to abandon mask ventilation should be made after the anesthesia practitioner has made an optimal attempt at mask ventilation.

The first component of an optimal attempt at conventional mask ventilation is that it should be a two-person effort (Fig. 3–2),[3] because a far better mask seal and jaw thrust and therefore greater tidal volume can be achieved with two people than with one person. Figure 3–2A shows a proper two-person mask ventilation effort when the second person knows how to perform a jaw-thrust maneuver. Figure 3–2B shows a proper two-person mask ventilation effort when the second person is capable only of squeezing the reservoir bag (i.e., is unfamiliar with airway maneuvers). The second component of the optimal attempt at conventional mask ventilation is to use large oral or nasal airways, or both. If mask ventilation is poor or nonexistent with a vigorous two-person effort in the presence of large artificial airways, then it is time to move on to a potentially organ- and lifesaving alternative plan (see Fig. 3–1 and the section Appropriate Options for the Cannot-Ventilate, Cannot-Intubate Situation).

DEFINITION OF OPTIMAL OR BEST ATTEMPT AT CONVENTIONAL LARYNGOSCOPY

The problem with multiple repeated attempts at conventional laryngoscopy is the creation of laryngeal edema and bleeding that will impair mask ventilation, as well as subsequent endotracheal intubation attempts, thereby creating a CVCI situation. Thus, it is imperative that anesthesia practitioners make their best attempt at laryngoscopy as

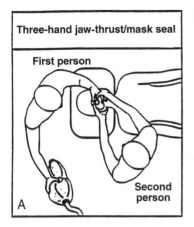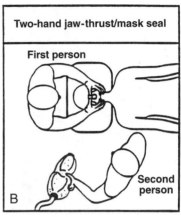

Figure 3–2 Optimal two-person mask ventilation. *A*, Two-person effort when second person knows how to perform jaw thrust. *B*, Two-person effort when second person can only squeeze the reservoir bag. (From Benumof JL: The ASA management of the difficult airway algorithm and explanation-analysis of the algorithm. *In* Benumof JL [ed]: Airway Management Principles and Practice. St. Louis, Mosby–Year Book, 1996, p 153.)

early as possible, and if that fails, a second plan of action should be activated so that no further risk, without likely benefit, will be incurred.

What is an optimal or best attempt at conventional laryngoscopy? First, a reasonably experienced person, that is, an anesthesia practitioner who has had at least 3 full years of experience, should perform the laryngoscopy.

Second, the patient should always be in an optimal sniffing position (slight flexion of the neck on the head and extreme extension of the head on the neck),[4] which aligns the oral, pharyngeal, and laryngeal axes into a fairly straight line. In some patients, such as obese ones, obtaining an optimal sniffing position takes a great deal of work (Fig. 3–3),[5] such as placing pillows and blankets under the scapulae, shoulders, nape of the neck, and head. These positioning maneuvers are extremely difficult to perform once anesthesia and paralysis have made the patient a massive (dead) weight. Thus, an attempt at endotracheal intubation should not be wasted because of failure to have the patient in an optimal sniffing position before the induction of GA.

Third, if the laryngoscopic grade is II (just arytenoids), III (just epiglottis), or IV (just soft palate), then optimal external laryngeal manipulation (OELM) should be used (Fig. 3–4).[4-6] OELM is not simply cricoid pressure but rather pressure applied in a posterior and cephalic direction over the thyroid (the best location in 9% of patients),[6] hyoid, and cricoid cartilages and can be achieved in 5 to 10 seconds. It can frequently improve the laryngoscopic view by at least a whole grade[6] and should be an inherent part of laryngoscopy and an instinctive response to a poor laryngoscopic view. Thus, an attempt at endotracheal intubation should not be wasted because of failure to use OELM.

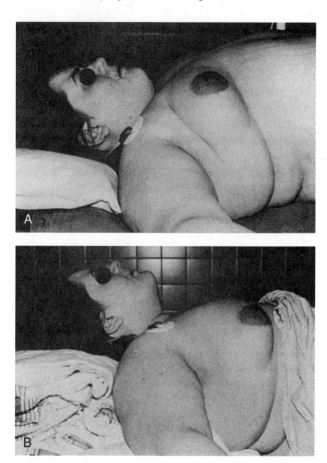

Figure 3–3 Getting the patient (especially the obese patient) into an optimal sniffing position before the induction of general anesthesia may take a great deal of effort. *A*, Head resting on pillow. *B*, Scapula, shoulder, nape of neck, and head support results in the sniffing position. (From Davis JM, Weeks S, Crone LA: Difficult intubation in the parturient. Can J Anaesth 36:668, 1989. Photo permission granted by Williams & Wilkins, Baltimore, MD.)

Fourth, the proper function of both a MacIntosh and a Miller blade is dependent on using an appropriate length of blade. In order to lift the epiglottis out of the line of sight, the MacIntosh blade must be long enough to put tension on the hyoepiglottic ligament, and the Miller blade must be long enough to trap the epiglottis against the tongue. Thus, in some patients it may be appropriate to change the length of the blade one time in order to obtain proper blade function.

Fifth, in some patients, a MacIntosh blade may provide superior intubating conditions compared with a Miller blade, and vice versa. A

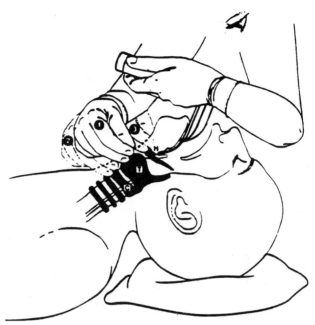

Figure 3–4 Determining optimal external laryngeal manipulation with free (right) hand. Optimal external laryngeal manipulation should be an inherent part of laryngoscopy and is performed when laryngoscopic view is poor. Ninety percent of the time, the best view is obtained by pressing over the thyroid cartilage (1) or the cricoid cartilage (2); pressing over the hyoid bone (3) may also be effective. (From Benumof JL: The ASA management of the difficult airway algorithm and explanation-analysis of the algorithm. *In* Benumof JL [ed]: Airway Management Principles and Practice. St Louis, Mosby–Year Book, 1996, p 152.)

MacIntosh blade is generally regarded as a better blade whenever there is little upper airway room to pass the ET (e.g., with a small narrow mouth, palate, or oropharynx), and a Miller blade is generally regarded as a better blade in patients with a small mandibular space, anterior larynx, large incisors, or a long, floppy epiglottis.

In summary, an optimal or best attempt at laryngoscopy can be defined as (1) performance by a reasonably experienced laryngoscopist, (2) the use of the optimal sniffing position, (3) the use of OELM, (4) one change in the length of the blade, and (5) one change in the type of blade. With this definition, and with no other confounding considerations, the optimal attempt at laryngoscopy may be achieved on the first attempt and should not take more than four attempts.[6]

USE OF REGIONAL ANESTHESIA AND THE DIFFICULT AIRWAY

The use of RA in patients with a recognized difficult airway does not solve the problem of the difficult airway; the difficult airway is still present. The danger of RA in a patient with a known or suspected difficult airway is that the failure of RA could result in the need for the precipitous induction of GA under suboptimal conditions, with a resultant loss of control of the airway.

RA is an acceptable choice in this patient population under two broadly defined circumstances: (1) if the surgery can be discontinued at any point by the surgeon without harm to the patient and (2) if the patient and the anesthesia practitioner are well prepared for the performance of an awake intubation *and* there is good access to the patient's airway. Further consideration should be given to the type of surgery (i.e., upper or lower extremity versus abdominal surgery) and the technique of RA (i.e., peripheral nerve block versus major conduction blockade). Common sense and experience should be applied. If surgery can be quickly terminated and if RA fails (irrespective of the patient's position), then the surgery can be canceled, the patient can be intubated awake (if cooperative and after proper preparation), or another attempt at RA can be made (*left panel* of Fig. 3–5).[3] No respiratory bridges are burned with these approaches.

When surgery cannot be quickly terminated, it is acceptable to perform RA in a patient with a known difficult airway if a preoperative contract (firm agreement) has been made with the patient that an awake intubation will be done if RA fails (*middle panel* of Fig. 3–5).[3] Obviously, in order for this plan to work, there must be good access to the patient's airway. In order for awake intubation to succeed under such conditions, it is essential that the patient be kept in meaningful contact with the anesthesia practitioner (i.e., rational, oriented, and responsive to commands), fully cooperative, and not oversedated or disinhibited. Finally, if GA is necessary in this situation, there must also be good access to the patient's airway, and another plan of action must be ready to be immediately used (e.g., the elective preinduction placement of an appropriate TTJV catheter, or immediate availability of an experienced surgeon and preparation of the patient's neck). *It is unacceptable to do RA with a known difficult airway when surgery cannot be terminated rapidly and there is poor access to the patient's airway or head (right panel* of Fig. 3–5).[3]

USE OF MUSCLE RELAXANTS AND THE DIFFICULT AIRWAY

In patients presenting for elective surgery who end up in a CVCI situation, the following is a common story. Preoperatively, the anesthesia practitioner does not recognize a difficult airway or believes the difficult airway is questionable, and GA is induced with an intravenous induction agent and succinylcholine. Mask ventilation is initiated without difficulty, but endotracheal intubation with conventional laryngoscopy fails (see Fig. 3–1).[3]

Appropriately, gas exchange is controlled by mask ventilation for a second time, and then, after some adjustments are made in positioning, conventional laryngoscopy and endotracheal intubation are reattempted but without success. Mask ventilation continues to control gas exchange for a third attempt, but it is now perceptibly more difficult

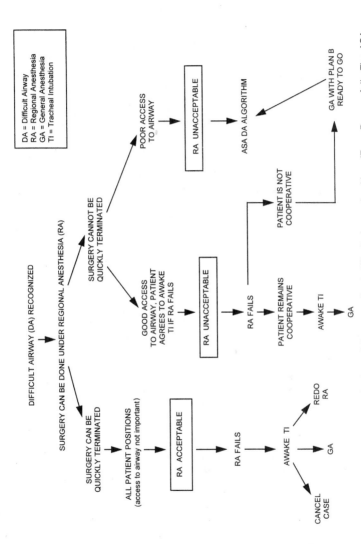

Figure 3–5 Regional anesthesia and the recognized difficult airway algorithm. (From Benumof JL: The ASA management of the difficult airway algorithm and explanation-analysis of the algorithm. *In* Benumof JL [ed]: Airway Management Principles and Practice. St Louis, Mosby–Year Book, 1996, p 150.)

than before. After further adjustment (see the section More Realistic Definition of Difficult Tracheal Intubation), conventional laryngoscopy and endotracheal intubation are attempted for the third time and again fail. At this point, approximately 5 to 8 minutes have passed since the administration of succinylcholine. Although the anesthesia practitioner may want to exercise the awake option, the patient is not breathing spontaneously, and mask ventilation is now attempted for a fourth time. However, mask ventilation is extremely difficult or impossible because the chest wall is rigid since the patient is sustaining a forceful exhalation mode and because of the presence of laryngospasm owing to the prior three laryngoscopic procedures and attempts at intubation. Now a race begins, and the question arises whether the patient will resume adequate spontaneous ventilation (awaken) before experiencing severe hypoxemia, possibly resulting in organ or body damage. The answer is not certain and depends on many pharmacologic and physiologic variables. From this common story in patients who have ended up in a CVCI situation, the advantages and disadvantages of muscle relaxants with different durations of action become obvious (Table 3–3).[3] With the induction of general anesthesia in an uncooperative patient with a recognized difficult airway, the practitioner should consider the relative merits of the preservation of spontaneous ventilation versus the use of muscle relaxants.

The use of succinylcholine in a patient with either a recognized or a questionable difficult airway may not be the best choice, particularly if it is thought that mask ventilation will be possible and a smooth transition to an alternative plan of action (e.g., fiberoptic bronchoscopy[7]) is desirable. The key element in the choice of using a nondepolarizing relaxant is the assumption that mask ventilation will be adequate (see the section Definition of Optimal or Best Attempt at Conventional Mask Ventilation) and preparations for rescue plans have been made. Alternatively, endotracheal intubation can be successfully accomplished without the use of any muscle relaxant, and this option should be considered in certain situations.[8] Also, if a small dose of succinylcholine (0.5 to 0.75 mg/kg) is used, good intubating conditions can be achieved

Table 3–3   Advantages and Disadvantages of Muscle Relaxants with Different Durations of Action

Relaxant	Advantage	Disadvantage
Succinylcholine	Permits the awaken option early	As the drug wears off, a period of poor ventilation may occur Poor transition to plan B
Short-acting nondepolarizers	Good transition to plan B if mask ventilation is adequate	Does not permit early-awaken options

From Benumof JL: The ASA management of the difficult airway algorithm and explanation—Analysis of the algorithm. *In* Benumof JL (ed): Airway Management Principles and Practice. St. Louis, Mosby–Year Book, 1996, p 151.

within 75 seconds for a duration of 60 seconds, thus allowing an early-awaken option.

Another consideration is that in a large majority of patients, prior administration of a small dose of a nondepolarizing neuromuscular blocker may slightly diminish the duration of action of succinylcholine,[9] and thus the time to spontaneous recovery of airway reflexes may be shortened.

Lastly, whether to administer a second dose of succinylcholine following a cannot-intubate situation in which the patient resumes spontaneous ventilation is debatable, depending on the situation. If the chances of achieving successful tracheal intubation are high (i.e., a fairly good laryngoscopic grade) yet it is difficult to accomplish intubation because of incomplete paralysis, the administration of a second dose of succinylcholine may be appropriate. It may also be considered appropriate in situations in which mask ventilation is possible, the laryngoscopist is highly skilled, and a simple change in either the patient's position or the type of laryngoscope is necessary. A small dose of glycopyrrolate (0.2 to 0.4 mg) should be administered in conjunction with the repeat dose of succinylcholine in order to prevent a bradycardic response.

APPROPRIATE OPTIONS FOR THE CANNOT-VENTILATE, CANNOT-INTUBATE SITUATION

Since 1992, anesthesia practitioners in the United States have become familiar with the LMA[10] and the ETC[11] and have found that the LMA works well in elective situations and that both the LMA and the ETC work well as ventilatory devices in CVCI situations.[10–12]

The LMA, in addition, has proved to be an excellent conduit to the larynx for a flexible fiberoptic bronchoscope.[10–12] Although the ASA Difficult Airway Algorithm lists these two devices, along with TTJV, as appropriate nonsurgical solutions for the CVCI situation (see Fig. 3–1),[3] they both deserve a higher prominence ranking in the minds of many anesthesia practitioners.

First, they will *probably* work as ventilatory mechanisms. Second, both can be inserted blindly, quickly, and with a relative low level of skill. Third, thus far, complications have been limited. Also, even though TTJV can also be rapidly instituted with a low level of skill and work well if the practitioner has prepared in advance, there is still a significant risk of barotrauma (delivery of too large a tidal volume, allowing too short or inadequate exhalation, letting go of the catheter with subsequent dislodgment).

Although the algorithm does not dictate the order of preference of these devices in the CVCI situation, the anesthesia practitioner must take into account (1) the practitioner's own experience and level of comfort in the use of these methods, (2) the availability of these devices, (3) the type of airway obstruction (upper versus lower), and (4) the benefits and risks involved. Although the LMA is easily inserted, even by inexperienced personnel,[13] it does not provide an airtight seal around the larynx or protect the trachea from aspiration. The ETC, on the other hand, prevents aspiration by sealing the esophagus rather than the trachea. The author is unaware of any cases of major aspiration.

However, it must be remembered that both the LMA and the ETC are *supraglottic* ventilatory devices (Chapter 8) and that is their inherent weakness. Thus they cannot solve a truly glottic (e.g., spasm, massive edema, tumor, abscess) or subglottic problem.[11] If a truly glottic or subglottic problem exists, the only solution will be to get the ventilatory mechanism below the level of the lesion (e.g., TTJV, ET, surgical airway).

Nonetheless, out of these options, the LMA is the one device that most anesthesia practitioners are accustomed to because it has gained so much familiarity as a routine airway for use during GA. Also, since its introduction, it has proved to serve as an excellent conduit for tracheal intubation. As such, the LMA fits into the ASA Difficult Airway Algorithm[14] in five places (Fig. 3–6).

CONFIRMATION OF ENDOTRACHEAL INTUBATION DURING CARDIAC ARREST

Cardiac arrest may occur in a CVCI situation. During cardiac arrest, there is no pulmonary blood flow and end-tidal partial pressure of carbon dioxide ($P_{ET}CO_2$) decreases to zero. Thus, methods that rely on CO_2 detection such as capnography or calorimetry cannot be used to confirm endotracheal intubation during this clinical scenario.

A variety of methods can be used to confirm tracheal intubation; they may be categorized under three main headings (Table 3–4).[15] If the ET cannot be visualized passing through the vocal cords (even with depression of the pharyngeal part of the ET posteriorly, which pulls the larynx posteriorly) and a flexible fiberoptic bronchoscope cannot quickly reveal endotracheal intubation, then no fail-safe method of confirming endotracheal intubation is available (all other methods during cardiac arrest and cardiopulmonary resuscitation are subject to considerable error, including combined auscultation of the epigastrium and both axillae). However, the esophageal detector device is a nearly fail-safe device for detecting esophageal and tracheal intubation that is easy to use and provides immediate results.[16] If the ET is in the esophagus, the previously collapsed bulb of the esophageal detector device *fails* to expand immediately, whereas if the ET is in the trachea, the bulb immediately expands. Although it is considered to be a reliable device, several conditions produce both false-negative and false-positive results (Table 3–5).[16] The presence of nasogastric tube or cuff deflation does not affect the performance of the device or contribute to the occurrence of false-positive results.[17]

Transtracheal illumination is also a useful method to differentiate esophageal from tracheal tube placement in the cardiac arrest situation. Typically, there is an intense circumscribed midline glow in the region of the laryngeal prominence and sternal notch when the ET is positioned in the trachea. If an esophageal intubation occurs, the illumination may be dull and diffuse or even absent. Although the reliability of

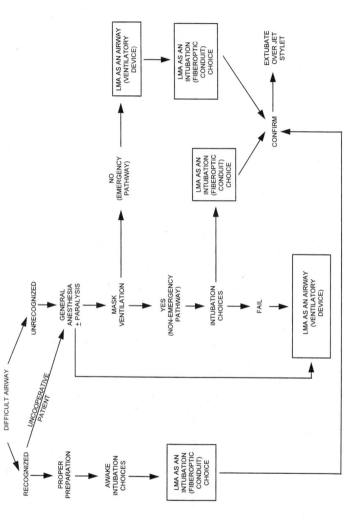

Figure 3-6 The laryngeal mask airway (LMA) fits into the ASA algorithm on the management of the difficult airway in five different places as either an airway (ventilation device) or a conduit for a fiberscope. (From Benumof JL: The laryngeal mask airway and the ASA difficult airway algorithm. Anesthesiology 84:686–699, 1996.)

Table 3–4   Signs of Tracheal Intubation

Non–fail-safe signs
1. Breath sounds over chest
2. No breath sounds over stomach
3. No gastric distention
4. Chest rise and fall
5. Intercostal spaces filling out during inspiration
6. Large spontaneous exhaled tidal volumes
7. Respiratory gas moisture disappearing on inhalation and reappearing on exhalation
8. Sound of air exit from the endotracheal tube when the chest is compressed
9. Reservoir bag having the appropriate compliance
10. Reciprocating pulsed pressures to and from suprasternal notch and to and from balloon on the pilot tube of the endotracheal tube
11. Progressive arterial desaturation by pulse oximetry

Near–fail-safe signs
1. Carbon dioxide excretion waveform
2. Rapid expansion of an esophageal or tracheal indicator bulb

Fail-safe signs
1. Endotracheal tube visualized between vocal cords
2. Fiberoptic visualization of cartilaginous rings of the trachea and tracheal carina

From Benumof JL: Conventional (laryngoscopic) orotracheal and nasotracheal intubation (single-lumen tube). *In* Benumof JL (ed): Airway Management Principles and Practice. St. Louis, Mosby–Year Book, 1996, p 534.

this technique in distinguishing esophageal from tracheal intubation has been demonstrated, false-negative results may occur in obese patients or in patients with neck swelling and dark skin, whereas false-positive results have occurred in thin patients.[18]

In summary, the ASA Difficult Airway Algorithm has worked well over the past 9 years. In fact, there has been a dramatic decrease (30% to 40%) in the number of respiratory-related malpractice lawsuits, brain damage, and death attributable to anesthesia since 1990.[19] However, a number of issues have emerged that indicate that the ASA Difficult Airway Algorithm can be improved. They include the role of regional anesthesia and muscle relaxants of different durations of action in difficult airway management; the definition of end points for the use of conventional laryngoscopy and mask ventilation; the definition of difficult endotracheal intubation; confirmation of endotracheal intubation during cardiac arrest; reconsideration of CVCI options; and dispensing MedicAlert bracelets to patients who have experienced a near–life-taking difficult airway experience so that future caretakers will not unwittingly reproduce the same experience and risk (see Chapter 17).[20] Consideration of these issues should make the ASA Difficult Airway Algorithm still more clinically specific and functional.

Table 3–5 Problems with Use of a Self-Inflating Bulb

FALSE-NEGATIVE RESULTS

Obstruction
    Tube
        Kinking, secretions, blood clots
    Upper airway (below the tube)
        Infants
        Tracheomalacia
        Tube at carina
        Main bronchus intubation
        Tumors and other abnormality
    Lower airway
        Bronchospasm
        COPD

Marked reduction in FRC
    Morbid obesity
    Pregnancy
    Pulmonary edema
    Atelectasis

FALSE-POSITIVE RESULTS

Massive gastric insufflation

Incompetent lower esophageal sphincter
    Hiatal hernia
    Pregnancy
    Gastroesophageal disease

COPD, chronic obstructive pulmonary disease; FRC, functional residual capacity.
Data from Salem R, Baraka A: Confirmation of tracheal intubation. *In* Benumof JL (ed): Airway Management Principles and Practice. St. Louis, Mosby–Year Book, 1996.

REFERENCES

1. Practice guidelines for management of the difficult airway. A report by the ASA Task Force on Management of the Difficult Airway. Anesthesiology 78:597–602, 1993.
2. Benumof JL: Management of the difficult airway. Anesthesiology 75:1087–1110, 1991.
3. Benumof JL: The ASA management of the difficult airway algorithm and explanation—Analysis of the algorithm. *In* Benumof JL (ed): Airway Management Principles and Practice. St Louis, Mosby–Year Book, 1996, p 147.
4. Benumof JL: Difficult laryngoscopy [editorial]. Can J Anaesth 41:361–365, 1994.
5. Davis JM, Weeks S, Crone LA: Difficult intubation in the parturient. Can J Anaesth 36:668, 1989.
6. Benumof JL, Cooper SD: Quantitative improvement in laryngoscopic view by optimal laryngeal manipulation. J Clin Anesth 8:136–140, 1996.
7. Ovassapian AK, Wheeler M: Fiberoptic endoscopy aided technique. *In* Benumof JL (ed): Airway Management Principles and Practice. St Louis, Mosby–Year Book, 1996.
8. Wong AKH, Teoh GS: Intubation without muscle relaxant: An alternative technique for rapid tracheal intubation. Anaesth Intensive Care 24:224–230, 1996.
9. Walts LF, Dillon JB: Clinical studies of the interaction between *d*-tubocurarine and succinylcholine. Anesthesiology 31:39–44, 1969.
10. White P, Smith I: Laryngeal mask airway. *In* Benumof JL (ed): Airway Management Principles and Practice. St Louis, Mosby–Year Book, 1996.

11. Frass M: The Combitube. *In* Benumof JL (ed): Airway Management Principles and Practice. St Louis, Mosby–Year Book, 1996.
12. Benumof JL: The laryngeal mask airway [editorial]. Anesthesiology 77:843–846, 1992.
13. Pennant JH, Walker MB: Comparison of the endotracheal tube and laryngeal mask airway in airway management by paramedical personnel. Anesth Analg 74:531–534, 1992.
14. Benumof JL: The laryngeal mask airway and the ASA difficult airway algorithm. Anesthesiology 84:686–699, 1996.
15. Benumof JL: Conventional (laryngoscopic) orotracheal and nasotracheal intubation (single-lumen tube). *In* Benumof JL (ed): Airway Management Principles and Practice. St Louis, Mosby–Year Book, 1996, p 534.
16. Salem R, Baraka A: Confirmation of tracheal intubation. *In* Benumof JL (ed): Airway Management Principles and Practice. St Louis, Mosby–Year Book, 1996.
17. Salem MR, Wafai Y, Joseph NJ, et al: Efficacy of the self-inflating bulb in detecting esophageal intubation: Does the presence of a nasogastric tube or cuff deflation make a difference? Anesthesiology 80:42–48, 1994.
18. Stewart RD, LaRose A, Stoy WA, et al: Use of a lighted stylet to confirm correct endotracheal tube placement. Chest 92:900, 1987.
19. Cheney FW: Committee on Professional Liability—Overview. Am Soc Anesth News June 1994.
20. Mark L, Schauble J, Gibby G, et al: Effective dissemination of critical airway information: The MedicAlert National Difficult Airway/Intubation Registry. *In* Benumof JL (ed): Airway Management Principles and Practice. St Louis, Mosby–Year Book, 1996, chap 44.

Chapter 4

Preparation of the Patient

for Awake Intubation

Antonio F. Sanchez and Debra E. Morrison

The first documented awake endotracheal intubation was performed in 1880 on a patient in extremis, suffering from glottic edema. Without the benefit of anesthesia and without topical or regional blocks, sedatives, or analgesics, the patient underwent an awake manual endotracheal intubation with a metallic endotracheal tube (ET). The ET was kept in place with the patient in an awake state for 35 hours.[1] Although we may perceive this as brutal, the anesthesia practitioner (Dr. E. M. Macewend) who performed the intubation was aware over 100 years ago that in spite of the patient's discomfort, the safest method for securing a difficult airway was to perform an awake intubation (AI) rather than to provide comfort at the risk of compromising the airway totally.[2]

PSYCHOLOGIC PREPARATION

Subsequent reports of AI with favorable results are myriad,[3–11] yet there still seems to be an overall general hesitancy within the anesthesia community to perform AI.[12] There are no surveys to verify this statement,[13] but general attitudes and concerns are summarized in Table 4–1.

The reservations represented by these statements are adequately

Table 4–1 Reasons for Avoiding Awake Intubation

Luck, or heretofore long and safe practice of anesthesia without having had to perform any AIs

Lack of training in AI

Time constraints: desire not to be cause of delay

Reluctance or refusal of AI by patients

Concern that AI is too stressful emotionally and physically for patient

Fear of litigation in event of patient recall

AI, awake intubation.

Table 4–2   Key Elements of Past Anesthetics

Intubation, especially most recent
Ease of mask ventilation
Tolerance of drugs
Evidence of reactions to local anesthetics
Apnea with minimal doses of narcotics
Surgical procedure involved
Postoperative respiratory problems

addressed elsewhere in the literature. However, luck (see Table 4–1) is unreliable, and we recommend accepting the necessity of and developing skill and efficiency in the techniques of AI.

Psychologic preparation for AI thus begins with the anesthesia practitioner. Practitioners must develop confidence commensurate with their technical skills and develop the ability to communicate. Skill, confidence, and the ability to communicate will allow practitioners to successfully address the issues of patient refusal and surgeon impatience, to minimize the patient's emotional and physical distress, and to mitigate the negative effect of any recall on the part of the patient.

We focus on patients having elective surgery, in whom there is time to evaluate the airway and communicate. Evaluation is the beginning of psychologic engagement with the patient. In an emergency, which in itself should alert the practitioner to the probability of airway difficulty, especially with a patient in extremis,[14] the practitioner may not have time, nor can he or she be expected to be able to conduct an investigation with the thoroughness described later.

Investigation: Review of Medical Records

Whenever possible, the practitioner should examine previous anesthetic records (records, not just a record!), because they may provide useful information.[15, 16] By checking as many anesthetic records as possible, the practitioner may discover that the last intubation was routine but the three previous ones were difficult, or the last intubation was routine but the operation rendered the airway difficult. Note key elements of past anesthetics (Table 4–2), and focus on important features of the endotracheal intubations (Table 4–3). Decide whether the intubation technique, if successful, is one that can be duplicated in the present setting (the practitioner should not attempt to learn a new technique on a difficult airway). In addition, the practitioner should scan the medical records for evidence of postoperative airway problems.

Investigation: Review of History

After reviewing the medical records, the practitioner should ask the patient about any memories of past anesthetics (here, recall of past AIs

Table 4–3   Important Features of Past Intubations

Degree of difficulty of endotracheal intubation (difficulty encountered, method used)

Positioning of patient during laryngoscopy (sniffing position, other position)

Equipment used (even if intubation was performed routinely in one attempt, a Bullard blade or a fiberoptic bronchoscope, neither of which requires alignment of the three axes, may have been used)

Whether technique used can be duplicated successfully

is an advantage) or of anything another anesthesia practitioner has told the patient about the airway, and any possible changes or events that may have occurred since the last anesthetic use, such as weight gain in the obese patient; laryngeal stenosis from previous airway intervention; a suicide attempt with lye ingestion; a motor vehicle accident; an outpatient plastic surgery procedure such as chin implants; worsening rheumatoid arthritis; or use of medications such as steroids.

Be alert for patients in whom AI is indicated[3, 11, 17–19] (Table 4–4) as well as for the presence of absolute contraindications[20] to AI (Table 4–5).

Communication Skills

Dorland's Medical Dictionary defines *empathy* as "intellectual and emotional awareness and understanding of another person's thoughts, feelings, and behavior, even those that are distressing and disturbing." Although the practitioner may participate in a thousand operations a year, few patients undergo more than five in a lifetime.[19] A patient's perception of the practitioner's empathy is the cornerstone of his or her acceptance of an AI. Communicate empathy: the practitioner may need to abandon the traditional interview format and the appearance of clinical detachment.[21, 22] One should focus on the patient, not the disease, in order to gather key data and recruit the patient's willing compliance.[23]

Recognize and abandon negative feelings toward an individual patient (such as the patient with morbid obesity, drug addiction, or simply the need to remain in control) that could be detrimental to effective communication and, ultimately, the patient's compliance.[24, 25] Acknowledge family members present at the interview. If convinced by the practitioner's manner that he or she has genuine concern for the patient, caring family members will be helpful allies.

After the practitioner performs the airway examination, he or she should explain to the patient, and to any family members present, any concerns and conclusions about the patient's anatomy. Once it has been determined that AI is in order, the practitioner should describe to the patient, in a careful, unhurried manner, the conventional intubation contrasted with AI. Focusing on the fact that the former is easier and less time-consuming but that the latter is safer in view of the patient's

Table 4–4 Indications for Awake Intubation

Previous history of difficult intubation
Anticipated difficult airway (assessment on physical examination)
    Prominent protruding teeth
    Small mouth opening (scleroderma, temporomandibular joint abnormality, anatomic variant)
    Narrow mandible
    Micrognathia
    Macroglossia
    Short muscular neck
    Very long neck
    Limited range of motion of neck
    Congenital airway anomalies
    Obesity
    Abnormality involving airway (tracheomalacia)
    Malignancy involving airway
    Upper airway obstruction
Trauma
    Face
    Upper airway
    Cervical spine
Anticipated difficult mask ventilation
Severe risk of aspiration
Respiratory failure
Severe hemodynamic instability

Data from Kopman AF, Wollman SB, Ross K, Surks SN: Awake endotracheal intubation: A review of 267 cases. Anesth Analg 54:323, 1975; Latto IP: Difficulties in tracheal intubation. *In* Latto IP, Rosen M (eds): Management of Difficult Intubation. London, Balliere Tindall, 1984; Miller RD: Anesthesia, 3rd ed. New York, Churchill Livingstone, 1990; Reed AF, Han DG: Preparation of the patient for awake intubation. Anesthesiol Clin North Am 9:69, 1991; and Thomas JL: Awake intubation: Indications, techniques and a review of 25 patients. Anaesthesia 24:28, 1969.

own anatomy or condition communicates to the patient that the knowledgeable, caring anesthesia practitioner is willing to take extra measures to ensure the patient's safety. The practitioner should present his or her recommendations to the patient with conviction, but at the same time allow the patient the option of the conventional method of intubation as a last resort.[17] One should lead, not push, the patient toward acceptance of the necessity for AI.

Table 4–5 Absolute Contraindications to Awake Intubation

Patient refusal
Patient unable to cooperate
    Most children
    Most mentally retarded patients
    Intoxicated, combative patient
Patient with documented true allergy to all local anesthetics

From Benumof JL: Management of the difficult airway. Anesthesiology 75:1087, 1991.

Table 4–6 Complications of Awake Intubation

Local anesthetic toxicity
Specific complications of technique planned
Discomfort
Recall

Present to the patient the possible complications of AI (Table 4–6) as well as the potential advantages (Table 4–7).[3, 11, 20] If the practitioner has developed sufficient skill in the techniques of AI, he or she will be able to communicate honestly to patients that they will experience a minimum of discomfort and unpleasantness, although they may or may not recall the intubation. Recall of deftly performed AI should not necessarily be considered undesirable.

Patient recall after AI using different methods of sedation, analgesia, or local anesthetics has not been studied in a controlled fashion. Although episodes of explicit awareness during general anesthesia are rare (the incidence is 0.2% to 3% and depends on both the depth of anesthesia and the specific agents administered),[19] it is logical to expect that the incidence of recall of AI using minimal levels of sedation will be higher.[3, 4, 7, 11, 19] The practitioner's technique and ability to communicate before, during, and after the AI will determine whether the experience will be recalled as unpleasant.

If the patient refuses AI, discuss the case with the primary care physician or the surgeon, or both, in order to recruit them in helping to convince the patient. If all attempts are unsuccessful, document this explicitly in the chart.

PREMEDICATION AND INTRAVENOUS SEDATION

In addition to the anesthesia practitioner's effective demonstration of empathy throughout the procedure, patients undergoing AI often re-

Table 4–7 Advantages of Awake Intubation

Patency of natural airway is preserved by maintaining upper pharyngeal muscle tone

Spontaneous breathing (oxygenation and ventilation) is maintained

Patient who is awake and well topicalized is easier to intubate than one in whom anesthesia has been induced, causing larynx to move to more anterior position

Patient can still protect airway from aspiration

Patients, in particular those with cervical abnormality, are able to monitor their own neurologic symptoms

Data from Benumof JL: Management of the difficult airway. Anesthesiology 75:1087, 1991; Kopman AF, Wollman SB, Ross K, Surks SN: Awake endotracheal intubation: A review of 267 cases. Anesth Analg 54:323, 1975; and Thomas JL: Awake intubation: Indications, techniques and a review of 25 patients. Anaesthesia 24:28, 1969.

quire medication to relieve anxiety and fear even after an effective preoperative visit. The primary goals of premedication are to relieve anxiety and to provide a clear, dry airway; to protect from aspiration and complications of aspiration; and to provide adequate topicalization of the airway.

In the preoperative period, the most commonly used medications for AI include sedatives, antisialagogues, aspiration prophylaxis agents, and mucosal vasoconstrictors.

Sedatives

Because the patient's cooperation is of utmost importance, one should use the minimal amount of medication needed to provide adequate relief from anxiety. Secure intravenous access before giving medication. Monitor the patient closely when using sedation. Titrate all sedatives carefully to the desired effect. The heavily sedated patient may not be able to protect the airway or to maintain adequate oxygenation and ventilation.

■ Benzodiazepines

The benzodiazepines (diazepam, midazolam, and lorazepam) are the drugs most commonly used to relieve anxiety and provide adequate amnesia. Oral diazepam (0.1 to 0.2 mg/kg) is rapidly absorbed with a peak effect in 55 minutes and an elimination half-life of 21 to 37 hours.[26] Parenteral midazolam (0.1 mg/kg intramuscularly [IM], 1 to 2.5 mg intravenously [IV]) has a rapid onset of action with an elimination half-life of 1 to 4 hours. Midazolam provides greater amnesia and less postoperative sedation compared with diazepam. Oral lorazepam is slowly absorbed from the gastrointestinal (GI) tract with peak effects in 2 to 4 hours.[27] All three agents provide adequate sedation and relief of anxiety for AI, but midazolam is preferable because of its rapid onset and short duration.

If a patient becomes heavily sedated, flumazenil, a specific and exclusive benzodiazepine antagonist, can reverse the effects of benzodiazepines in doses of 8 to 15 μg/kg IV without major side effects.[28]

■ Other Medications

Other medications less commonly used for sedation are narcotics, ketamine, and droperidol.

Fentanyl and alfentanil are excellent narcotic agents that can provide mild sedation and adequate analgesia even in low doses but can be associated with respiratory depression and chest wall rigidity. Respiratory depression can easily be reversed with an opioid-specific antagonist (naloxone 1 to 5 μg/kg IV). Chest wall rigidity can be relieved by a small dose of short-acting muscle relaxant (succinylcholine 0.2 to 0.3 mg/kg IV), but respiration may need to be supported, and awareness of paralysis must be treated.[29] The newer opioid agent remifentanil has a rapid onset of action and an elimination half-life of 3 to 5 minutes. It provides sedation with excellent analgesia. This drug has not been studied extensively, but it appears that it may be an excellent drug for shorter procedures.[30]

Ketamine in low doses (0.2 to 0.5 mg/kg IV) may be used for sedation, but side effects include excessive secretions and hallucinations, which may be recalled, and the possibility of mild respiratory depression.[31] Droperidol (50 to 70 μg/kg IV), a butyrophenone derivative with a longer duration of action, used alone or with fentanyl, can provide sedation but causes respiratory depression, extrapyramidal symptoms, and confusion.[32]

Antisialagogues

Anticholinergic drugs (scopolamine, glycopyrrolate, and atropine) are excellent agents for drying airway secretions in order to facilitate AI.

Scopolamine produces excellent antisialagogue effects with good sedation. Glycopyrrolate, which does not cross the normal blood-brain barrier, provides a moderate antisialagogue effect with no sedation. Atropine provides a mild antisialagogue effect and mild sedation but is the most likely to cause tachycardia.[33]

The anticholinergics are not benign pharmacologic agents and can cause delirium, restlessness, confusion, tachycardia, relaxation of lower esophageal sphincter tone, mydriasis, and cycloplegia.[34] Each of the three agents provides satisfactory drying of the airway.

Aspiration Prophylaxis

A small percentage of patients requiring AI may be categorized as "full stomachs" (i.e., a history of gastroesophageal reflux, hiatal hernia, diabetes with gastroparesis) and require aspiration prophylaxis. Drugs that can be administered preoperatively include the following:

Nonparticulate antacids such as Bicitra (sodium citrate and citric acid) provide effective buffering of gastric acid pH.[35] Polycitra (sodium citrate, potassium citrate, and citric acid) is also a nonparticulate antacid with better buffering capacity than Bicitra.[36] A single dose of antacid increases the gastric volume but also increases the pH of gastric fluid, so that if aspiration occurs, the morbidity and mortality are usually significantly lower.[37]

The H_2-receptor antagonists (cimetidine, ranitidine) are selective and competitive antagonists that block hydrogen ion (H^+) secretion by gastric parietal cells and decrease the secretion of gastric fluid. With intravenous administration of cimetidine (100 mg) or ranitidine (50 mg), peak effects are achieved within 30 to 60 minutes, increasing the gastric pH and decreasing the gastric volume.[38]

Metoclopramide, a dopamine antagonist, stimulates motility of the upper GI tract and increases lower esophageal sphincter tone. The net effect is accelerated gastric clearance of liquids and solids in the patent GI tract.[39]

For complete aspiration prophylaxis, a combination of a nonparticulate antacid, an H_2-receptor blocking agent, and metoclopramide may be used.

Nasal Mucosal Vasoconstrictors

The nasal mucosa and nasopharynx are highly vascular. When a patient requires nasal AI, adequate anesthesia and vasoconstriction of this area are essential. Agents commonly used are 4% cocaine and 2% lidocaine with 1% phenylephrine.[40]

Once these agents are applied appropriately to the nasal area, adequate anesthesia and vasoconstriction can be achieved in 10 to 15 minutes, which will facilitate nasal AI.

The process of vasoconstriction is begun preoperatively with nasal decongestants. A nasal solution of 0.025% to 0.05% oxymetazoline hydrochloride (Afrin spray) can be applied on call to the operating room (OR), by the floor nurse, or by the outpatient on arrival at the hospital. Two sprays in each nostril should vasoconstrict the anterior half of the nasal cavity. When the patient arrives in the holding area, the process should be repeated, allowing the solution to reach the posterior half of the nasal cavity.

STRATEGIC PREPARATION

The preparation of the patient for an AI begins, as discussed, with verbal communication to allay fear, followed by appropriate premedication. Additional preparation for AI includes assembling the necessary equipment, as discussed later, and arranging in advance for needed assistance.

Transport

The urgency of the case must be considered when arranging transport to the OR. Various scenarios may include, in decreasing order of urgency, the following: (1) a need to secure the airway at once (the patient in extremis who warrants a bedside emergency airway procedure) before transportation to the OR; (2) sufficient time to transport the patient to the OR in order to apply the appropriate monitors (electrocardiogram, pulse oximeter, automated blood pressure cuff) and supplemental oxygen, with the patient accompanied by an anesthesia practitioner or surgeon, or both; and (3) no requirement of immediate attention, with the patient able to be transported in a routine manner to the OR.

Patients with a difficult airway may be asymptomatic, scheduled for outpatient surgery unrelated to the airway, and may simply walk in from the waiting area. With an increasing number of patients being seen for the first time on the day of surgery, the anesthesia practitioner must be on constant alert for a patient with a possible difficult airway and must be prepared to both recruit the patient's cooperation and perform AI with little advance notice. We try to see patients at risk for a possible difficult airway (with obesity, a history of sleep apnea, previous trauma or burns, previous or scheduled head and neck surgery) in our outpatient preoperative clinic before the day of surgery in order to detect the potential difficult airway in advance and introduce the patient to the idea of AI before the morning of surgery. This aids in psychologic preparation of the patient, the surgeon, and the anesthesia practitioner, as well as in planning the OR schedule. However, patients with an unsuspected difficult airway may still be seen for the first time on the day of surgery.

In the elective scenario, supplemental O_2 should be provided during transport if appropriate (high-dose O_2 may be detrimental in some patients, such as those who rely on hypoxic respiratory drive),[19] and the patient's position should be considered (the morbidly obese patient may experience dramatic physiologic changes when supine and should be transported in a wheelchair or on a gurney in a semirecumbent position).[41–43]

Staff

There should be "at least one additional individual who is immediately available to serve as an assistant in difficult airway management."[15] Whenever possible, it is preferable to have another anesthesia practitioner who can assist in monitoring and ventilation (two-person ventilation, and assistance in mask ventilation while the primary anesthesia practitioner performs fiberoptic intubation). In cases of the patient in extremis or a patient who refuses AI, a surgeon trained in establishing a surgical airway should be available with the appropriate equipment, ready to obtain an emergent surgical airway.

Monitors

During AI, the routine use of electrocardiography, noninvasive blood pressure monitoring, pulse oximetry, capnography, and a precordial stethoscope is required as part of standard basic intraoperative monitoring. Depending on the complexity of the surgery and the patient's condition, invasive monitoring may be required before airway management.[44–48]

Supplemental Oxygen

Administration of supplemental O_2 should be considered during the entire process of difficult airway management, which includes topicalization, intubation, and extubation.[15] Arterial hypoxemia has been well documented during bronchoscopy (an average decrease in PaO_2 of 20 to 30 mm Hg in patients breathing room air) and has been associated with cardiac dysrhythmias.[49] In an animal study, the use of supplemental O_2 has been shown to delay circulatory arrest secondary to local anesthetic toxicity but did not in a statistically significant way decrease the incidence of respiratory arrest.[50] Considering the advantage of improving the patient's safety, the use of supplemental O_2 must be encouraged in all patients undergoing AI.

In addition to the standard methods of supplementing O_2 (nasal prongs, face mask, binasal airways), there are several nonconventional methods for increasing FIO_2, including delivering O_2 through the suction port of the fiberoptic bronchoscope,[20] delivering O_2 through the atomizer during topicalization,[51] or elective transtracheal jet ventilation in the patient in extremis.[20, 41, 51–53]

Airway Equipment

Consultants of the ASA Difficult Airway Task Force agreed strongly that "preparatory efforts enhance success and minimize risk to the patient" (fewer adverse outcomes).[15] The concept of preassembled carts for emergency situations is not new (there are "crash carts" for cardiac arrest on every floor and malignant hyperthermia carts in every operating room area). Difficult Airway Task Force recommendations are that every anesthetizing location be equipped with a difficult airway cart (if the main operating room is in a different location from the outpatient surgical center, two carts are necessary). The difficult airway cart should be a portable storage unit that contains specialized equipment for managing the difficult airway. This cart should be customized to the individual group of anesthesia practitioners who will be using it. For example, only one practitioner in the group may be familiar with a specific cricotome for establishing a surgical airway. The options are to either train the rest of the staff in the mechanics of that particular instrument or supply the cart with various types of equipment sufficient to satisfy all individuals' preferences and expertise. At our institution we have chosen the latter approach.

On top of our cart we have a dedicated capnograph and pulse oximeter because we are frequently asked to participate in difficult airway management outside the OR setting in locations such as the burn unit or the intensive care unit. The top surface of the cart is used as a work station for the preparation of fiberoptic equipment as well as for laying out equipment for topicalizing the airway and for nerve blocks. The drawers contain drugs (including flumazenil and naloxone), ancillary fiberoptic equipment, specialized blades, lighted stylets, and laryngeal mask airways. The fiberoptic bronchoscopes themselves are suspended on the outside of the cart, with tubes designated for clean or used bronchoscopes. Below the drawers, space is available for the fiberoptic light source, different sizes of ETs, and other ancillary equipment. On the outer wall of the airway cart we hang, on clips, emergency airway equipment such as cricotomes, retrograde kits, jet stylets, Combitubes, and portable jet ventilator equipment.

In addition to the equipment on the cart, we have a designated Combitube, gum elastic bougie, and jet ventilator with preassembled transtracheal kit in every OR. Several acceptable transtracheal jet ventilation systems are available. We are currently using an injector (blowgun) powered by a regulated central wall oxygen pressure unit with a universal adapter to the oxygen wall outlet.[52] Taped to the jet ventilator is a kit containing a 14-gauge angiocatheter (for adult patients), an 18-gauge angiocatheter (for pediatric patients), and a 20-mL syringe. As part of our machine check the jet ventilator is set at 40 to 50 psi[20, 52, 54] for adults and 5 psi[28] for pediatric patients as starting pressures in order to minimize the incidence of barotrauma.[20, 21, 55, 56]

TOPICALIZATION

AI with airway instrumentation causes discomfort unless adequate topical anesthesia of the respiratory tract is obtained, rendering the process painless.

Local Anesthetics

Local anesthetics can be used alone or in combination, in various forms, in order to topicalize the airway in the performance of airway nerve blocks. Appropriate knowledge of each of the local anesthetics should be obtained, including the mechanism and onset of action; metabolism; available formulations; optimal concentration; usual dosage and maximal amount of a drug that can be used safely; and toxicity.[57]

The rate and amount of topical drug absorption usually vary depending on the site of application, the amount of the drug applied locally, the hemodynamic status of the patient, and individual patient variation.[56] The rate at which the drug is absorbed in the respiratory tract is higher from the alveoli than from the tracheobronchial tree, and the rate from the tracheobronchial tree is higher than that from the pharynx. It is still controversial whether the addition of a vasoconstrictor really prolongs the duration of action or slows the rate of absorption of these drugs.[57]

The most commonly used drugs for topical anesthesia are cocaine, benzocaine, lidocaine, and tetracaine.

Cocaine is a natural alkaloid that causes local anesthesia and vasoconstriction when applied topically; thus cocaine is widely used in otolaryngologic surgical procedures.[58] The vasoconstrictive properties of cocaine result from interference with the reuptake of circulating catecholamine by the adrenergic nerve endings.[59] After topical application of cocaine to the nasal mucosa, the peak plasma level is achieved within an hour, and the drug persists in plasma for 5 to 6 hours.[60] The metabolism of cocaine is mainly by plasma cholinesterase, with hepatic and renal excretion. Cocaine is available in two preparations, 4% and 10% solutions, for topical application. The 10% solution is not used for this purpose because of a very high incidence of toxicity.

The dosage varies and depends on the area to be anesthetized, the vascularity of the tissue, individual tolerance, and the anesthetic technique employed. The dosage should be reduced in children and elderly and debilitated patients. The maximal dose in an average adult should not exceed 200 mg.

In addition, cocaine should be used with caution in patients with known hypersensitivity, coronary artery disease, hypertension, pseudocholinesterase deficiency, pregnancy with hypertension (preeclampsia), or hyperthyroidism and in patients taking monoamine oxidase inhibitors. The signs and symptoms of cocaine overdose include tachycardia, cardiac dysrhythmias, hypertension, and fever. It is important to remember that cocaine does have addictive properties due to cortical stimulation resulting in euphoria, excitement, feeling "high," and increased muscle activity. Severe complications include convulsions, respiratory failure, coronary spasm, stroke, and death.

Benzocaine (ethyl aminobenzoate) is a water-insoluble ester-type local anesthetic agent that is mainly useful for topical application. The onset of action is rapid (less than 1 minute) with an effective duration of about 10 minutes. Benzocaine is hydrolyzed by plasma and liver cholinesterases. It is available as 10%, 15%, and 20% solutions. To prolong its duration of action, it is usually mixed with 2% tetracaine. The 20% spray (Hurricaine, Beutlich Pharmaceuticals) contains 200 mg/mL; thus 0.5 mL is equal to the toxic dose, which is 100 mg. A half-second spray delivers approximately 0.15 mL, or 30 mg.

Cetacaine is a topical application spray containing benzocaine 14%, tetracaine 2%, butyl aminobenzoate 2%, benzalkonium chloride, and cetyldimethyl ethyl ammonium bromide, which have been shown to be effective for topicalizing the airway. Combining these agents hastens the onset and prolongs the duration of their action.

Topical application of benzocaine is usually nontoxic, although methemoglobinemia has been reported in adult patients taking sulfonamides and in pediatric patients.[61] There are case reports of methemoglobinemia occurring immediately after the application of Cetacaine spray. Of the compounds in the mixture, only benzocaine has been implicated. In the patient who develops this complication, cyanosis appears first (at a methemoglobin level of as low as 2.5%) and clinical symptoms (fatigue, weakness, headache, dizziness, and tachycardia) appear later (at methemoglobin levels of 20% to 50%). Treatment is with intravenous methylene blue (1 mg/kg of body weight).[62-64]

Lidocaine is an amide local anesthetic agent that is widely used. Its onset is rapid and its duration after infiltration is approximately 60 to 120 minutes. Once in the plasma, lidocaine is metabolized mainly by the hepatic microsomal system. It is available in various preparations including aqueous (1%, 2%, 4%) and viscous (1%) solutions, ointment (1%), and aerosol preparation. Xylocaine 10% metered-dose oral spray (Astra-Zeneca) delivers 10 mg per spray, rapidly anesthetizes the upper airway, and is excellent for quick topicalization before nerve blocks using the internal approach.

In awake patients, the toxic plasma level of lidocaine is 5 μg/mL.[48] In most of the clinical situations in which lidocaine is used as a local anesthesic agent for topicalization, the peak plasma level measured has been far below 5 μg/mL,[64, 65] and thus severe toxic reactions from lidocaine use are uncommon in the context of airway management. Symptoms of severe lidocaine toxicity include convulsions, respiratory failure, and circulatory collapse.

Tetracaine is an amide local anesthetic agent with a longer duration of action than lidocaine and cocaine. It is metabolized by hydrolysis by plasma cholinesterase. It is available as 0.5%, 1%, and 2% solutions for local use. Tetracaine has been shown to have higher toxic effects when used as an aerosol with doses as small as 40 mg, because absorption of the drug from the respiratory tract and GI tract is fast.[66] The maximal dose for topical use in the adult is 100 mg. Severe toxic reactions after tetracaine overdose include convulsions, respiratory arrest, and circulatory collapse.[67] Fatalities have been reported with the topical application of 100 mg of tetracaine to anesthetize mucous membranes.[68]

Application Techniques (Fig. 4–1)

Atomizers: Sprays and atomizers with long delivery systems are available to deliver local anesthetic to the larynx and trachea. Place tetracaine (0.3% to 0.5% with epinephrine 1:200,000), maximum 20 mL, or lidocaine (4%), maximum 10 mL, in an atomizer (see Fig. 4–1) and connect to the O_2 tank (flow rate 8 to 10 L/min) and then spray in the oropharynx for 10-second periods with 20-second rest intervals for a total of about 20 minutes. Suction out any residual agents from the oropharynx to reduce absorption from the GI tract. This is a relatively safe and simple method to provide adequate anesthesia of the airway.

Nebulizers: Either 5 mL of 4% lidocaine or 4 mL of 0.5% tetracaine can be nebulized with oxygen (6 to 8 L/min) using an ultrasonic nebulizer. The size of the droplet depends on the flow of oxygen. With an oxygen flow of less than 6 L/min, a droplet size of 30 to 60 μm can be achieved, which coats the mucosa up to the trachea. This technique is safe and easy to apply in all but small children and uncooperative patients. This approach is especially advantageous in patients with increased

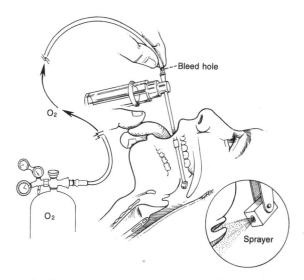

Figure 4–1   Atomizer hooked up to an oxygen tank. A bleed hole is made close to the operator's hand, allowing intermittent spraying. The inset shows the tip of the atomizer as it is angulated to spray toward the glottic opening. (From UCI Department of Anesthesia: DA Teaching Aids.)

Table 4–8 Anatomy for Nerve Block: Nasal Cavity and Nasopharynx

The nasal cavity is innervated by a plethora of sensory fibers with multiple origins. The majority of the innervation is derived from two sources: the sphenopalatine ganglion and the anterior ethmoidal nerve.

The sphenopalatine ganglion (pterygopalatine, nasal, or Meckel's ganglion) is located in the pterygopalatine fossa, posterior to the middle turbinate. It is covered by a 1- to 5-mm layer of connective tissue and mucous membrane. The ganglion is a 5-mm triangular or heart-shaped structure constituted of branches primarily from the gasserian ganglion via the trigeminal nerve (V2). Although it sends out multiple branches, two nerves in particular, the greater and lesser palatine nerves, provide sensory innervation to the nasal turbinates as well as two thirds of the posterior nasal septum (including the periosteum).

The anterior ethmoidal nerve is one of the branches of the ciliary ganglion, the other of which is located within the orbital cavity and is inaccessible to nerve blocks. The anterior ethmoidal nerve gives sensory innervation to one third of the anterior portion of the nares.

intracranial pressure, open eye injury, and severe coronary artery disease.[69]

AIRWAY NERVE BLOCKS

Even though in the majority of patients topicalization of the mucosa adequately anesthetizes the entire airway, some patients require supplementation to ablate sensation in those nerve endings running deep to the mucosal surface such as the periosteal nerve endings of the nasal turbinates and the stretch receptors at the base of the tongue that are involved in gagging.

Because of the multitude of nerves innervating the airway, there is no single anatomic site where one nerve block can anesthetize the entire airway. The following nerve blocks are remarkable for their ease of performance, their minimal risk to the patient, the density of the block (complete ablation of sensory fibers), and the speed of onset.

Nasal Cavity and Nasopharynx
(Table 4–8) (Figs. 4–2, 4–3, and 4–4)[16–18, 67, 70–77]

Regardless of which technique is used to anesthetize the nasal cavity, first inspect the nares for a deviated septum using a nasal speculum, asking the patient to breathe deeply through each individual naris (occluding the opposite naris). Determine patency by passing multiple applicators along the floor of the nasal cavity.

■ Sphenopalatine Nerve Block: Oral Approach
  (see Fig. 4–3A and B)[16, 18, 67, 71–73, 77]

  Equipment
  2% viscous lidocaine on cotton-tipped applicators

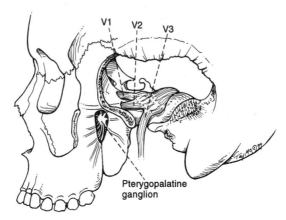

Figure 4–2 Left lateral view of the skull with the temporal bone removed depicting the gasserian ganglion with the three branches (V1 to V3) of the trigeminal nerve. V2 is the major contributor to the pterygopalatine ganglion (shown as it sits in the pterygopalatine fossa). (From UCI Department of Anesthesia: DA Teaching Aids.)

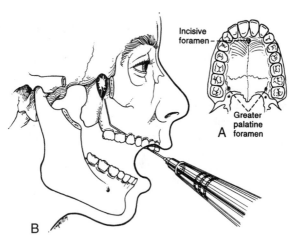

Figure 4–3 *A,* Inferior view of the hard palate showing the location of the greater palatine foramen. *B,* Right lateral view of the head with the zygomatic arch and coronoid process of the mandible removed, exposing the pterygopalatine fossa (containing the pterygopalatine ganglion) with an angulated spinal needle in place. (From UCI Department of Anesthesia: DA Teaching Aids.)

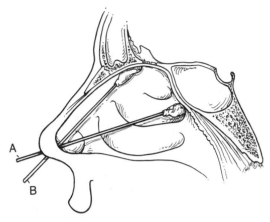

Figure 4–4   Left lateral view of the right nasal cavity, showing long cotton-tipped applicators soaked in local anesthetic with vasoconstrictors. *A,* Applicator angled 45 degrees to the hard palate with a cotton swab over the mucosal surface overlying the sphenopalatine ganglion. The angiocatheter should be placed in the same position. *B,* Applicator placed parallel to the dorsal surface of the nose, blocking the anterior ethmoidal nerve. (From UCI Department of Anesthesia: DA Teaching Aids.)

    25-gauge spinal needle, bent 2 to 3 cm proximal to the tip, to an
       angle of 120 degrees
    Syringe containing 2 to 4 mL of 2% lidocaine with epinephrine
       1:100,000

With the patient in the supine position, stand facing the patient on the contralateral side of the nerve to be blocked. Using the left index finger, identify the greater palatine foramen, which is located between the second and third maxillary molars approximately 1 cm medial to the palatogingival margin and usually can be palpated as a small depression near the posterior edge of the hard palate. In approximately 15% of the population the foramen is closed and inaccessible. Apply 2% viscous lidocaine with a cotton-tipped applicator for 1 to 2 minutes, or digital pressure over the foramen to avoid pain on insertion of the needle. Insert the 25-gauge spinal needle into the greater palatine foramen in a superior and slightly posterior direction (to a depth of 2 to 3 cm). Perform an aspiration test to ascertain that the sphenopalatine artery has not been cannulated, and then inject 1 to 2 mL of the lidocaine solution. The epinephrine is used to vasoconstrict the sphenopalatine artery running parallel to the nerves and further decreases the incidence of epistaxis. Inject the local anesthetic slowly and continuously (preventing acute increases in pressure within the fossa) in order to decrease sympathetic stimulation. This injection anesthetizes the anterior, middle, and posterior palatine nerves, as well as the nasociliary and nasopalatine nerves. Repeat, if appropriate, on the opposite side. Complications are bleeding, infection, nerve trauma, intravascular injection of local anesthetics, and hypertension.

■ Sphenopalatine Nerve Block: Nasal Approach (see Fig. 4–4)[18, 75–80]

Two noninvasive nasal approaches to the sphenopalatine ganglion have been described, both of which take advantage of the ganglion's shallow position beneath the nasal mucosa

Direct Application (see Fig. 4–4A)

Equipment
Long cotton-tipped applicators (or neuropledgets held in bayonet forceps), soaked in either 4% lidocaine with epinephrine 1:200,000 or 4% cocaine

Apply the applicator or the neuropledget held in bayonet forceps over the mucosal surface overlying the ganglion. Pass along the upper border of the middle turbinate (at an approximately 45-degree angle to the hard palate) and direct the applicator or neuropledget back and down until it reaches the upper posterior wall of the nasopharynx (sphenoid bone). Leave it in place for approximately 5 to 10 minutes.

Spray (see Fig. 4–4A)

Equipment
Plastic sheath of a 20-gauge angiocatheter
5-mL syringe containing anesthetic solution (4 mL of 4% lidocaine containing 3 mg of phenylephrine)

Attach the angiocatheter sheath to the syringe and place it along the same path as described in the first method; then rapidly inject. Allow about 2 minutes for the anesthetic to take effect.

■ Nasal Pledgets and Trumpets[17, 18, 70, 75–77]

Equipment
Long cotton-tipped applicators soaked in either 4% cocaine or 4% lidocaine with epinephrine 1:200,000
Nasal trumpets soaked in 2% viscous lidocaine

Insert the applicators to the level of the posterior nasal pharyngeal wall. This technique provides additional airway topicalization, helps to predict the angle of ET insertion, and begins dilation of the nasal cavity. To further dilate the nasal cavity, remove the applicators and serially place nasal trumpets of increasing diameters. This also helps to approximate the ET size (a 36 Fr nasal trumpet predicts easy passage of a 7.0 internal diameter ET).

■ Anterior Ethmoidal Nerve Block (see Fig. 4–4B)[17, 73, 75, 77]

Equipment
Long cotton-tipped applicators, soaked in either 4% cocaine or 4% lidocaine with epinephrine 1:200,000

The anterior ethmoidal nerve is blocked by the insertion of the applicator, placed parallel to the dorsal surface of the nose until it meets the anterior surface of the cribriform plate (see Figure 4–4B). The applicator is held in position for approximately 5 to 10 minutes.

Table 4–9   Anatomy for Nerve Block: Oropharynx

The somatic and visceral afferent fibers of the oropharynx are supplied by a plexus derived from the vagus, facial, and glossopharyngeal nerves. The glossopharyngeal nerve emerges from the skull through the jugular foramen and passes forward between the internal jugular and carotid vessels, traveling anteriorly along the lateral wall of the pharynx. It supplies sensory innervation to the posterior third of the tongue (lingual branch); anterior surface of the epiglottis; posterior and lateral walls of the pharynx; and tonsillar pillars. Its only motor innervation in the pharynx is to the stylopharyngeus muscle (one of the muscles of deglutition).

Oropharynx (Table 4–9) (Figs. 4–5 and 4–6)[18–20, 49, 67, 71, 73, 77–89]

In the majority of patients, topicalizing the mucosa of the oropharynx is sufficient to allow instrumentation of the airway, as in the placement of a fiberoptic oral airway. In some patients, the gag reflex is so pronounced that no amount of topicalization allows a stationary, quiet field for intubation. The gag arises from stimulation of deep pressure receptors in the posterior third of the tongue that cannot be reached by the diffusion of local anesthetics through the mucosa. There are various measures for minimizing this problem. Instructing the patient to breathe in a nonstop panting fashion helps to minimize pressure on the tongue during nasal intubation. Administration of narcotics helps to suppress the response to pressure on the posterior tongue but also suppresses respiration. We recommend the glossopharyngeal nerve block.[18, 87] This block is easy to perform and highly effective in abolishing the gag

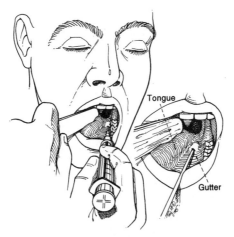

Figure 4–5   Anterior approach, left-sided glossopharyngeal nerve block. The tongue is displaced medially, forming a gutter (glossogingival groove) that ends distally in a cul-de-sac. A 25-gauge spinal needle is placed at the base of the palatoglossal fold. (From UCI Department of Anesthesia: DA Teaching Aids.)

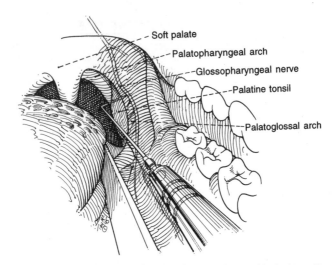

Figure 4–6   Posterior approach, left glossopharyngeal nerve block. A tonsillar needle (or a 25-gauge spinal needle bent at a right angle) is placed behind the midportion of the palatoglossal fold, allowing blocking of the glossopharyngeal nerve at a more proximal position. (From UCI Department of Anesthesia: DA Teaching Aids.)

reflex as well as decreasing the hemodynamic response to laryngoscopy, including awake laryngoscopy. Two approaches are described: the anterior and the posterior approach.

■ Glossopharyngeal Nerve Block: Anterior Approach (Palatoglossal Fold) (see Fig. 4–5)

Equipment
Tongue blade
25-gauge spinal needle (attached to a 5-mL syringe of 1% to 2% lidocaine)

Topicalize the oropharynx as previously described. Place the patient in the sitting position and stand facing the patient on the contralateral side of the nerve to be blocked. Ask the patient to open the mouth wide and to protrude the tongue anteriorly. Hold the tongue blade with the nondominant hand and displace the tongue medially, forming a gutter or trough along the floor of the mouth between the tongue and the teeth. The gutter ends in a cul-de-sac formed by the base of the palatoglossal arch (in its tented state it resembles a hammock or U-shaped structure). Insert the spinal needle at the base of the cul-de-sac (where the gutter meets the base of the palatoglossal arch) and advance 0.25 to 0.5 cm. Perform an aspiration test: if air is aspirated, the needle has been advanced too deeply (the tip has gone all the way through the thin membrane) and should be withdrawn until no air can be aspirated. If blood is aspirated, redirect the needle more medially. Inject 2 mL of the lidocaine, and repeat the procedure on the other side. Using a spinal needle allows an unobstructed view of the very narrow field of view in the oral cavity, which would be obstructed by the syringe were a shorter needle to be used.

The block is intended to isolate the lingual branch of the glossopharyngeal nerve, although in one study using methylene blue it was shown that in some cases retrograde submucosal tracking occurs, blocking the primary trunk of the nerve (pharyngeal and tonsillar branches).[20]

■ Glossopharyngeal Nerve Block: Posterior Approach
(Palatopharyngeal Fold) (see Fig. 4–6)

Equipment
Tongue blade
23-gauge tonsillar needle attached to a three-ring syringe containing 3 mL of 2% lidocaine with epinephrine 1:200,000

The posterior approach is a technique used frequently by the otolaryngologist for tonsillectomies and blocks the nerve more proximally, closer to its origin, than the anterior approach. It blocks both the sensory fibers (pharyngeal, lingual, and tonsillar branches) and the motor branch innervating the stylopharyngeus muscle.

Place the patient in the sitting position and stand facing the patient on the ipsilateral side of the nerve to be blocked. Ask the patient to open the mouth wide. Using a tongue blade held in the nondominant hand, displace the tongue caudad and medially, exposing the soft palate, uvula, palatoglossal arch, tonsillar bed, and palatopharyngeal arch. This maneuver stretches both the palatoglossal arch and the palatopharyngeal arch, making them more accessible. Hold the tonsillar needle in the dominant hand. Place it behind the palatopharyngeal arch at its midpoint and insert it into the lateral wall of the oropharynx to the maximal depth allowed by the 1-cm needle shaft. Perform an aspiration test to prevent intravascular injection. Give a test dose of 0.25 to 0.5 mL, looking for hemodynamic changes as well as signs of local anesthetic toxicity. If blood is aspirated or the patient complains of headache, remove and reposition the needle. If the position is appropriate, inject the remainder of the local anesthetic and repeat the procedure on the opposite side.

Potential complications have been cited, including headache; pharyngeal abscess; paralysis of the pharyngeal muscles with airway obstruction; hematoma; dysrhythmias; seizures; and intraarterial injection. There have been no reported complications with the anterior approach. One would expect potential complications to be bleeding, infection, and intravascular injection of local anesthetics. There is greater potential for intraarterial injection using the posterior approach because of the proximity of the carotid artery in this region. In a study of 823 patients who had blocks by the posterior approach, two had self-limited hematomas.[78] A second study using the posterior approach reported an 0.8% incidence of headache, believed to be due to intravascular injection,

Table 4–10   Anatomy for Nerve Block: Larynx

The general nerve supply of the laryngeal inlet is primarily via the superior laryngeal nerve (SLN). The SLN supplies sensory innervation to the base of the tongue; vallecula; epiglottis; aryepiglottic folds; and arytenoids; and down to but excluding the vocal cords. The SLN originates as a branch of the vagus nerve, lying deep to the carotid artery. It then travels anteriorly and at the level of the cornu of the hyoid bone branches into the internal branch, which is sensory, and the external branch, which is motor (cricothyroid muscle). The internal branch subsequently pierces the thyrohyoid ligament (membrane) along with the accompanying superior laryngeal artery and vein. The nerve then enters the space just beneath the mucosa covering the piriform fossa and preepiglottic space.

an 0.4% incidence of seizures, and a 1% incidence of dysrhythmias (supraventricular tachycardia, bigeminy). Of the patients with dysrhythmias, one required treatment with propranolol.[83] Some believe that the tachycardia may result from blocking the afferent nerve fibers of the glossopharyngeal nerve, which arise from the carotid sinus.[79] There have been no reported cases of airway obstruction secondary to laxity of the pharynx resulting from paralysis of the pharyngeal musculature.

Larynx (Table 4–10) (Fig. 4–7)[3, 7, 14, 16–20, 49, 67, 70, 72, 77, 78, 83, 86–94]

Sensation to the larynx can be blocked by the superior laryngeal nerve (SLN) block. Place the patient in the supine position, head slightly extended, and stand on the ipsilateral side of the neck. Identify two main anatomic structures: the cornu of the hyoid bone and the superior cornu of the thyroid cartilage. The cornu of the hyoid bone lies beneath the angle of the mandible and anterior to the carotid artery. Palpate it transversely with the thumb and index finger on the sides of the neck as a bilateral rounded structure. To make one side more prominent, displace the contralateral side toward the side being blocked. To identify the superior cornu of the thyroid cartilage, palpate the thyroid notch (Adam's apple) and trace the upper edge of the thyroid cartilage posteriorly until reaching a smaller bilateral rounded structure lying just underneath the superior cornu of the hyoid bone.

Four approaches to the block have been described: three external approaches and one internal approach. When performing the block from the external approaches, use aseptic technique. Exercise caution in order not to insert the needle into the thyroid cartilage, since there is a possibility of injecting the solution at the level of the vocal cords, causing edema and airway obstruction. Identify the carotid artery and displace it posteriorly in order to minimize the risk of intravascular injection; even small amounts of local anesthetics (0.25 to 0.5 mL) can induce seizures. On rare occasions (reported incidence of 2.7%), hypotension and bradycardia have been associated with SLN blocks. A number of possible causes of this reaction have been postulated (Table

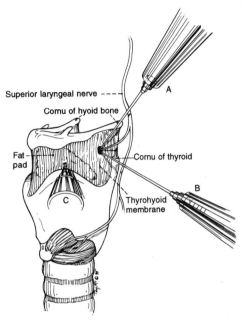

Figure 4–7 Superior laryngeal nerve block, external approach. *A*, Using the cornu of the hyoid bone as a landmark. *B*, Using the cornu of the thyroid cartilage as a landmark. *C*, Using the thyroid notch as a landmark (a fat pad is found in the pre-epiglottic space). (From UCI Department of Anesthesia: DA Teaching Aids.)

4–11). It is therefore recommended that anticholinergics be administered before the block is performed.

Complications of the external approach also include hematoma (reported incidence of 1.4%), pharyngeal puncture, and rupture of the ET cuff in patients already intubated.

Contraindications to the external approach are poor anatomic landmarks, local infections, local tumor growth, coagulopathy, and patients at risk for aspiration of gastric contents. The last is also a relative contraindication to the internal approach.

With the external approaches, SLN block can be achieved in approxi-

Table 4–11 Hypotension and Bradycardia with Superior Laryngeal Nerve Block

Apprehension and subsequent vasovagal reaction due to painful stimulation
Digital pressure on sensitive carotid sinus
Excessive manipulation of larynx causing vasovagal reaction
Large doses or accidental intravascular administration of local anesthetic drugs
Direct neural stimulation of branch of the vagus nerve by needle

mately 1 minute after administration of the local anesthetic. The internal approach takes longer. The success rate of the SLN blocks has been reported to be as high as 92%.[93]

■ External Approach (Cornu of the Hyoid) (see Fig. 4–7A)

Equipment
    23-gauge tonsillar needle attached to a three-ring syringe containing 3 to 4 mL of 2% lidocaine with epinephrine 1:200,000

Use the nondominant index finger to depress the carotid artery laterally and posteriorly. With the dominant hand, walk the needle off the cornu of the hyoid bone in an anterior-caudad direction aiming toward the middle of the thyrohyoid ligament. A slight resistance can be felt as one advances the needle through the ligament usually at a depth of 1 to 2 cm (2 to 3 mm deep to the hyoid bone). The needle at this point has entered a closed space between the thyrohyoid membrane laterally and the laryngeal mucosa medially. Attempt aspiration through the needle. If air is aspirated, the needle has gone too deep and may have entered the pharynx; withdraw slowly until no air can be aspirated. If blood is aspirated, the needle has cannulated either the superior laryngeal artery or vein or the carotid artery; withdraw slightly and direct it more anteriorly. Inject the space, when found, with 1.5 to 2.0 mL while withdrawing the needle. Repeat the block on the opposite side.

■ External Approach (Cornu of the Thyroid) (see Fig. 4–7B)

Equipment
    4-cm 25-gauge needle (attached to a syringe containing 3 to 4 mL of 2% lidocaine with epinephrine 1:200,000)

This is the same technique as described previously but uses the cornu of the thyroid as the landmark. The benefit of this technique is that in many patients this structure is easier to palpate and the procedure is less painful for the patient. Walk the needle off the cornu of the thyroid cartilage in a superior-anterior direction aiming toward the lower third of the thyroid ligament and taking the same precautions as before. Inject the space, when found, with 1.5 to 2.0 mL while withdrawing the needle. Repeat the block on the opposite side.

■ External Approach (Thyroid Notch) (see Fig. 4–7C)

Equipment
    2.5-cm 25-gauge needle
    Two syringes containing 2 mL of 2% lidocaine with epinephrine 1:200,000

The easiest identifiable landmark in many of the patients, especially males, is the thyroid notch (Adam's apple). Palpate the thyroid notch and trace the upper border of the thyroid cartilage posteriorly for approximately 2 cm. Direct the thyrohyoid ligament posterior and cephalad and enter the needle (attached to one of the syringes) to a depth of 1.0 to 1.5 cm. This corresponds to the preepiglottic space, which normally contains the terminal branches of the SLN embedded in a fat pad. Inject the area with the anesthetic solution using precautions as previously described, but inject the entire 1 to 2 mL into the preepiglottic space before withdrawing the needle. Repeat the block on the opposite side with an additional 1 to 2 mL. An added benefit of this approach is the decreased likelihood of blocking the motor branch of the SLN.

■ Internal Approach (Piriform Fossa) (Figs. 4–8 and 4–9)

Equipment
Gauze pads
Tongue blade
Jackson (Krause) forceps armed with Cottonoids soaked in 4%
    cocaine or 4% lidocaine

A noninvasive SLN block can be performed by applying local anesthetic to the piriform fossa (the internal branch of the SLN lies just superficial to the mucosa). After applying local anesthetic topically to the tongue and pharynx, place the patient in the sitting position and stand on the contralateral side of the nerve to be blocked. Ask the patient to open the mouth wide with tongue protruded. Grasp the tongue with the nondominant hand using a gauze pad and gently pull it anteriorly (or just try depressing the tongue with a tongue blade). Advance the forceps slowly over the lateral posterior curvature of the tongue (along the downward continuation of the tonsillar fossa) with the dominant hand until the tip meets resistance and cannot be ad-

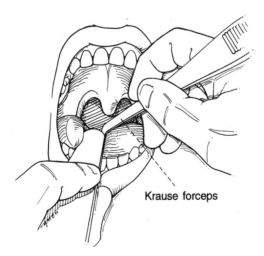

Krause forceps

Figure 4–8 Superior laryngeal nerve block, internal approach. Krause forceps are advanced over the tongue toward the piriform sinus. (From UCI Department of Anesthesia: DA Teaching Aids.)

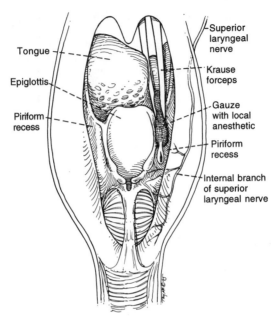

Figure 4–9 Superior laryngeal nerve block, internal approach. A posterior view of the larynx shows the tip of Krause forceps at the level of the piriform sinus. (From UCI Department of Anesthesia: DA Teaching Aids.)

vanced any farther; at this point, the handle of the forceps should be in a horizontal position. Check the position of the tip of the forceps by palpating the neck lateral to the posterior-superior aspect of the thyroid cartilage. Hold the forceps in this position for at least 5 minutes, and then repeat the process on the opposite side.

Trachea and Vocal Cords (Table 4–12)[3, 4, 7, 14, 16, 17, 19, 20, 49, 72, 77, 84–89, 94–97]

Because the sensory and the motor fibers run together, nerve blocks cannot be performed since this would result in bilateral vocal cord paralysis and complete airway obstruction. The only alternative is topi-

---

Table 4–12 Anatomy for Nerve Block: Trachea and Vocal Cords

The sensory innervation of the trachea and vocal cords is supplied by the vagus nerve via the recurrent laryngeal nerves (RLNs). The right RLN originates at the level of the right subclavian artery and the left originates at the level of the aortic arch (distal to the ligamentum arteriosum). Both ascend along the tracheoesophageal groove to supply sensory innervation to the tracheobronchial tree (up to and including the vocal cords) as well as supplying motor nerve fibers to the intrinsic muscles of the larynx (except the cricothyroid muscle).

calization of the mucosa. In addition to the use of nebulizers and atomizers to topicalize the trachea, there are three other techniques: translaryngeal (transtracheal) anesthesia, "spray as you go" via the fiberoptic bronchoscope, and Labat's technique.

■ Translaryngeal (Transtracheal) Anesthesia (Fig. 4–10)

Equipment
Tuberculin syringe with small amount of 1% lidocaine
20-gauge angiocatheter
10-mL syringe containing 4 to 5 mL of 2% to 4% lidocaine

The ideal position for translaryngeal anesthesia is the supine position with the neck hyperextended. In this position the cervical vertebrae push the trachea and cricoid cartilage anteriorly and displace the strap muscles of the neck laterally. As a result, the cricoid cartilage and the structures above and below it are easier to palpate.

The practitioner should stand on the left side of a supine patient if the practitioner is right-hand dominant, and vice versa. Ask the patient not to talk, swallow, or cough until instructed. Following aseptic technique, use a tuberculin syringe to raise a small skin wheal over the intended puncture site, but not through the cricothyroid membrane. The practitioner should use the nondominant hand to stabilize the trachea by placing the thumb and third digit on either side of the thyroid cartilage. Use the index finger to identify the midline of the cricothyroid membrane as well as the upper border of the cricoid cartilage. With the dominant hand, the practitioner should grasp the angiocatheter[16] and syringe like a pencil with the fifth digit used to brace the hand on the patient's lower neck. Aim the needle at a 45-degree angle in a caudad direction. As the needle passes through the cricothyroid membrane, the practitioner should feel resistance. Attempt aspiration for air to verify placement in the lumen of the airway (do not advance the needle any farther). Advance only the sheath of the angiocatheter, remove the needle, and carefully reattach the syringe and again perform the aspiration test. Ask the patient to take a vital capacity breath, and at the end of inspiration, inject 4 mL of 2% to 4% lidocaine. Leave the sheath of the angiocatheter in place until the intubation is completed in case more local anesthetic is needed, and to decrease the likelihood of subcutaneous emphysema. The coughing helps to nebulize the local anesthetic so that the inferior and superior surfaces of the vocal cords can be anesthetized.[87, 89]

Whether the entry site is above or below the cricoid cartilage, a significant amount of local anesthetic bathes the tracheobronchial tree, false cords, true cords, epiglottis, vallecula, tongue, and posterior pharyngeal wall.[98] The success of translaryngeal anesthesia has been found to be as high as 95% and is attributed to both topicalization of the airway and systemic absorption.[17, 98–101] Serum levels of lidocaine after translaryngeal anesthesia using 5 mg/kg of a 10% lidocaine solution have been measured and found to be in the therapeutic range (over 1.4 μg/mL) in a mean time of 5.1 minutes (±3.2 minutes).[99]

The technique has been described using a 25-gauge needle, but we

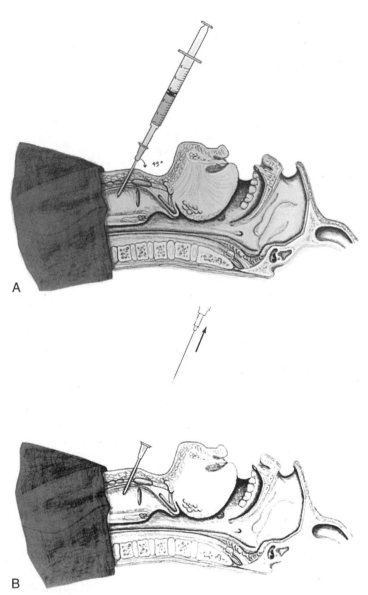

Figure 4–10   Translaryngeal anesthesia, midsagittal view of the head and neck. *A*, Angiocatheter aimed 45 degrees to the cricothyroid membrane. An aspiration test is performed to verify the position of the tip of the needle in the tracheal lumen. *B*, The needle is removed from the angiocatheter. The aspiration test is repeated with the syringe reattached to the angiocatheter. The patient is then asked to take a vital capacity breath and to cough. At end inspiration the local anesthetic is injected, resulting in coughing and nebulization of the local anesthetic. (From UCI Department of Anesthesia: DA Teaching Aids.)

discourage this because of the possibility of breaking the needle as a result of the cricoid cartilage's moving cephalad when the patient is coughing.[97] The tip of the needle should not be aimed in a cephalad direction since the tip of the angiocatheter sheath would then be advanced above the level of the vocal cords, resulting in local anesthetic above but not below the vocal cords. Coughing is a known factor in elevation of the mean arterial pressure, heart rate, intracranial pressure, and intraocular pressure. Potential complications are bleeding (subcutaneous and intratracheal), infection, subcutaneous emphysema, pneumomediastinum, pneumothorax, vocal cord damage, and esophageal perforation. These complications are rare, as illustrated by a study of 17,500 cases of translaryngeal punctures with an incidence of complications of less than 0.01%.[97] Translaryngeal anesthesia is relatively contraindicated in patients at risk for elevated intracranial pressure and intraocular pressure, those with severe cardiac disease, chronic cough, or unstable cervical fracture (unless adequate stabilization has been achieved), and patients at risk for aspiration of gastric contents.

■ "Spray as You Go"[17, 20, 75, 102]

In addition to using a nebulizer or atomizer to anesthetize the vocal cords and trachea, a technique called "spray as you go" by the fiberoptic bronchoscope can be performed. The technique is noninvasive and involves injecting local anesthetics through the suction port of the fiberoptic bronchoscope. Two methods have been described.

Oxygen Spray Technique

Equipment
Three-way stopcock
Oxygen tubing from a regulated O_2 tank set at 2 to 4 L/min flow
5-mL syringe with 2% to 4% lidocaine

Attach a three-way stopcock to the proximal portion of the suction port, connect oxygen tubing, and set at 2 to 4 L/min flow. Under direct vision through the bronchoscope, spray targeted areas with aliquots of 0.2 to 1.0 mL of lidocaine. Wait 30 to 60 seconds before advancing to deeper structures and repeat the maneuver. The flow of oxygen allows a higher FIO_2 delivery, keeps the fiberoptic bronchoscope lens clean, disperses mucous secretions away from the lens allowing a better view, and aids in nebulizing the local anesthetic.

Catheter Technique

Equipment
Long angiographic or epidural catheter (internal diameter 0.5 to 1.0 mm) with proximal Luer-Lok connection
5-mL syringe with 2% to 4% lidocaine

Pass the catheter through the suction port of an adult fiberoptic bronchoscope. Cut the catheter short of the end of the fiberoptic insertion cord by 5 mm in order to prevent obstruction of the fiberoptic lens and allow more accurate placement of the local anesthetic (which flows as a stream instead of dribbling on the field).

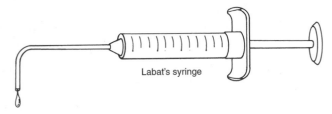

Figure 4–11   Labat's needle for dripping local anesthetic over the vocal cords. (From UCI Department of Anesthesia: DA Teaching Aids.)

These techniques are especially useful in those patients who are at risk for aspirating gastric contents, since the topical anesthetic is applied only seconds before the intubation is accomplished and allows the patient to maintain the airway reflexes as long as possible.

■ Labat's Technique[103–105]

Labat's technique is an antiquated method of anesthetizing the vocal cords and trachea (Fig. 4–11).

Equipment
Headlamp
Laryngeal mirror
Gauze pad
Labat's needle attached to a syringe with 4 mL of 2% lidocaine

Place the patient in the sitting position and ask the patient to open the mouth wide. Pull the tongue out and ask an assistant to hold the tongue with a gauze pad. With the nondominant hand, hold the laryngeal mirror over the oropharynx in order to identify the vocal cords. Hold the Labat needle and syringe with the dominant hand, and drip local anesthetic over the vocal cords. We use this technique only to illustrate to our residents that ear, nose, and throat surgeons frequently claim an easy direct laryngoscopy because they were indeed able to visualize the vocal cords using this same method. This is misleading, because it does not take into account the three-axis alignment required for direct laryngoscopy using a standard anesthesia laryngoscope.

ACKNOWLEDGMENT

With special thanks to Tay McClellan for her outstanding medical illustrations.

REFERENCES

1. Macewend EM: Clinical observations on the introduction of tracheal tubes by the mouth instead of performing tracheostomy or laryngotomy. BMJ 24:122, 1880.
2. Sanchez A, Trivedi NS, Morrison DE: Preparation of the patient for awake intubation. *In* Benumof JL (ed): Airway Management: Principles and Practice. St. Louis, Mosby–Year Book, 1996, p 159.
3. Thomas JL: Awake intubation: Indications, techniques and a review of 25 patients. Anaesthesia 24:28, 1969.

4. Ovassapian A, Yelich SJ, Dykes MH, Brunner EE: Blood pressure and heart rate changes during awake fiberoptic nasotracheal intubation. Anesth Analg 62:951, 1983.
5. Dundee JW, Haslett WHK: The benzodiazepines: A review of their actions and uses relative to anesthetic practice. Br J Anaesth 42:217, 1970.
6. Sidhu VS, Whitehead EM, Ainsworth QP, et al: A technique of awake fibreoptic intubation: Experience in patients with cervical spine disease. Anaesthesia 48:910, 1993.
7. Mongan PD, Culling RD: Rapid oral anesthesia for awake intubation. J Clin Anesth 4:101, 1992.
8. Meschino A, Devitt JH, Koch JP, et al: The safety of awake tracheal intubation in cervical spine injury. Can J Anaesth 39:114, 1992.
9. Ovassapian A, Krejcie TC, Yelich SJ, Dykes MH: Awake fibreoptic intubation in the patient at high risk of aspiration. Br J Anaesth 62:13, 1989.
10. Sinclair JR, Mason RA: Ankylosing spondylitis: The case for awake intubation. Anaesthesia 39:3, 1984.
11. Kopman AF, Wollman SB, Ross K, Surks SN: Awake endotracheal intubation: A review of 267 cases. Anesth Analg 54:323, 1975.
12. Latto IP: Awake intubation. First International Symposium on the Difficult Airway, Newport Beach, Calif, Sept 16, 1993.
13. Le P, Ovassapian A, Benumof JL: Survey of university training programs: Residency training in airway management (unpublished data).
14. Norton ML, Brown ACD: Atlas of the Difficult Airway. St Louis, Mosby–Year Book, 1991.
15. American Society of Anesthesia Practitioners Task Force: Practice guidelines for management of the difficult airway. Anesthesiology 78:597, 1993.
16. Barash PG, Cullen BF, Stoelting RK: Clinical Anesthesia. Philadelphia, JB Lippincott, 1989.
17. Reed AF, Han DG: Preparation of the patient for awake intubation. Anesthesiol Clin North Am 9:69, 1991.
18. Latto IP: Difficulties in tracheal intubation. *In* Latto IP, Rosen, M (eds): Management of Difficult Intubation. London, Balliere Tindall, 1984.
19. Miller RD: Anesthesia, 3rd ed. New York, Churchill Livingstone, 1990.
20. Benumof JL: Management of the difficult airway. Anesthesiology 75:1087, 1991.
21. Evans BJ, Stanley RO, Burrows GD: Measuring medical students' empathy skills. Br J Med Psychol 66:121, 1993.
22. Block MR, Coulehan JL: Teaching the difficult interview in a required course on medical interviewing. Education 62:35, 1987.
23. Farsad P, Galliguez P, Chamberlin R, Roghmann KJ: Teaching interviewing skills to pediatric house officers. Pediatrics 61:384, 1978.
24. Breytspraak LM, McGee J, Conger JC, et al: Sensitizing medical students to impression formation processes in the patient interview. J Med Educ 52:47, 1977.
25. Smith RC: Teaching interviewing skills to medical students: The issue of 'countertransference'. J Med Educ 59:582, 1984.
26. Frumin MJ, Herekar VR, Jarvik ME. Amnestic actions of diazepam and scopolamine in man. Anesthesiology 45:406, 1976.
27. Fragan RJ, Caldwell N: Lorazepam premedication: Lack of recall and relief of anxiety. Anesth Analg 55:792, 1976.
28. White PF, Shafer A, Boyle WA, et al: Benzodiazepine antagonism does not provoke a stress response. Anesthesiology 70:636, 1989.
29. Shafer SL, Varvel JR: Pharmacokinetics, pharmacodynamics, and rational opioid selection. Anesthesiology 74:53, 1991.
30. Egan TD, Lemmens HJM, Fiset P, et al: The pharmacokinetics of the new short acting opioid remifentanil in healthy adult male volunteers. Anesthesiology 79:881, 1993.
31. White PF, Way WL, Trevor AJ: Ketamine: Its pharmacology and therapeutic uses. Anesthesiology 56:119, 1982.
32. Tornetta FJ: A comparison of droperidol, diazepam and hydroxyzine hydrochloride as premedication. Anesth Analg 56:496, 1977.

33. Mirakhur RK: Anticholinergic drugs and anesthesia. Can J Anaesth 35:443, 1988.
34. Mirakhur RA, Clarke RSJ, Dundee JW, et al: Anticholinergic drugs in anesthesia: A survey of their present position. Anesthesia 33:133, 1978.
35. Eyler SW, Cullen BF, Murphy ME, Welch WD: Antacid aspiration in rabbits: A comparison of Mylanta and Bicitra. Anesth Analg 61:288, 1982.
36. Conklin KA, Ziadlou-Rad F: Buffering capacity of citrate antacids. Anesthesiology 58:391, 1983.
37. James CF, Modell JH, Gibbs CP, et al: Pulmonary aspiration effects of volume and pH in the rats. Anesth Analg 63:665, 1984.
38. Feldman M, Burton ME: Histamine receptor antagonists. N Engl J Med 323:1672, 1990.
39. Schulze-Delrieuer RT: Drug therapy: Metoclopramide. N Engl J Med 305:28, 1981.
40. Gross JB, Hartigan ML, Schaffer DW: A suitable substitute for 4% cocaine before blind nasotracheal intubation: 3% lidocaine–0.25% phenylephrine nasal spray. Anesth Analg 63:915, 1984.
41. Tsueda K, Debrand M, Zeok SS, et al: Obesity supine death syndrome: Reports of two morbidly obese patients. Anesth Analg 58:4, 1979.
42. Paul DR, Hoyt JL, Boutros AR: Cardiovascular and respiratory changes in response to change of posture in the very obese. Anesthesiology 45:73, 1976.
43. Vaughan RW: Obesity: Implications in Anesthetic Management and Toxicity. ASA Refresher Course in Anesthesiology, vol 9. Philadelphia, JB Lippincott, 1981.
44. Slogoff S, Keats AS, David Y, et al: Incidence of perioperative myocardial ischemia detected by different electrocardiographic systems. Anesthesiology 73:1074, 1990.
45. Bertrand CA, Steiner NV, Jameson AG, et al: Disturbances of cardiac rhythm during anesthesia and surgery. JAMA 216:1615, 1971.
46. Ramsey M: Blood pressure monitoring: Automated oscillometric devices. J Clin Monit 7:56, 1991.
47. Barker SJ, Tremper KK: Pulse oximetry: Applications and limitations. Int Anesthesiol Clin 25:155, 1987.
48. Bhavani-Shanker K, Mosely H, Kumar AY, et al: Capnometry and anesthesia. Can J Anaesth 39:617, 1992.
49. Zupan J: Fiberoptic bronchoscopy in anesthesia and critical care. In Benumof JL (ed): Clinical Procedures in Anesthesia. Philadelphia, JB Lippincott, 1992.
50. Daos FG, Lopez L, et al: Local anesthetic toxicity modified by oxygen and by combination of the agents. Anesthesiology 23:755, 1962.
51. Boucek CD, Gunnerson HB, Tullock WC: Percutaneous transtracheal high-frequency jet ventilation as an aid to fiberoptic intubation. Anesthesiology 67:247, 1987.
52. Benumof JL, Scheller MS: The importance of transtracheal jet ventilation in the management of the difficult airway. Anesthesiology 71:769, 1989.
53. Ravussin P, Bayer-Berger M, Monnier P, et al: Percutaneous trans-tracheal ventilation for laser endoscopic procedures in infants and small children with laryngeal obstruction. Can J Anaesth 34:83, 1987.
54. Yealy DM, Stewart RD, Kaplan RM: Myths and pitfalls in emergency translaryngeal ventilation: Correcting misimpresssions. Ann Emerg Med 17:690, 1984.
55. Benumof JL: First International Symposium on the Difficult Airway, Newport Beach, Calif, Sept 16, 1993.
56. Perry LB: Topical anesthesia for bronchoscopy. Chest 73:691, 1978.
57. Adriani J, Zepernick R, Arens J, et al: The comparative potency and effectiveness of topical anesthetics in man. Clin Pharmacol Ther 5:49, 1964.
58. Schenck NL: Local anesthesia in otolaryngology. Ann Otol Rhinol Laryngol 84:65, 1975.
59. Anderton JM, Nassar WY: Topical cocaine and general anesthesia: An investigation of the efficacy and side effects of cocaine on the nasal mucosa. Anaesthesia 30:809, 1975.
60. Van Dyke C, Barash PG, Jatlow P, et al: Cocaine: Plasma concentrations after intranasal application in man. Science 191:859, 1976.
61. Murphy TM: Somatic blockade of head and neck. In Cousins MJ, Bridenbaugh

PO (eds): Neural Blockade in Clinical Anaesthesia and Management of Pain, 2nd ed. Philadelphia, JB Lippincott, 1988, p 533.

62. Sandza JG, Roberts RW, et al: Symptomatic methemoglobinemia with a commonly used topical anesthetic, Cetacaine. Ann Thorac Surg 30:187, 1980.

63. Douglas WW, Fairbanks VF: Methemoglobinemia induced by a topical anesthetic spray (Cetacaine). Chest 71:587, 1977.

64. Kotler RL, Hansen-Flaschen J, et al: Severe methemoglobinemia after flexible fibre optic bronchoscopy. Thorax 44:234, 1989.

65. Rosenberg PH, Heinonen J, et al: Lidocaine concentration in blood after topical anesthesia of the upper respiratory tract. Acta Anesthesiol Scand 24:125, 1980.

66. Weisel W, Tella RA: Reaction to tetracaine used as topical anesthetic in bronchoscopy: A study of 1000 cases. JAMA 147:218, 1951.

67. Roberts JT: Anatomy and patient positioning for fiberoptic laryngoscopy. Anesthesiol Clin North Am 9:53, 1991.

68. Adriani J, Campbell D: Fatalities following topical application of local anesthetic to the mucous membrane. JAMA 162:1527, 1956.

69. Bourke DL, Katz J, Tonneson A: Nebulized anesthesia for awake endotracheal intubation. Anesthesiology 63:690, 1985.

70. Reed AF: Preparation for Awake Fiberoptic Intubation: ASA Refresher Course: Workshop on the Management of the Difficult Airway. Orlando, Fla, Nov 5, 1994.

71. Raj PP: Handbook of Regional Anesthesia. New York, Churchill Livingstone, 1985.

72. Katz J: Atlas of Regional Anesthesia, 2nd ed. New York, Appleton & Lange, 1994.

73. Adriani J: Nerve Blocks: A Manual of Regional Anesthesia for Practitioners of Medicine. Springfield, Ill, Charles C Thomas, 1954.

74. Boudreaux AM: Simple technique for fiberoptic bronchoscopy. Am Soc Crit Care Anesth Pract 6:8, 1994.

75. Ovassapian A: Fiberoptic airway endoscopy in anesthesia and critical care. New York, Raven Press, 1990.

76. Reed AP: Preparation of the patient for awake flexible fiberoptic bronchoscopy. Chest 101:244, 1992.

77. Clemente CD: Gray's Anatomy, 13th ed. Philadelphia, Lea & Febiger, 1985.

78. Cooper M, Watson RL: An improved regional anesthetic technique for peroral endoscopy. Anesthesiology 43:372, 1975.

79. Kazuhisa K, Norimasa S, Takanori M, et al: Glossopharyngeal nerve block for carotid sinus syndrome. Anesth Analg 75:1036, 1992.

80. Rovenstein EA, Papper EM: Glossopharyngeal nerve block. Am J Surg 75:713, 1948.

81. Platzer W: Atlas of topographical anatomy. Stuttgart, Georg Thieme, 1985.

82. Bedder MD, Lindsay D: Glossopharyngeal nerve block using ultrasound guidance: A case report of a new technique. Reg Anesth 14:304, 1989.

83. Demeester TR, Skinner DB, et al: Local nerve block anesthesia for peroral endoscopy. Ann Thorac Surg 24:278, 1977.

84. Snell RS, Katz J: Clinical Anatomy for Anesthesia Practitioners. New York, Appleton & Lange, 1989.

85. Wildsmith JAW, Armitage EN: Principles and practices of regional anaesthesia. New York, Churchill Livingstone, 1987.

86. Byron J, Bailey J: Head and Neck Surgery-Otolaryngology. Philadelphia, JB Lippincott, 1993.

87. Prakash UB: Bronchoscopy: A Text Atlas. New York, Raven Press, 1994.

88. Finucane TF, Santora HS: Principles of airway management. Philadelphia, FA Davis, 1988.

89. Paparella MM, Shumrick DA, Gluckman JL (eds): Otolaryngology. Philadelphia, WB Saunders, 1991.

90. Gotta AW, Sullivan CA: Superior laryngeal nerve block: An aid to intubating the patient with fractured mandible. J Trauma 24(1):83, 1984.

91. Hunt LA, Boyd GL: Superior laryngeal nerve block as a supplement to total intravenous anesthesia for rigid laser bronchoscopy in a patient with myasthenic syndrome. Anesth Analg 75:458, 1992.

92. Wiles JR, Kelly J, Mostafa SM: Hypotension and bradycardia following superior laryngeal nerve block. Br J Anaesth 63:125, 1989.

93. Gotta AW, Sullivan CA: Anaesthesia of the upper airway using topical anaesthetic and superior laryngeal nerve block. Br J Anaesth 53:1055, 1981.

94. Hast M: Anatomy of the larynx. XIV. *In* English GM (ed): Otolaryngology, vol 3. Philadephia, Harper & Row, 1987.

95. Bonica JJ: Transtracheal anesthesia for endotracheal intubation. Anesthesiology 10:736, 1949.

96. Walts LF, Kassity KJ: Spread of local anesthesia after upper airway block. Arch Otolaryngol 81:77, 1965.

97. Gold MI, Buechael DR: Translaryngeal anesthesia: A review. Anesthesiology 20:181, 1959.

98. Hamill JF, Bedford RF, et al: Lidocaine before endotracheal intubation: Intravenous or laryngotracheal? Anesthesiology 5:578, 1981.

99. Boster SR, Danzl DF, Madden RJ, Jarboe CH: Translaryngeal absorption of lidocaine. Ann Emerg Med 11:461, 1982.

100. Viegas O, Stoelting RK: Lidocaine in arterial blood after laryngotracheal administration. Anesthesiology 43:491, 1975.

101. Chu SS, Rah KH, Brannan MD, Cohen JL: Plasma concentration of lidocaine after endotracheal spray. Anesth Analg 54:438, 1975.

102. Hill AJ, Feneck RO, et al: The hemodynamic effects of bronchoscopy: Comparison of propofol and thiopentone with and without alfentanil pretreatment. Anaesthesia 46:266, 1991.

103. Adriani J (ed): Labat's Regional Anesthesia, 4th ed. St Louis, Warren HJ Green, 1985, p 650.

104. Snow JC (ed): Anesthesia in Otolaryngology and Ophthalmology. London, Prentice-Hall, 1982, p 104.

105. Eriksson E: Illustrated Handbook in Local Anaesthesia. London, Lloyd Luke, 1979.

Chapter 5

Flexible Fiberoptic

....

Tracheal Intubation

....

Andranik Ovassapian and
Melissa Wheeler

Tracheal intubation is one of the most common medical procedures performed in tertiary care hospitals. On one hand, it is highly successful and easy to perform using a rigid laryngoscope. On the other hand, hypoxic brain damage and death may result rapidly if it is unsuccessful. This disastrous outcome happens when the airway cannot be secured by intubation and face mask ventilation becomes extremely difficult or impossible. To avoid these major complications, one should be careful in selection of the technique applied for tracheal intubation.

Over the past 40 years, different techniques of tracheal intubation have been introduced, the most effective under difficult conditions being fiberoptic intubation.[1, 2] It is interesting that the fiberoptic bronchoscope (FB) was not developed for this purpose, nor was it used for the first fiberoptic intubation.[3, 4] The first recorded fiberoptic tracheal intubation was performed in 1967 by Murphy, using a flexible fiberoptic choledochoscope through the nose on a patient with Still's disease.[4] The value of the FB as an airway management tool was recognized by anesthesia practitioners, and they played an important role in expanding its use in the management of the difficult airway.[5–10]

Since the introduction of the FB in 1964, continuous improvements have been made in the design and quality of these instruments. New applications of fiberoptic bronchoscopy have been identified in many aspects of medicine, such as anesthesiology, otolaryngology, emergency and intensive care medicine, thoracic surgery, and trauma. Intubating patients while they are conscious and spontaneously breathing provides safety for those with a difficult airway. Flexible fiberoptic bronchoscopy facilitates awake tracheal intubation, which when performed under topical anesthesia is painless and well tolerated.[11]

The value of fiberoptic airway endoscopy and tracheal intubation is so great that no anesthesia practitioner can afford not to master this technique. The major barrier in its use is a lack of training and experience; to overcome this, the art of fiberoptic airway management should be a routine in anesthesia training programs, and those in practice should learn the technique by attending hands-on workshops.[1, 12, 13] Successful performance of fiberoptic intubation requires training and practice. Learning the technique is easy, provided a stepwise approach is taken,[12] yet only practice brings skill and expertise.

A common statement regarding management of the difficult airway is that one should apply the technique that one is most familiar or experienced with. However, this statement should not and could not be used as an excuse to avoid learning new techniques that are superior for the management of difficult intubation. Under nonemergency situations, a health care provider who is not skillful in fiberoptic techniques should not accept the management of a patient with a very difficult airway and risk the patient's well-being. Unfortunately, under emergency situations, the choice is limited and the patient is more likely to suffer from the consequences of airway mismanagement.

Fiberoptic intubation has proved itself to be the technique of choice for the management of the difficult airway under most circumstances.[1, 2, 14] The appropriate selection and efficient use of the FB minimizes disastrous outcomes and increases the safety of airway management. Fiberoptic tracheal intubation is critical in airway management and should be mastered by all individuals involved in airway management.

INDICATIONS FOR FIBEROPTIC INTUBATION

Any indication for tracheal intubation is an indication for fiberoptic intubation. The routine use of the FB in tracheal intubation provides the first step in learning this fascinating airway management skill.[1] Under many circumstances, the FB provides a superior technique for tracheal intubation compared with conventional techniques (Table 5–1).

Fiberoptic intubation is usually fast and easily accomplished when appropriate preparatory steps are taken. Many patients who might be denied a general anesthetic or subjected to tracheostomy because intubation by rigid laryngoscopy appeared difficult may be safely and easily intubated with the help of the FB.[1, 15–18]

There are no specific contraindications to fiberoptic intubation, but under certain circumstances, such as major bleeding in the airway and massive facial injury, successful use of the FB is almost impossible. In an uncooperative and combative patient, tracheal intubation is difficult without the aid of pharmacologic agents, and the chance of instrument

Table 5–1 Indications for Fiberoptic Intubation

Routine intubation
Difficult intubation
   Anticipated
     History of difficult intubation
     Physical evidence of difficult intubation
   Unanticipated
     Ignored, rushed, or missed evidence of difficult intubation
     Hidden causes of difficult intubation (hypertrophy of lingual tonsils)
Compromised airway
   Upper airway abnormality
   Lower airway abnormality (tracheal compression)
Extension of neck not desirable
   Unstable neck
   Vertebral artery insufficiency
High risk of dental damage
   Poor, loose, or fragile teeth
   Extensive dental restoration
Awake intubation with topical anesthesia

From Ovassapian A: Fiberoptic Endoscopy and the Difficult Airway. Philadelphia, Lippincott-Raven, 1996.

damage is high. In the pediatric age group, a lack of the appropriately sized FB limits its use, and special techniques need to be applied for fiberoptic intubation.[19, 20] Patients with severe airway obstruction due to edema or tumor should be handled with extreme caution in order to avoid complete airway obstruction and emergency intervention.[1]

Tracheal Intubation Under Topical Anesthesia

Successful fiberoptic intubation in conscious patients depends on the expertise of the endoscopist, proper preparation of the patient, and setup of a well-functioning fiberscope with the necessary supplies (Fig. 5–1).

■ Preparation of the Fiberscope

Before its use, the FB, light source, and ancillary equipment must be checked and inspected to ensure that they are in proper working order

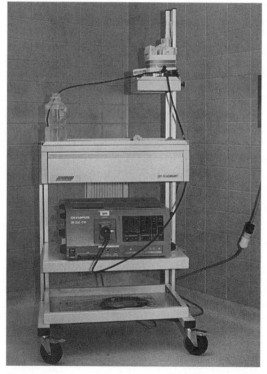

Figure 5–1 Simple fiberoptic cart arrangement. The top surface of the cart is cleaned with disinfectant solution after each use and is covered with a clean towel. The fiberscope is placed on the top of the cart and is covered with clean towels ready for the next use. The supplies for awake fiberoptic intubation are stored in the drawer. (From Ovassapian A: Fiberoptic Endoscopy and the Difficult Airway. Philadelphia, Lippincott–Raven, 1996.)

(Table 5–2). The insertion cord is checked for defects. The angulation lever is manipulated to see that it functions smoothly. By holding the tip of the FB a few millimeters away from written words, one adjusts the diopter ring to ensure a clear and focused view. The suction line is connected to the FB. The insertion cord of the FB and the endotracheal tube (ET) are placed in warm water.[1] This prevents fogging of the lens and softens the ET, thus easing its passage through the intubating airway or nasal passage. The insertion cord of the FB and the distal part of the ET should be lubricated with a water-soluble lubricant.

The body of the FB is held by the tip of the fingers, so that the thumb position remains perpendicular to the angulation lever. The index finger controls the suction button, and the thumb adjusts the angulation lever, controlling movement of the FB tip in an up-and-down direction (Fig. 5–2). The tip of the FB moves in the direction opposite to that of the angulation lever. An upward movement of the lever moves the tip of FB downward; a downward movement moves the tip upward. To view to the right or left, the body of the FB is rotated in the desired direction while the tip is tilted up or down by movement of the lever. The insertion cord should move freely within the lumen of the ET to make this maneuver possible. The insertion cord should also be kept straight to avoid loop formation on its longitudinal axes. If a loop is formed, the tip of the insertion cord will not follow the directional changes transferred by rotating the body of the FB. The nonscope hand helps guide the insertion cord into the airway and controls the advancement and withdrawal of the FB.[1]

■ Preparation of the Patient

The patient with a history of a failed intubation, an expected difficult intubation, or a distorted upper airway can benefit from awake fiberoptic intubation (Table 5–3). The application of good topical anesthetic

Table 5–2 Preparation and Inspection of Fiberscope

Attach fiberscope to light source

Adjust light intensity to desired level

Check insertion cord for dents, wrinkles, or bite marks

Check function of tip control lever

Focus lens to your eyes

Connect suction line to suction valve

Place tip of fiberscope in warm water bath to prevent fogging

Place endotracheal tube in warm water bath to soften tube, ease passage, and minimize tissue trauma

Lubricate fiberscope and endotracheal tube

Modified from Ovassapian A: Fiberoptic Endoscopy and the Difficult Airway. Philadelphia, Lippincott-Raven, 1996.

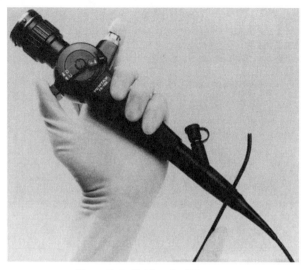

Figure 5–2 Holding the fiberscope.

and conscious sedation makes fiberoptic intubation relatively easy in the awake patient. Spontaneous ventilation keeps the airway open, and the patient can swallow and clear secretions. Phonation or deep breathing by the patient can assist the endoscopist in locating the glottis when airway anatomy is distorted.[1, 21]

Conscious sedation is desirable in awake intubation to minimize psychologic trauma, provided that the patient's safety is not compromised. Depending on the patient's condition and the indication for awake intubation, an opioid, a sedative, or a combination is used.[1, 22]

Table 5–3 Tracheal Intubation in Conscious Patient

Advantages
- Safest approach in patients with difficult airway
- Maintains spontaneous ventilation
- Keeps airway open
- Time of intubation not limited
- Patient can swallow secretions
- Deep breaths on command assist exposure of glottis
- Allows postintubation neurologic examination

Disadvantages
- Patient cooperation needed
- Possible patient discomfort
- Gagging with poor topical anesthesia
- Difficult in children and uncooperative patients

From Ovassapian A: Fiberoptic Endoscopy and the Difficult Airway. Philadelphia, Lippincott-Raven, 1996.

Opioids produce profound analgesia, are strong depressants of the airway reflexes, and facilitate oropharyngeal instrumentation, yet the patient should remain capable of following verbal commands. However, patients are more susceptible to aspiration of gastric contents if regurgitation or vomiting occurs. A combination of fentanyl and midazolam (1.5 μg/kg and 30 μg/kg, respectively) has been used successfully for sedation before arrival in the operating room. If the patient has a compromised airway, premedication should be avoided because of the possibility of airway obstruction.

Drying agents are essential when intubation is carried out before the induction of anesthesia. Excessive secretions interfere with the effectiveness of topical anesthesia, thereby leaving airway reflexes active, and are a major cause of discomfort and failure of the technique. In addition, instrumentation of the airway increases the flow of saliva, and increased secretions add to the difficulty of fiberoptic intubation.[1, 22]

The patient at high risk for aspiration will benefit from premedications that increase the gastric pH, reduce the gastric volume, and enhance gastric emptying. Ranitidine 150 mg orally is given the night before surgery. A β_2-blocking agent increases the gastric pH and reduces the gastric volume. Metoclopramide is a dopamine antagonist and has three different effects: it accelerates gastric emptying, increases the tone of the lower esophageal sphincter, and depresses the vomiting center in the medulla. The danger of regurgitation and aspiration is increased in patients with a difficult airway and at risk of aspiration if tracheal intubation is attempted after the induction of anesthesia. Breathing against an obstructed airway in an anesthetized patient opens the gastroesophageal sphincter, thus promoting regurgitation. Pushing air into the stomach during a difficult mask ventilation causes distention of the stomach, which also promotes regurgitation of gastric contents. Intubation of the trachea before the induction of anesthesia avoids these possibilities, reducing the chance for regurgitation and aspiration.

Oral Approach

Five or six sprays (50 to 60 mg) of 10% aerosolized lidocaine are applied to the palate, base of the tongue, and lateral pharyngeal walls. Translaryngeal injection of 3 mL of 4% lidocaine (120 mg) through the cricothyroid membrane provides topical anesthesia to the larynx and the trachea (Table 5–4).[11, 22]

To test its adequacy and supplement the topical anesthesia of the oropharynx, a local anesthetic jelly is spread on the base of the tongue using a tongue blade. In 94% of the cases, the topical anesthesia achieved is good to excellent for performing tracheal intubation.[11] Additional topical anesthetic may be applied to the oropharynx if the patient reacts to the presence of the airway. Laryngeal topical anesthesia can be supplemented, if necessary, by spraying an additional 2 mL of 4% lidocaine (80 mg) through the fiberscope.

The establishment of topical anesthesia before laryngoscopy prevents coughing, swallowing, laryngeal spasm, and excessive salivation, all of which add to the difficulty of fiberoptic intubation. With experience, the practitioner can achieve topical anesthesia of the larynx and trachea

Table 5-4   Steps of Awake Fiberoptic Orotracheal Intubation

Titrate sedation

Apply topical anesthesia

    Spray oropharynx with 10% lidocaine (5 to 8 sprays)

    Inject 3 ml of 4% lidocaine through cricothyroid membrane or spray as you go through fiberscope

    Apply lidocaine jelly to base of tongue

Place intubating airway in patient's mouth

Suction oropharynx gently through airway

Place endotracheal tube in intubating airway about 5 cm

Introduce fiberscope through endotracheal tube; make sure to pass through distal lumen; identify epiglottis and vocal cords; advance fiberscope in trachea

Pass endotracheal tube over fiberscope into trachea; avoid further advancement of fiberscope into main stem bronchi

Confirm correct position of endotracheal tube (3 cm above carina)

Attach breathing system; reconfirm correct tube placement

Perform neurologic examination when indicated

Tape tube, induce anesthesia

From Ovassapian A: Fiberoptic Endoscopy and the Difficult Airway. Philadelphia, Lippincott-Raven, 1996.

by spraying local anesthetic through the working channel of the FB. Inhalation of local anesthetics through a nebulizer also provides topical anesthesia of the upper airway[23] and can be used in patients in whom severe coughing should be avoided.[1]

After topical anesthesia is established, the head is placed in the normal intubating position. An airway intubator is placed in the mouth (Fig. 5–3), the oropharynx is suctioned, and the lubricated ET is placed 4 to 5 cm inside the airway. The fourth and fifth fingers of the right hand (for right-handed operators) hold the ET, preventing premature advancement of the tube, while the index finger and thumb advance the FB through it (Fig. 5–4). The endoscopist should look through the FB in order to avoid passing it through the Murphy eye of the ET.

As the FB is advanced toward the oropharynx, the white pharyngeal surface of the airway, soft palate, and uvula come into view (Fig. 5–5). With further advancement, the FB enters into the oropharynx and its tip is deflected anteriorly to expose the epiglottis and vocal cords. In the presence of a large floppy epiglottis, the tip of the FB should be manipulated under the tip of the epiglottis in order to visualize the vocal cords. By extending the patient's head at the atlantooccipital joint, keeping the mouth closed, one keeps the epiglottis away from the posterior pharyngeal wall. Occasionally, a jaw-thrust maneuver or pulling the tongue forward by an assistant may be required to facilitate glottic exposure.

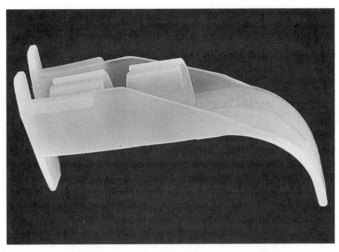

Figure 5–3 Ovassapian fiberoptic intubating airway.

In the obese patient and in most difficult airways, the use of the sitting position during the application of topical anesthetic and intubation should be considered, since it allows the sniffing position to be maintained more easily and the local anesthetics to gravitate toward the larynx and trachea.[21]

After the vocal cords are exposed, they are maintained in the center of the field of view by fine manipulations of the control lever, as the FB is advanced. Without such maneuvering, the tip of the FB often impinges on the anterior commissure or the anterior laryngeal wall. The flexing of the tip of the FB posteriorly at this point brings the laryngeal and tracheal lumen into view. The FB is then advanced into the lower trachea, and the ET is slipped over the firmly held stationary FB and advanced with a twisting motion into the trachea. The endoscopist should remove his or her eye from the FB eyepiece and observe the ET during this maneuver. It is important to ensure that the FB is not advanced farther into the tracheobronchial tree during advancement of the ET. The tip of the ET should be positioned 3 to 4 cm above the carina.

If an intubating airway is not used, the ET is fitted onto the FB, the tongue is pulled out, and the FB is placed in the mouth at midline position. With this approach, the problem of the FB inadvertently being passed through the Murphy eye of the ET is avoided, but FB deviation off the midline is common. Patients may also bite and damage the FB.

The oral approach is slightly more difficult than the nasal approach, because of the sharp curve leading from the oral cavity into the larynx.[1] In 20% to 30% of patients, even though the FB has entered the trachea, the ET impinges on laryngeal anatomy and cannot be advanced into the trachea.[1, 8] When this happens, the ET is pulled back over the FB, rotated 90 degrees clockwise or counterclockwise to change the position

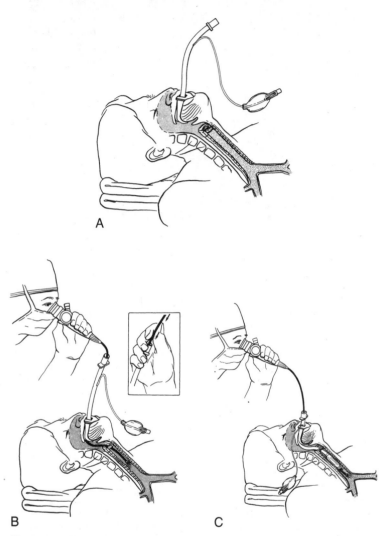

Figure 5–4 Fiberoptic orotracheal intubation in a conscious patient. *A*, Ovassapian intubating airway and endotracheal tube position. *B*, The fiberscope is advanced through the endotracheal tube into the midtrachea. *Inset*, Position of hand for holding the tracheal tube and advancing the fiberscope. *C*, The tube is advanced over the fiberscope into the trachea. (*A–C*, From Ovassapian A: Fiberoptic Endoscopy and the Difficult Airway. Philadelphia, Lippincott–Raven, 1996.)

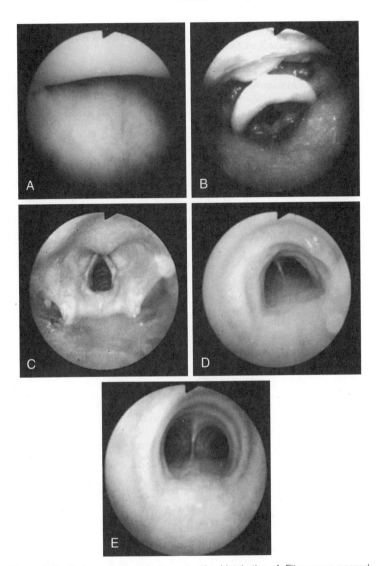

Figure 5–5 Endoscopic view during orotracheal intubation. *A,* Fiberscope passed just beyond the tracheal tube. The laryngeal surface of the Ovassapian airway is shown in white. The soft palate is seen in the lower half of the photograph. *B,* Tip of the fiberscope in the oropharynx. The distal end of the Ovassapian airway covers the base of the tongue. The epiglottis is in view. *C,* Tip of the fiberscope passed beneath the tip of the epiglottis. The glottis is in view. *D,* Tip of the fiberscope passed just beyond the vocal cords. The anterior wall of the larynx shows the entry site of the translaryngeal injection needle. *E,* Tip of the fiberscope in the lower third of the trachea. The carina is in view. (*A–E,* From Ovassapian A: Fiberoptic Endoscopy and the Difficult Airway. Philadelphia, Lippincott–Raven, 1996.)

of the bevel of the tube in relation to the larynx,[1, 24, 25] and readvanced during deep inspiration. In some patients, this maneuver may have to be repeated two or three times.

The larger the gap between the FB and the ET, the more the chance that the tube may not easily slide into the trachea.[1, 8] Laryngospasm due to poor topical anesthesia may also prevent ET advancement. Additional topical anesthetic applied through the FB before intubation frequently remedies the problem.[11]

Nasal Approach

Fiberoptic nasotracheal intubation is somewhat easier than the oral approach, because the FB remains midline. In addition, the FB is usually directed straight at the glottic opening as it enters the oropharynx, and the vocal cords are usually visualized from a distance (Table 5–5).[1, 7]

After selection of the more patent nostril, 4% or 5% cocaine is applied to the nasal mucosa with cotton-tipped applicators. This agent provides excellent topical anesthesia and shrinkage of mucosal tissue. The cotton-tipped applicators are gradually worked posteriorly along the floor of the nose until the applicator encounters the bony resistance of the cervical spine. Spraying the nasal passages with 10% lidocaine (Xylocaine) before advancing the applicators may minimize the discomfort. However, most patients dislike the burning sensation and the taste of the lidocaine.[26] If cocaine is unavailable, another successful approach is using a combination of Neo-Synephrine 1% and 4% lidocaine (1 mL of Neo-Synephrine and 3 mL of 4% lidocaine mixture). Afrin spray may be applied to achieve vasoconstriction, followed by application of 4% lidocaine for topical anesthesia.

Laryngotracheal anesthesia is achieved as described earlier. There is

Table 5–5   Advantages and Disadvantages of Nasotracheal Intubation

Advantages	Disadvantages
Easier fiberoptic technique	Takes more time to prepare
Gag reflex not stimulated, no need for oropharyngeal topical anesthesia	Longer and smaller tube
	Submucosal tunneling
Mouth opening not required	Trauma and epistaxis common
Easier mouth care	Pressure necrosis of septum and nasal alae
Biting of fiberscope and tube not possible	Bacteremia, sinusitis, otitis likely
Less laryngeal damage on short term	Basilar skull fracture a possible contraindication
Greater patient comfort	

Modified from Ovassapian A: Fiberoptic Endoscopy and the Difficult Airway. Philadelphia, Lippincott-Raven, 1996.

no need to apply topical anesthetic to the tongue and oropharynx, as the gag reflex is not stimulated by the nasal approach.[7]

The appropriately sized ET, softened in warm water, is lubricated generously and gently inserted through the prepared nostril, until the bend at the posterior nasopharynx is reached. If it does not make the bend, it is pulled back, rotated 90 degrees to the right or left, and reintroduced. If this maneuver is unsuccessful, the ET is pulled back and the lubricated FB is inserted into the ET and used to direct it into the nasopharynx.

It is important to avoid passing the ET too far distally into the oropharynx, as it may direct the FB away from the midline, interfering with laryngeal exposure. The oropharynx is suctioned through the ET, and the lubricated FB is inserted through it into the oropharynx. In 80% to 85% of patients, the epiglottis and vocal cords are seen with minimal or no manipulation of the FB tip.[7] In heavily sedated patients or edentulous patients, the tongue and pharyngeal tissue may block exposure of the larynx and vocal cords. Extension of the head, the application of a jaw thrust, or pulling the tongue forward aids in visualizing the vocal cords. The FB is advanced into the midtrachea, followed by the ET. In nasotracheal fiberoptic intubation, the problem of the ET's meeting resistance and not entering the trachea is much less common compared with orotracheal intubation.

The advantage of placing the ET first in the nasopharynx is to avoid contamination of the tip of the FB with secretions that can obscure the view. In addition, a tight nasal passage can be recognized when the FB is being advanced. Once the FB has passed through the ET and into the trachea, advancement of the ET over the FB is easily accomplished. The main disadvantage is the greater possibility of causing nasal bleeding because of trauma to the nasal mucosa.[1]

If the ET is loaded over the FB and the FB is passed first, advancement of the ET into the trachea may not be possible if the passage of the nose is inadequate. In this case, the procedure will have to be repeated using a smaller tube or using the other naris. Anterior septal deviation does not interfere with intubation, since the problem usually involves cartilaginous, not bony, tissues. Nasal spurs may be bony or cartilaginous, and either type may compress the ET, preventing its passage. Movement of the ET over bony spurs can damage the ET cuff or cause epistaxis.[1]

The presence of large polyps and adenoidal tissues interferes with nasal intubation. Large osteophytes of the cervical spine can deflect the ET and FB away from the glottic opening.

Tracheal Intubation Under General Anesthesia

In patients with normal upper airway anatomy, tracheal intubation under general anesthesia (GA) is as easily achieved with the FB as it is with the rigid laryngoscope. Compared with intubation in awake patients, the two major disadvantages of intubation under GA are the time limitation imposed by an apneic patient and the loss of tonicity of the tongue and pharyngeal tissues. This loss of tone closes down the pharyngeal space, blocking visualization of the larynx.[1]

To minimize apnea time and facilitate laryngeal exposure, an assistant is necessary. An assistant can have the FB ready, pass it to the endoscopist, apply a jaw thrust, and observe the apnea time. The endoscopy cart is placed at the head of the table on the left side of the patient, while the assistant stands on the patient's left side facing the endoscopist.

■ Oral Approach

After GA and muscle relaxation are established, the anesthesia mask is removed, the intubating airway is placed inside the mouth, and the oropharynx is suctioned (Table 5–6). Ventilation by mask is resumed for 30 to 60 seconds. The anesthesia mask is then removed, and the anesthesia practitioner grasps the FB from an assistant with the left hand and the tip of the insertion cord with the right. The tip of the insertion cord is placed inside the intubating airway and advanced into the oropharynx.[1]

The assistant then applies a jaw-thrust maneuver. This maneuver is vital and constitutes the most important step in fiberoptic intubation under GA. If an intubating airway is not available, the assistant may pull the tongue forward away from the palate and posterior pharyngeal wall to assist in exposure of the vocal cords. Care must be taken since forceful pulling of the tongue over the lower teeth may cause trauma and laceration of the tongue.[27] Lung forceps, a mouth gag with a tongue holder, and a malleable tongue retractor have been used to keep the tongue forward.[28]

The intubating airway helps ensure that the FB will remain in the

Table 5–6   Steps of Asleep Fiberoptic Intubation

Establish general anesthesia and paralysis
Place intubating airway into mouth
Suction oropharynx
Ventilate by mask, mild hyperventilation
Assistant hands fiberscope to intubator
Assistant exerts jaw thrust and monitors apnea time
Pass fiberscope through airway and glottic opening and into trachea
Thread endotracheal tube over fiberscope through airway and into trachea
Check position of tip of tube and remove fiberscope
For nasotracheal intubation, apply vasoconstrictor to nasal mucosa
For spontaneously breathing patient, apply topical anesthesia before advancing fiberscope into trachea to minimize risk of laryngospasm

From Ovassapian A: Fiberoptic Endoscopy and the Difficult Airway. Philadelphia, Lippincott-Raven, 1996.

midline position, thereby facilitating exposure of the vocal cords. After the FB is positioned in the midtrachea, the ET is advanced with a rotating motion. If the ET encounters resistance, it is pulled back, rotated 90 degrees to the left or right, and then readvanced while the assistant continues to apply a jaw thrust.

■ Nasal Approach

The general preparation, technique of intubation, and assistant duties are similar to those for orotracheal intubation. An oropharyngeal airway or intubating airway is placed to keep the tongue off the posterior pharyngeal wall. The application of a vasoconstrictor to the naris before intubation, before or after the induction of anesthesia, is recommended to minimize the incidence of bleeding.

The tip of the FB is inserted into the selected naris and advanced under direct vision toward the larynx and trachea. The assistant applies a jaw-thrust maneuver to maintain the oropharyngeal space open. After midtracheal placement of the FB, the ET is threaded into the trachea. Force should not be applied in passing the ET, as removal of the FB could be difficult or impossible, possibly owing to a narrow nasal passage that was not identified during passage of the FB.

Modified Endoscopy Mask Technique

To perform fiberoptic intubation by endoscopy mask technique, an assistant capable of administering anesthesia and maintaining mask ventilation is required.[14, 29, 30] Anesthesia is induced and ventilation is maintained with a regular face mask, and an intubating airway is placed inside the mouth. For smoother passage of the ET through the endoscopy mask (Fig. 5–6) and intubating airway and to maintain the ability to provide positive-pressure ventilation, a modified endoscopy

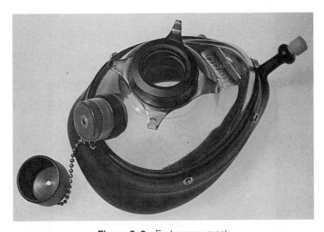

Figure 5–6   Endoscopy mask.

mask technique has been described.[1] With this modification, the breathing system of the anesthesia machine remains closed until the completion of intubation.

A lubricated ET is prepared with its 15-mm adapter loosely attached. A bronchoscopy swivel adapter is then mounted on the ET, and its 15-mm side arm is blocked with tape. The lubricated ET is passed through the diaphragm of the endoscopy mask port to about 10 cm (Fig. 5–7). Additional lubrication is then applied to the distal end of the ET.

After achieving the appropriate depth of anesthesia and relaxation, the regular anesthesia mask is removed. An oral intubating airway is then placed and the oropharynx is suctioned. The endoscopy mask mounted with the ET is positioned over the face by first inserting the tip of the ET inside the intubating airway. Anesthesia is continued with the endoscopy mask in place. The FB is advanced through the swivel adapter and ET into the oropharynx and trachea. The ET is threaded over the FB and into the trachea. The FB with the ET adapter and bronchoscopy adapter are removed together, leaving the ET in place. The endoscopy mask is then disengaged from the ET. The 15-mm ET adapter is then firmly reattached, completing the procedure.

In nasotracheal intubation, the ET with its loosely attached adapters is mounted over the FB before intubation. The breathing circuit remains closed when the ET passes through the endoscopy port, because of the seal provided by the swivel adapter.

One of the shortcomings of the endoscopy mask is the danger of tearing its diaphragm and pushing it into the trachea.[31] Diaphragm replacement is expensive, and segments remaining in the tracheobronchial tree may produce major problems.

Intubation Using the Nasal Airway

In the anesthetized, spontaneously breathing patient, anesthesia may be maintained through a nasopharyngeal airway in order to allow time

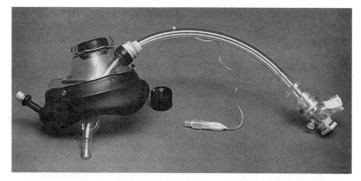

Figure 5–7 Modified endoscopy mask. The endoscopy mask is mounted with an endotracheal tube with a loosely attached tracheal tube and bronchoscopy swivel adapters. (From Ovassapian A: Fiberoptic Endoscopy and the Difficult Airway. Philadelphia, Lippincott–Raven, 1996.)

for unhurried tracheal intubation. Binasal airways with double-lumen tube adapters or a single nasopharyngeal airway with a regular ET adaptor is used for orotracheal intubation and connected to the anesthesia breathing system. An intubating airway is placed, and the FB is mounted with an ET and inserted through the airway before intubation.[29]

In performing nasotracheal intubation, a nasopharyngeal airway mounted with an ET adapter is inserted in one naris. The breathing circuit of the anesthesia machine is attached to the 15-mm adapter inserted into the nasal airway. The FB mounted with an ET is passed through the other naris to perform tracheal intubation.

Both the oral and the nasal approaches allow the patient to breathe spontaneously, thus maintaining an adequate depth of anesthesia and allowing time for an unhurried intubation. The FB also allows the option of spraying local anesthetic on the larynx to minimize laryngeal reaction and spasm. This may become necessary if the depth of anesthesia proves inadequate for airway manipulation.

Combining Fiberoptic and Other Intubation Techniques

The FB can be used in combination with the laryngeal mask, retrograde intubation, and blind nasal and rigid laryngoscopic intubation.

■ Fiberoptic Intubation Through the Laryngeal Mask

A number of case reports attest to the value of the laryngeal mask airway in failed intubations and in restoring ventilation when it could not be achieved by a face mask. Tracheal intubation through the laryngeal mask airway has been reported in awake and anesthetized patients, using blind or fiberoptic-aided techniques.[32-37]

■ Fiberoptic-Aided Retrograde Intubation

In the case of a failed retrograde intubation, a guide wire introduced through the cricothyroid membrane may be used to direct the FB toward the glottic opening and trachea to assist the passage of the ET into the trachea. Two different approaches are applied.[38-40]

The ET that cannot be advanced over the guide wire into the larynx is left in place. The FB is inserted into the ET, alongside the inserted guide wire, and out the distal end of the ET. The FB is then further advanced securely into the trachea. The guide wire is removed, and the ET is threaded over the FB and into the trachea.[38]

In the second approach, the guide wire is passed in a retrograde fashion through the suction channel of the FB, loaded with an ET.[39, 40] The FB is advanced over the guide wire into the trachea. The guide wire is removed, and the ET is threaded over the FB and into the trachea.

■ Fiberoptic and Blind Nasal Intubation

If the size of the nasal passage prevents the passage of the FB through the nasotracheal tube, the FB may be introduced through the contralateral naris. It can now be used to visualize the position of the tip of the ET and assist in its passage through the vocal cords.[19] Under visual observation, the nasotracheal tube and patient's head are manipulated in order to direct the nasotracheal tube toward the larynx (Fig. 5–8).

In patients with a distorted and compromised airway, blind nasotracheal intubation, as well as fiberoptic exposure of the glottis, may fail. A combination of blind nasal and fiberoptic intubation techniques may prove successful.[41]

The practitioner gently and slowly advances the nasotracheal tube through the prepared nostril while listening to breath sounds of the spontaneously breathing patient. Advancement of the ET is discontinued when breath sounds are the loudest. In this position, the tip of the nasotracheal tube is a short distance from the glottic opening, and the tube has passed beyond the distorted obstructed airway.

The passage of a lubricated FB through the nasotracheal tube brings the tip of the FB close to the glottic opening, allowing easy identification of the epiglottis and the glottic opening. After the application of topical anesthesia to the vocal cords and trachea, the FB is positioned into the trachea, followed by the nasotracheal tube.

■ Fiberoptic Intubation Aided by Rigid Laryngoscopy

In patients with an oropharyngeal mass, upper airway edema, or posteriorly displaced epiglottis (Fig. 5–9), the passage of an FB beneath the

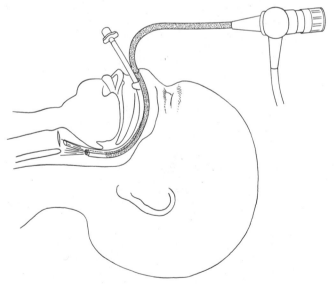

Figure 5–8 Tracheal intubation under fiberoptic observation. The fiberscope is introduced through the contralateral nostril to expose the larynx and the tip of the nasotracheal tube. Manipulation of the nasotracheal tube to pass through the vocal cords is performed under visual observation. (From Ovassapian A: Fiberoptic Endoscopy and the Difficult Airway. Philadelphia, Lippincott–Raven, 1996.)

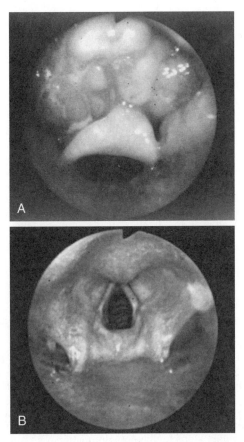

Figure 5–9   *A,* Large, benign lymphoid mass at the base of the tongue compressing the epiglottis. The fiberscope was advanced into the trachea, but the endotracheal tube would not pass into the trachea. Rigid laryngoscopy was necessary to retract the tongue and assist passage of the tube into the trachea. *B,* Normal glottis. (From Ovassapian A: Fiberoptic Endoscopy and the Difficult Airway. Philadelphia, Lippincott–Raven, 1996.)

epiglottis and into the glottic opening may prove difficult. Combining rigid laryngoscopy with fiberoptic intubation is helpful under these circumstances.[42–44]

The epiglottis is exposed by a second anesthesia practitioner using a rigid laryngoscope. The endoscopist looking directly inside the mouth (not through the FB) passes the tip of the FB under the epiglottis. This combined maneuver allows easy exposure of the vocal cords and completion of the intubation by the FB.

CAUSES OF FAILURE OF FIBEROPTIC INTUBATION

Failure of fiberoptic intubation can happen in each of the three steps of intubation: an inability to identify the laryngeal structures, an inability to guide the FB through the cords after exposure of the vocal cords, and an inability to advance the ET into the trachea after the FB is positioned in the trachea (Table 5–7).[1]

Lack of Training and Experience

Lack of experience in the use of the FB is the major factor contributing to failure of this technique. A simple mistake such as too-deep advancement of the FB before looking through it directs the FB into the esophagus. Moving the FB off the midline also contributes to the difficulty of exposing the larynx. The distance from the teeth to the vocal cords averages 16 cm in adults.[45] If the FB is advanced 20 cm and laryngeal structures are not identified, the FB is most likely in the esophagus. With the FB in the larynx or trachea, it is still possible not to identify these structures because acute flexion of the tip of the FB causes it to be positioned against the tracheal wall. Simple maneuvers such as tilting the tip in the opposite direction or rotating the body of the FB bring the tracheal rings into view.

Presence of Secretions and Blood

Airway secretions and blood are common causes of failure in identifying the laryngeal structures. Although the presence of a large amount of secretions or blood is an obstacle to the successful completion of fiberoptic intubation, in the hands of an inexperienced person, any amount of secretions will interfere with the success of the technique. A lack of technical skill in suctioning the secretions through the FB adds to the problem and to failure of the technique. For successful suctioning of secretions, the tip of the FB should be placed very close to the secretions. The administration of an adequate dose of antisialagogue and the proper suctioning of secretions before intubation are two important preparatory steps to fiberoptic intubation. The conscious patient can be asked to swallow or breathe deeply to clear secretions. High-flow insufflation of oxygen through the suction channel in order to keep

---

Table 5–7   Causes of Failure of Fiberoptic Intubation

Lack of experience
Presence of secretions and blood
Tip of epiglottis against posterior pharyngeal wall
  Large, floppy epiglottis
  Supraepiglottic cyst or mass
  Inflammation or edema of oropharynx
  Severe flexion deformity of cervical spine
Distorted airway anatomy
Inability to advance endotracheal tube
Inability to withdraw endotracheal tube

From Ovassapian A: Fiberoptic Endoscopy and the Difficult Airway. Philadelphia, Lippincott-Raven, 1996.

secretions away is not recommended, especially for the inexperienced endoscopist. Insufflation of oxygen can cause gastric distention and rupture of the stomach[46, 47] and has the potential to cause barotrauma to the lungs.[1] In cases of unexpected difficult rigid laryngoscopy and tracheal intubation, fiberoptic intubation should be instituted as soon as possible, before inducing trauma and bleeding. This simple principle is often ignored by those who are inexperienced in this technique, as a lack of skill prevents the early application of the FB in the management of a difficult or failed intubation.

Distorted Airway Anatomy

Distorted upper airway anatomy caused by prior surgery, a mass, edema, or soft tissue contraction may contribute to the difficulty of vocal cord exposure (Fig. 5–10). A deviated nasal septum may direct a nasotracheal tube away from the glottic opening.

Fogging of the lens also interferes with exposure of the laryngeal structures, and special antifog solutions are available. Also, insertion of the FB tip in warm water before its use prevents this problem.

Inability to Advance the Endotracheal Tube

Difficulty in advancing the ET over the FB into the trachea is common during fiberoptic orotracheal intubation. Contributing factors to this problem include (1) a large gap between the FB and the ET (a large ET used with a small-size FB), (2) the curve and rigidity of the ET, (3) intubation without the use of an intubating airway, (4) laryngeal spasm during intubation, and (5) limited or a lack of expertise of the endoscopist.

The right arytenoid cartilage and epiglottis are common sites at which the ET can "hang up" when being threaded over the FB.[1, 7, 24, 25] A 90-degree counterclockwise rotation of the tube turns the bevel of the tube to the 6 o'clock position, and the Murphy eye to the 12 o'clock position, respectively, permitting the ET to avoid the right arytenoid and enter the trachea without resistance.[24]

Rotating the ET to place its bevel at the 12 o'clock position may help with advancement under the epiglottis.[25] If the tip of the epiglottis is pushed down against the posterior pharyngeal wall, advancement of the ET may be possible only by using rigid laryngoscopy to elevate the tip of the epiglottis.

In order to minimize the gap between a large ET and a small FB, the placement of an uncuffed 5- or 5.5-mm internal diameter ET inside the larger adult tube has been suggested. The tip of the 5-mm tube should protrude beyond the distal end of the larger tube, thereby filling the gap between the larger tube and the 4-mm FB.[48, 49] The placement of a smaller tube inside the larger tube also prevents the accidental passage of an FB through the Murphy eye of the larger ET.[48]

An ET with a tapered tip and without a bevel was designed to overcome the gap between a large-sized ET and a smaller-sized FB (Fig. 5–11).[50] Sixty fiberoptic intubations were performed in anesthetized,

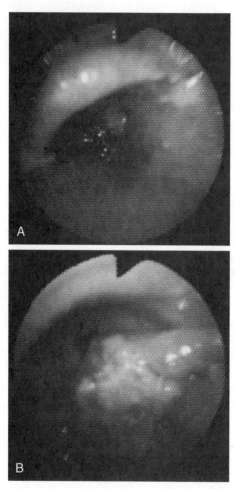

Figure 5–10 Large squamous cell carcinoma of right aryepiglottic fold. *A*, Tip of the epiglottis in view. The lower portion of the tumor is also visible. *B*, Fiberscope beyond the tip of the epiglottis. Tumor mass blocks the view of the glottis. The fiberscope was maneuvered to the upper left side over the mass and advanced toward the glottis. (*A* and *B*, From Ovassapian A: Fiberoptic Endoscopy and the Difficult Airway. Philadelphia, Lippincott–Raven, 1996.)

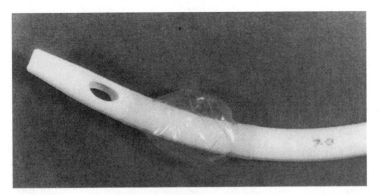

Figure 5–11   Tapered-tip Moore endotracheal tube. (From Jones HE, Pearce AC, Moore P: Fiberoptic intubation. Influence of tracheal tube tip design. Anaesthesia 48:672, 1993.)

paralyzed patients to compare a tapered-tip tube with a standard ET. In the orotracheal group, 4 of 15 regular ETs entered the trachea on the first attempt, compared with 14 of 15 of the tapered-tip tubes. In the nasotracheal group, 4 of 14 standard ETs entered smoothly on the first attempt, compared with all 16 of the tapered tubes. The results indicate that the removal of the gap between the ET and the FB eliminated most of the difficulty encountered during advancement of the ET during fiberoptic intubation.[50]

The flexometallic (anode) tubes are easier to pass[51, 52] and less damaging to the tissues and to the FB. In a prospective study, the ease of fiberoptic tracheal intubation was compared between regular ETs and flexometallic ETs.[53] Nineteen of 20 flexometallic intubations were successful on the first pass, compared with 7 of 20 of the regular ETs. Placing polyvinyl chloride ETs into warm water baths makes those tubes more flexible, thus allowing easier passage into the trachea. The pliable tube behaves like a flexometallic tube.

Fiberoptic orotracheal intubation without the use of an intubating airway tends to increase the FB deviation from the midline. The advancing ET has a greater tendency to catch the epiglottis or enter into the piriform sinus, contributing to the difficulty or failure of the technique.[1] Multiple attempts at ET advancement can cause airway trauma. Any degree of laryngeal trauma can become significant in patients with a difficult airway.

Inadequate Topical Anesthesia

Laryngospasm caused by inadequate topical anesthesia during awake intubation and light GA leads to resistance in the passage of the ET. With the fiberoptic technique, the FB is advanced into the trachea before the ET. In a lightly anesthetized, unparalyzed patient, the advancement of the FB can induce laryngeal spasm preventing passage of the ET into the trachea.

Limited Space Between the Epiglottis and the Posterior Pharyngeal Wall

When the epiglottis is pushed posteriorly against the posterior pharyngeal wall by a supraepiglottic mass, such as hypertrophied lingual tonsils or a vallecular cyst, it contributes to the difficulty of advancing the tip of the FB under the epiglottis. A large floppy epiglottis (Fig. 5–12), the tip of which touches the posterior pharyngeal wall, may also interfere with the passage of the FB beneath the tip of the epiglottis. A jaw thrust or pulling the tongue forward moves the epiglottis away from the posterior pharyngeal wall, correcting the problem in most patients. If the problem is secondary to a supraepiglottic mass or to inflammation and edema of the upper airway, the problem may not resolve with these maneuvers. In these circumstances, even if the FB is advanced into the trachea, threading the ET over the FB into the trachea may fail. Anterior displacement of the base of the tongue with a rigid laryngoscope may be required to assist passage of the ET.

Inability to Remove the Fiberoptic Bronchoscope

If the FB is passed through the Murphy eye of the ET, rather than through the distal lumen, withdrawal of the FB may prove difficult or

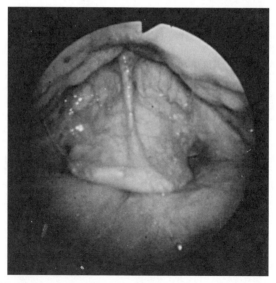

Figure 5–12 Large, floppy epiglottis blocks the view of the glottis. A jaw thrust or pulling the tongue forward will move the tip of the epiglottis away from the posterior pharyngeal wall, making exposure of the glottis possible. (From Ovassapian A: Fiberoptic Endoscopy and the Difficult Airway. Philadelphia, Lippincott–Raven, 1996.)

damage the instrument.[54] In this case, the FB and ET should be withdrawn together as a unit. The procedure may then be repeated. Careful advancement of the FB through the distal opening of the ET, or loading of the ET over the FB insertion cord before endoscopy, eliminates this error.

Poor lubrication of the FB may make removal from the ET difficult. If the FB's plastic cover is loose and force is applied, it may intussuscept over itself and occlude the ET lumen, causing obstruction.[55] Difficulty in removing the instrument from the ET may cause removal of the tube along with the FB. On one occasion, the author was forced to remove the FB and the ET together because of the drying of the water-soluble lubricant that had been applied to the FB, which made movement of the FB inside the ET impossible.

In a large series of fiberoptic intubations, the success rate is reported to be 96% [8] and 98.8%.[7]

ADVANTAGES OF FIBEROPTIC INTUBATION

The most important advantage of fiberoptic intubation is its role in the management of difficult intubation (Table 5–8). The FB offers an effective, safe, and easy approach in patients who are difficult to intubate with conventional techniques. Whenever movement of the head and neck is limited and the opening of the mouth is restricted, the FB provides an excellent approach for securing the airway. Fiberoptic intubation is tolerated well by awake patients under topical anesthesia, is less stressful, and is associated with lesser degrees of hypertension and

Table 5–8   Advantages of Fiberoptic Tracheal Intubation

Provides best success in difficult intubation

Can be applied orally and nasally in all age groups

Provides evaluation of airway before intubation

Avoids unrecognized esophageal and endobronchial intubation

Provides definitive check of tube position

Intubation can easily be performed with patient in sitting or lateral position

Only approach in patients with no access to anterior neck

Excellent patient acceptance of awake intubation

Less cardiovascular response during awake intubation

Ability to apply topical anesthetic, suction secretions, and insufflate oxygen for application of topical anesthesia

Excellent visualization of airway

Less traumatic

Teaching attachment and video system

From Ovassapian A: Fiberoptic Endoscopy and the Difficult Airway. Philadelphia, Lippincott-Raven, 1996.

tachycardia.[23, 56, 57] The cardiovascular response to fiberoptic intubation under GA has not been shown to be more favorable compared with rigid laryngoscopy.[58-62]

Visualization of the airway provides the opportunity to evaluate the airway before ET placement, and it allows precise placement of the ET in patients with tracheal compression.[63] After completion of intubation, the position of the ET is checked visually by reference to the carina, thus avoiding inadvertent bronchial intubation.

Fiberoptic intubation can easily be carried out with the patient in the supine, sitting, lateral, or even prone position. The FB provides the only hope for securing the airway in patients in whom access to the anterior neck is not possible.[64] Other advantages include less trauma and complete avoidance of tooth damage, which is a common complication with rigid laryngoscopy.[65, 66]

DISADVANTAGES OF FIBEROPTIC INTUBATION

The FBs are expensive, delicate instruments and require a separate light source for illumination during endoscopy. They occupy a large space and need their own cart and setup. The cost and size of the FB limit its practical availability in every place in a hospital (Table 5–9).

Cleaning, disinfecting, and sterilizing consume time and resources. A lack of expertise and skills in the use of the FB continues to be a problem for anesthesia practitioners. Secretions and blood can completely obscure the endoscopist's view, interfering with airway evaluation and tracheal intubation. Also, airway resistance is increased when the FB is advanced through the ET, thus compromising the effective lumen for air exchange.

COMPLICATIONS

Some complications of tracheal intubation are related to the presence of the ET, whereas others are technique-specific. Laceration of the oropharyngeal mucosa, damage to gums or teeth, and perforation of the pharynx and esophagus are rare with fiberoptic intubation. Repeated vigorous attempts at passing the ET over the FB can cause trauma to the larynx. One case of the development of a laryngeal cyst attributed to fiberoptic nasotracheal intubation has been reported.[67] A 16-year-old boy with juvenile chronic arthritis was fiberoptically intubated under

Table 5–9   Disadvantages of Fiberoptic Tracheal Intubation

Expensive instrument
Delicate instrument
More difficult to clean and disinfect
Vision obscured easily by secretions and blood
Size of instrument and light source

From Ovassapian A: Fiberoptic Endoscopy and the Difficult Airway. Philadelphia, Lippincott-Raven, 1996.

GA while breathing spontaneously, and some firm manipulation was required to advance the ET over the FB into the trachea. One month later the patient developed dysphagia and weight loss, followed by the development of a vocal cord mucosal cyst. The cyst was subsequently removed and his condition improved.[67]

Complications in 2031 patients in our series of fiberoptic intubations were limited to laryngospasm in 51 patients (due to inadequate topical anesthesia); pain or hematoma, or both, at the translaryngeal injection site in 33 patients; gagging or vomiting, or both, in 8; and mild epistaxis in 70 who were nasotracheally intubated.[42] None of the patients with epistaxis required treatment by nasal packing.

In one patient who underwent awake orotracheal fiberoptic intubation, a small amount of gastric juice was noticed in the oropharynx before tracheal intubation as the FB had entered the esophagus on the first attempt. There were no radiologic signs or clinical signs or symptoms of aspiration pneumonitis postoperatively. The FB passed into the esophagus on 49 occasions at least once during an intubation attempt. Although this is usually harmless, it may relax the cricopharyngeus muscle and facilitate regurgitation of gastric contents into the oropharynx if the esophagus contains gastric juice.

Respiratory depression and hypoxemia are relatively common with intravenous sedation during awake intubation. We recorded several instances of major respiratory depression necessitating assisted ventilation. Since the oximeter was introduced into clinical practice, we have routinely administered oxygen and used it continuously during conscious sedation.

The endoscopy mask diaphragm can be pushed inside the oropharynx. This is a potential danger, and care should be exercised to avoid it.[31]

Passage of the ET when threaded off the FB is a blind technique, and its tip may impinge on laryngeal structures. Error in measurement of the ET tip distance from the carina may lead to high tube placement. If the cuff is inflated in the hypolarynx, the possibility of recurrent laryngeal nerve palsy may increase. Endobronchial intubation is also possible by mistaking upper and lower lobe bifurcations of the lung for the carina.

WHICH FIBEROPTIC BRONCHOSCOPE TO USE

Several varieties of FBs are available, depending on the particular manufacturer and model. The basic components are similar and consist of a handle, an insertion cord, and a universal cord.[1]

The handle or control section contains the tip control lever or knob that flexes the tip of the insertion cord in one plane. It also contains a suction valve, the access port to the suction (working) channel, and the eyepiece. The handle is held in one hand in such a way that the thumb can maneuver the control lever and the index finger can activate the suction (see Fig. 5–2). This allows the operator's other hand to be free to advance the insertion cord or the endotracheal tube. The handle allows coordinated rotation of the FB by rotation of the handle along the longitudinal axis of the insertion cord. To look to the right, the handle is rotated to the right and the tip of the FB is tilted up.

The eyepiece contains optical lenses and a diopter adjustment ring to focus the transmitted image to the viewer's eye. There is a mark at the 12 o'clock position that can be seen along the margin of the picture. This mark helps the endoscopist determine what plane he or she is looking at during endoscopy.

Tip control of the lever type is preferred to the knob control type as it is easier to maneuver. Most new models of FBs have incorporated a lever-type control mechanism.

The insertion cord is the flexible part of the FB and is inserted into the patient during fiberoptic intubation. It contains one or two light guides (incoherent) and one image transmission (coherent) bundle, the suction (working) channel, and the tip-bending control wires. The outside diameter of the insertion cord determines the size of the ET that can be used. The insertion cord is flexible, such that it will tolerate gentle bending to accommodate the bends of the airways and the patient's anatomy. The delicate nature of the insertion cord and coating makes this a very easily damaged part of the FB, which is extremely expensive to repair.

The working or suction channel extends from the handle of the FB to the tip of the insertion cord and can be used to suction secretions, inject drugs, insufflate oxygen, or pass various biopsy and brush instruments.

Since the overall diameter of the insertion cord is dependent on the component parts, the size of the working channel is sacrificed for smaller-diameter FBs to maintain reasonable image clarity. FBs with outer diameters less than 2 mm do not have a working channel, and those with outer diameters less than 3.6 mm have working channels of 1.5 mm or less.

The larger the insertion cord in relation to the ET, the easier the passage of the ET into the trachea. A larger suction channel is desirable for effective suctioning of the secretions. For adult patients, a 5-mm FB with a suction channel of 2 mm or larger is a good choice for tracheal intubation.

Accessory Instruments

A variety of accessories and attachments are available for the FB. Some of these accessories, such as the light source and the leak tester, are integral parts of the FB that are necessary for viewing, cleaning, or testing. Most of the remaining attachments are used either for teaching or for photography.

Cleaning and Sterilization

Specific recommendations for cleaning, disinfecting, and sterilizing that were made by the manufacturer or each health care facility should be followed.

The FB should be washed immediately after its use, and the suction

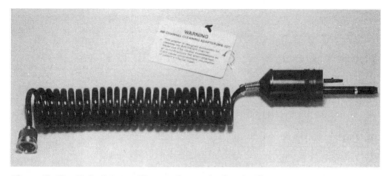

Figure 5–13 Air leak tester. The cap is attached to the fiberscope venting connector. The adapter is attached to the light source. The air pumped by the light source pressurizes the fiberscope. When the fiberscope is immersed in water, any defect in the fiberscope plastic cover is identified by leaking air bubbles.

channel should be flushed with water to remove secretions. Before being soaked in disinfecting solution or placed in a washing or disinfecting machine, the FB should be tested for leaks using a leakage tester and pressurized air (Fig. 5–13). It should be promptly sent to the manufacturer for appropriate repair when leaks or other defects are noted.

If the patient has tuberculosis or other transmissible illnesses, the FB should be sterilized. FB sterilization is also important before use on patients with immune deficiencies. It should not be autoclaved or placed in boiling water. Complete sterilization can be accomplished with ethylene oxide gas. The ethylene oxide cap should be securely attached to the venting connector on the light transmission cord to avoid pressure buildup inside the FB during gas sterilization.

Fiberoptic Cart

The immediate availability of an FB, a light source, ancillary equipment, and supplies is critical for easy accessibility and use. A properly equipped fiberoptic cart with large wheels is a must. The cart can be moved to the operating room or to the bedside at short notice in order to allow easy access to the FB and all the accessories used for fiberoptic intubation (see Fig. 5–1).

SUMMARY

Fiberoptic intubation is the technique of choice in the management of a difficult intubation and should be used initially, and not as a last resort after repeated attempts using conventional techniques have failed. Fiberoptic tracheal intubation is critical to modern airway management and should be mastered by all caregivers who are involved in airway management.

REFERENCES

1. Ovassapian A: Fiberoptic Endoscopy and the Difficult Airway. Philadelphia, Lippincott-Raven, 1996.
2. Messeter KH, Petersson KI: Endotracheal intubation with the fiberoptic bronchoscope. Anaesthesia 35:294–298, 1980.
3. Ikeda S: Atlas of Flexible Bronchofiberscopy. Baltimore, University Park, 1974.
4. Murphy P: A fibre-optic endoscope used for nasal intubation. Anaesthesia 22:489–491, 1967.
5. Taylor PA, Towey RM: The broncho-fiberscope as an aid to intubation. Br J Anaesth 44:611–612, 1972.
6. Conyers AB, Wallace DH, Mulder DS: Use of the fiberoptic bronchoscope for nasotracheal intubation: A case report. Can Anaesth Soc J 19:654–656, 1972.
7. Ovassapian A, Yelich SJ, Dykes MHM, Brunner EA: Fiberoptic nasotracheal intubation—Incidence and causes of failure. Anesth Analg 62:692–695, 1983.
8. Stiles CM, Stiles QR, Denson JS: A flexible fiberoptic laryngoscope. JAMA 221:1246–1247, 1972.
9. Raj PP, Forestner J, Watson TD, et al: Technics for fiberoptic laryngoscopy in anesthesia. Anesth Analg 53:708–714, 1974.
10. Aps C, Towy RM: Expreiences with fiberoptic bronchoscopic positioning of single-lumen endobroncheal tubes. Anaesthesia 36:415–418, 1981.
11. Ovassapian A: Flexible bronchoscopic intubation of awake patients. J Bronchol 1:240–245,1994.
12. Ovassapian A, Yelich SH, Dykes MHM, et al: Learning fiberoptic intubation: Use of simulators. V: Traditional teaching. Br J Anaesth 61:217–220, 1988.
13. Dykes MHM, Ovassapian A: Dissemination of fiberoptic airway endoscopy skills by means of a workshop utilizing models. Br J Anaesth 63:595–597, 1989.
14. Rogers SN, Benumof JL: New and easy techniques for fiberoptic endoscopy–aided tracheal intubation. Anesthesiology 59:569–572, 1983.
15. Benumof JL: Management of the difficult adult airway. Anesthesiology 75:1087–1110, 1991.
16. Rucker RW, Silva WJ, Worcester CC: Fiberoptic bronchoscopic nasotracheal intubation in children. Chest 76:56–58, 1979.
17. Fuhrman TM, Farina RA: Elective tracheostomy for a patient with a history of difficult intubation. J Clin Anesth 7:250–252, 1995.
18. Ovassapian A, Mesnick PS: Elective tracheostomy in an obstetric patient. J Clin Anesth 8:337–338, 1996.
19. Alfery DD, Ward CF, Harwood IR, Mannino FL: Airway management for a neonate with congenital fusion of the jaws. Anesthesiology 51:340–342, 1979.
20. Berthelsen P, Prytz S, Jacobsen E: Two-stage fiberoptic nasotracheal intubation in infants: A new approach to difficult pediatric intubation. Anesthesiology 63:457–458, 1985.
21. Norton ML: Atlas of the Difficult Airway, 2nd ed. St Louis, Mosby-Year Book, 1996.
22. Reed AP, Han DG: The basics of awake intubation. In Roberts JT (ed): Clinical Management of the Airway. Philadelphia, WB Saunders, 1994, pp 147–157.
23. Southerland AD, Sale JP: Fiberoptic awake intubation—A method of topical anaesthesia and orotracheal intubation. Can Anaesth Soc J 33:502–504, 1986.
24. Schwartz D, Johnson C, Roberts J: A maneuver to facilitate fiberoptic intubation. Anesthesiology 71:470–471, 1989.
25. Katsnelson T, Frost EAM, Farcon E, Goldiner PL: When the endotracheal tube will not pass over the flexible fiberoptic bronchoscope. Anesthesiology 76:152–152, 1992.
26. Randell T, Yli-Hankala A, Valli H, Lindgren L: Topical anesthesia of the nasal mucosa for fiberoptic airway endoscopy. Br J Anaesth 66:164–167, 1991.
27. El-Ganzouri, El-Baz N, Ford E, et al: Training residents in fiberoptic intubation in the operating room [abstract]. Anesthesiology 69:a805, 1988.
28. Childress WF: New method for fiberoptic endotracheal intubation of anesthetized patients. Anesthesiology 55:595–596, 1981.
29. Patil V, Stehling LC, Zauder HL: Fiberoptic endoscopy in anesthesia. Chicago, Year Book, 1983.

30. Mallios C: A modification of the Laerdal anesthesia mask for nasotracheal intubation with the fiberoptic laryngoscope. Anaesthesia 35:599–600, 1980.

31. Zorrow MH, Mitchell MM: Foreign body aspiration during fiberoptic assisted intubation. Anesthesiology 64:303, 1986.

32. Brain AIJ: Three cases of difficult intubation overcome by use of the laryngeal mask. Anaesthesia 40:353–355, 1985.

33. Calder I, Ordman AJ, Jackowski A, et al: The Brain laryngeal mask airway. An alternative to emergency tracheal intubation. Anaesthesia 45:137–139, 1990.

34. Nath G, Major V: The laryngeal mask in the management of a paediatric difficult airway. Anaesth Intensive Care 20:518–520, 1992.

35. Heath ML, Allagain J: Intubation through the laryngeal mask. A technique for unexpected difficult intubation. Anaesthesia 46:545–548, 1991.

36. Chadd GD, Ackers JW, Bailey PM: Difficult intubation aided by the laryngeal mask airway. Anaesthesia 45:1015, 1990.

37. McCrirrick A, Pracilio A: Awake intubation: A new technique. Anaesthesia 46:661–663, 1991.

38. Tobias R: Increased success with retrograde guide for endotracheal intubation. Anesth Analg 62:366–367, 1983.

39. Lechman MJ, Donahoo JS, McVaugh M III: Endotracheal intubation using percutaneous retrograde guide wire insertion followed by antegrade fiberoptic bronchoscopy. Crit Care Med 14:589–590, 1986.

40. Gupta B, McDonald JS, Brooks JHJ, Mendenhall J: Oral fiberoptic intubation over a retrograde guidewire. Anesth Analg 68:517–519, 1989.

41. Ovassapian A, Mesnick PS: The art of fiberoptic intubation. Anesthesiol Clin North Am 13:395–409, 1995.

42. Ovassapian A: Fiberoptic Airway Endoscopy in Anesthesia and Critical Care. New York, Raven, 1990.

43. Johnson C, Hunter J, Ho E, Bruff C: Fiberoptic intubation facilitated by a rigid laryngoscope. Anesth Analg 72:713, 1991.

44. Russell SH, Hirch NP: Simultaneous use of two laryngoscopes. Anaesthesia 48:918, 1993.

45. Ovassapian A, Rudy NW, Krejcie TC, Avram MJ: Variability in upper airway length: Its significance to tracheal intubation [abstract]. Anesthesiology 79:a1053, 1993.

46. Hershey MD, Hannenberg AA: Gastric distention and rupture from oxygen insufflation during fiberoptic intubation. Anesthesiology 85:1479–1480, 1996.

47. Richardson MG, Dooley JW: Acute facial, cervical, and thoracic subcutaneous emphysema: A complication of fiberoptic laryngoscopy. Anesth Analg 82:878–880, 1996.

48. Marsh NJ: Easier fiberoptic intubation. Anesthesiology 76:860–861, 1992.

49. Rosenblatt WH: Overcoming obstruction during bronchoscopic-guided intubation of the trachea with the double setup endotracheal tube. Anesth Analg 83:175–177, 1996.

50. Jones HE, Pearce AC, Moore P: Fiberoptic intubation. Influence of tracheal tube tip design. Anaesthesia 48:672–674, 1993.

51. Hodgkin JE, Rosenow EC, Stubbs SE: Diagnostic and therapeutic techniques in thoracic medicine. Oral introduction of the flexible bronchoscope. Chest 68:88–90, 1975.

52. Calder I: When the endotracheal tube will not pass over the flexible fiberoptic bronchoscope. Anesthesiology 77:398, 1992.

53. Brull SJ, Wiklund R, Ferris C, et al: Facilitation of fiberoptic orotracheal intubation with a flexible tracheal tube. Anesth Analg 78:746–748, 1994.

54. Ovassapian A: Failure to withdraw flexible laryngoscope after nasotracheal intubation. Anesthesiology 63:124–125, 1985.

55. Siegel M, Coleprate P: Complication of fiberoptic bronchoscope. Anesthesiology 61:214–215, 1984.

56. Ovassapian A, Yelich SJ, Dykes MHM, Brunner EA: Blood pressure and heart rate changes during awake fiberoptic nasotracheal intubation. Anesth Analg 62:951–954, 1983.

57. Schrader S, Ovassapian A, Dykes MHM, Avram M: Cardiovascular changes during awake rigid and fiberoptic laryngoscopy [abstract]. Anesthesiology 67:a28, 1987.
58. Finfer SR, Mackenzie JM Saddler, Watkins TG: Cardiovascular responses to tracheal intubation: A comparison of direct laryngoscopy and fibreoptic intubation. Anaesth Intensive Care 17:44–48, 1989.
59. Smith JE, Mackenzie AA, Scott-Knight, VCE: Comparison of two methods of fibrescope-guided tracheal intubation. Br J Anaesth 66:546–550, 1991.
60. Schaefer HG, Marsch SCU: Comparison of orthodox with fibreoptic orotracheal intubation under total IV anaesthesia. Br J Anaesth 66:608–610, 1991.
61. Schaefer HG, Marsch SCU, Strebel SP, Drewe J: Cardiovascular effects of fibreoptic oral intubation. Anaesthesia 47:1034–1036, 1992.
62. Smith JE, Mackenzie AA, Sanghera SS, Scott-Knight VCE: Cardiovascular effects of fibrescope-guided nasotracheal intubation. Anaesthesia 44:907–910, 1989.
63. Prakash UBS, Abel MD, Hubmayr RD: Mediastinal mass and tracheal obstruction during general anesthesia. Mayo Clin Proc 63:1004–1011, 1988.
64. Ovassapian A, Land P, Schafer MF, et al: Anesthetic management for surgical correction of severe flexion deformity of the cervical spine. Anesthesiology 58:370–372, 1983.
65. Wright RB, Manfield FFV: Damage to teeth during the administration of general anesthesia. Anesth Analg 53:405–408, 1974.
66. Burton JF, Baker AB: Dental damage during anaesthesia and surgery. Anaesth Intensive Care 15:262–268, 1987.
67. Smith BL: Laryngeal cyst following fiberoptic intubation. Anaesthesia 41:430–431, 1986.

Chapter 6

Retrograde Intubation

Antonio F. Sanchez and Debra E. Morrison

Among the techniques cited in the American Society of Anesthesiologists (ASA) Practice Guidelines, retrograde intubation (RI) is an invasive technique for accessing the airway via the cricothyroid membrane (CTM).[1] RI requires special equipment (Table 6–1) that can be assembled in advance and maintained in a portable storage unit for difficult airway management.

Table 6–1   Equipment for Retrograde Intubation

17-gauge Tuohy needle
18-gauge angiocatheter
10- to 20-mL syringe
Scalpel blade (no. 11)
Epidural catheter with removable stylet
J-tip guide wire (0.038-inch OD, 110- to 120-cm long)
Guide catheter (Cook Critical Care; Ellettsville, Ind)
Nerve hook (V. Mueller no. NL2490; Baxter, Deerfield, Ill)
30-inch length of silk suture (3–0) on cutting needle

ANATOMY

Basic knowledge of the anatomy of the cricoid cartilage (Fig. 6–1) and the structures above and below it is required in order to minimize complication and failure when performing RI. Indeed, regardless of the intubation technique planned, the cricoid cartilage and cricothyroid membrane (CTM) should be identified preoperatively in every patient.[2] Cartilage and membrane, vasculature, and the thyroid gland are relevant anatomy.

Cartilage and Membrane

The signet ring–shaped cricoid cartilage consists of a broad, flat plate posteriorly called the *lamina* and a narrow, convex structure anteriorly called the *arch*.[3, 4] The CTM connects the superior border of the arch to the inferior border of the arch to the inferior border of the thyroid cartilage. The cricotracheal ligament (CTL) connects the inferior border of the arch to the upper border of the first tracheal ring.[5]

Vasculature

There are paired major blood vessels above and below the cricoid cartilage: the cricothyroid artery and the superior thyroid artery.

The cricothyroid artery, a branch of the superior thyroid artery, runs along the anterior surface of the CTM, usually close to the inferior border of the thyroid cartilage.[3, 6–9] The cricothyroid arteries may anastomose in the midline and give rise to a descending branch that feeds the pyramidal lobe of the thyroid gland when it is present. The cricothyroid artery becomes insignificant in size as it approaches the midline.[9]

The bilateral anterior branches of the superior thyroid artery run along the upper border of the thyroid isthmus and anastomose in the midline.[3, 6–9] The inferior thyroid artery anastomoses with the anterior branch of the superior thyroid artery at the level of the isthmus. The arteries are remarkable for their large size and frequent anastomoses. In less than 10% of the population, an unpaired thyroid ima artery, which can be large, ascends ventral to the trachea (from either the

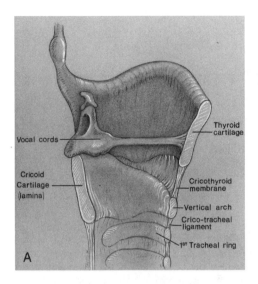

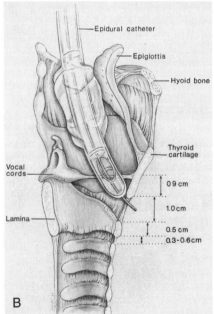

Figure 6–1 Anatomy. *A*, Anatomy of the cricoid cartilage. *B*, Midsagittal view of the larynx and trachea showing the distance between the vocal cords and the upper border of the first tracheal ring. Note that only a small portion of the endotracheal tube Murphy eye is below the vocal cords. (*A* and *B*, From University of California at Irvine, Department of Anesthesia, The Retrograde Cookbook.)

aortic arch or the brachiocephalic artery) to anastomose at the level of the isthmus. A rich venous plexus is formed in and around the isthmus.

Thyroid Gland (Isthmus, Pyramidal Lobe)

The isthmus of the thyroid gland is rarely absent and generally located anterior to the trachea between the first and the fourth tracheal rings.[3–5, 7–9] Extending from the isthmus, the highly vascular pyramidal lobe is well developed in one third of the population. It is found more frequently on the left of the midline and may extend into a thyromuscular continuation up to the hyoid bone.[3–5, 7–9]

PHYSIOLOGY

A sympathetic stress response (increased heart rate, blood pressure, intraocular pressure, intracranial pressure, and catecholamine levels) has been reported with laryngoscopy, endotracheal intubation, coughing, translaryngeal local anesthesia, laryngotracheal anesthesia, and fiberoptic intubation. Concern is therefore appropriate when performing any airway maneuver in patients with coronary artery disease, elevated intraocular pressure, or elevated intracranial pressure.[10–16] RI, performed skillfully, need not be more stimulating than any other technique for managing the airway, including direct laryngoscopy,[9, 17–27] and can be performed safely in patients with coronary artery disease,[17–27] elevated intraocular pressure,[28, 29] or elevated intracranial pressure.

INDICATIONS AND CONTRAINDICATIONS

RI has been used in a variety of clinical scenarios (Table 6–2) as a backup technique following failed attempts at laryngoscopy or fiberoptic intubation, or both; as a first technique for emergent establishment of an airway when visualization of the vocal cords is prevented by blood, secretions, or anatomic derangement; and electively, when clinically deemed necessary, in patients with an unstable cervical spine, mandibular fracture, or anatomic anomaly.

Contraindications (Table 6–3) to RI have been cited, often anecdotally. Most contraindications are relative.

TECHNIQUES

Preparation

Antisialogogue: An appropriate antisialogogue (see Chapter 4) may be indicated, especially if the fiberoptic bronchoscope (FB) is to be employed.

Positioning: The ideal position for RI is the supine sniffing position with the neck hyperextended.[30, 31] In this position the cricoid cartilage and the structures above and below it are easier to palpate.

Table 6–2   Indications for Retrograde Intubation*

Oral cavity
  Cancrum oris (27)
  Mandibular or maxillary fracture (31)
  Perimandibular abscess (1)
  Ankylosis TMJ (5)
  Microstomia (1)
  Macroglossia (1)
  Carcinoma of tongue (8)
  Oral myxoma (1)

Cervical
  Spinal cord injury (66)
  Ankylosing spondylitis (11)
  Rheumatoid arthritis (32)

Pharynx and larynx
  Laryngeal carcinoma (70)
  Pharyngeal abscess (1)
  Epiglottitis (1)
  Pharyngeal edema (1)
  Laryngeal edema after burn (2)

Others
  Pediatric anomalies (24)
  Obesity (11)
  CABG (failure to intubate) (28)
  Tracheostomy stoma (16)
  Trauma (failure to intubate) (33)
  Abnormality not specified (failure to intubate) (12)
  Cadaver studies (117)†

*Numbers in parentheses indicate the number of patients.
†Number of cadavers.
TMJ, temporomandibular joint; CABG, coronary artery bypass graft.
From University of California at Irvine, Department of Anesthesia Teaching Aids.

Table 6–3   Contraindications to Retrograde Intubation

Unfavorable anatomy
  Lack of access to CTM (severe flexion deformity of the neck)
  Poor anatomic landmarks (obesity)
  Pretracheal mass (thyroid goiter)
Laryngotracheal abnormality
  Malignancy
  Stenosis
Coagulopathy
Infection (pretracheal abscess)

CTM, cricothyroid membrane.
From University of California at Irvine, Department of Anesthesia Teaching Aids.

RI can also be performed with the patient in a sitting position,[2] which may be the only position in which some patients can breathe comfortably.

Potential cervical spine injury or limited range of motion of the cervical spine, or both, may necessitate RI with the neck in a neutral position.

Asepsis: Although most documented retrograde intubations have not been elective, every effort should be made to perform RI using aseptic technique. A standard sterile preparation should be used.

Anesthetic: If time permits, the airway should be anesthetized to prevent discomfort, sympathetic stimulation, and laryngospasm (see Chapter 4).

An awake RI with oral intubation can be performed with translaryngeal anesthesia (4 mL of 2% lidocaine injected through the CTM), which provides anesthesia for the vocal cords, lower larynx, and trachea, supplemented with topicalization (nebulized or sprayed local anesthetics) of the pharynx and hypopharynx. A 10% lidocaine metered-dose spray (Astra-Zeneca) is available and is quick and very effective for topicalization.

If the FB is to be employed as part of the technique, the airway should be prepared accordingly (see Chapter 4). If nasal intubation is planned, the nose should be prepared (see Chapter 4).

Puncture: The transtracheal puncture site for RI can be made either above or below the cricoid cartilage. Both CTM puncture and CTL puncture have been used successfully. Each entry site has advantages and disadvantages, as follows:

The CTM is relatively avascular and has less potential for bleeding. The disadvantages of the CTM are that initially only 1 cm of the endotracheal tube (ET) is actually placed below the vocal cords, and the angle of entry of the ET into the trachea is more acute.

A CTL puncture site allows a longer initial length of ET below the vocal cords. The disadvantage is that this site has more potential for bleeding (although none has been reported). In cadaver studies, the success rate for RI was higher and vocal cord trauma less frequent when the CTL rather than the CTM was used.[32, 33] Vocal cord trauma has not been reported in living patients.

Classic Technique (Fig. 6–2)

> **Equipment**
> 17-gauge Tuohy needle
> Epidural catheter with removable stylet
> Scalpel blade (no. 11)
> 10- to 20-mL syringe partially filled with saline
> Nerve hook (V. Mueller no. NL2490; Baxter, Deerfield, Ill.)
> ET

The classic RI is simple and is performed percutaneously using a standard 17-gauge Tuohy needle and a standard epidural catheter (EC).

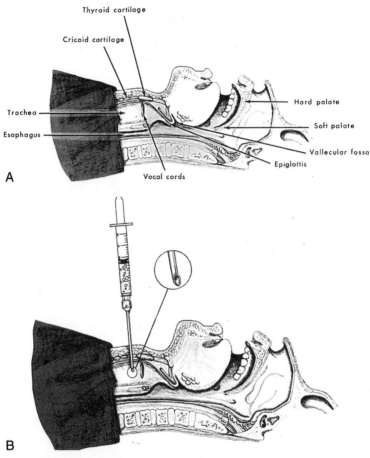

Figure 6–2 Classic technique. *A*, Midsagittal view of the head and neck. *B*, Advance a standard no. 17 Tuohy needle (with a saline-filled syringe) (with the bevel pointing sideways) through the cricothyroid membrane (CTM) at a 90-degree angle (trying to stay as close as possible to the upper border of the cricoid cartilage). Verify entrance into the trachea by the aspiration of air.

Illustration continued on following page

After preparation and anesthesia of the patient, stand at the side of the supine (or otherwise positioned) patient; position yourself at the same side as your dominant hand. Use the nondominant hand to stabilize the trachea: place the thumb and the third digit on opposite sides of the thyroid cartilage. Use the index finger of the nondominant hand to identify the midline of the CTM and the upper border of the cricoid cartilage.

The Tuohy needle is blunt; after ascertaining that the skin is anesthe-

Text continued on page 126

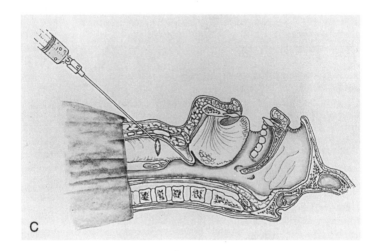

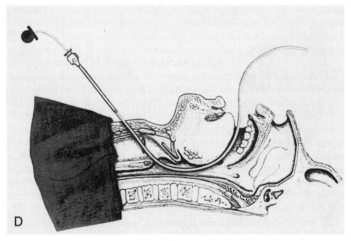

Figure 6–2 *Continued.* *C*, Change the Tuohy angle to 45 degrees with the bevel pointing cephalad (again verifying the position by aspirating air). *D*, Advance the epidural catheter (EC) through the vocal cords and into the pharynx. During this time, either ask the patient to stick the tongue out or pull the tongue out manually. The EC will usually come out of the mouth on its own. Withdraw the Tuohy needle to hang at the caudal end of the EC.

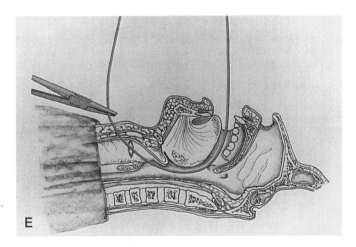

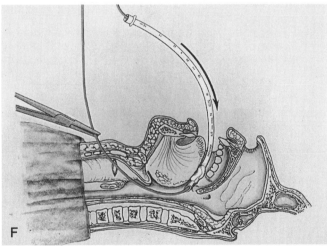

Figure 6–2 *Continued.*   *E,* Pull the EC out of the mouth to an appropriate length and then clamp a hemostat flush with the skin. *F,* Thread a well-lubricated endotracheal tube (ET) over the EC. Maintain a moderate amount of tension on the EC as you advance the ET *(arrow)* forward. You will feel a small click as the ET travels through the vocal cords.

Illustration continued on following page

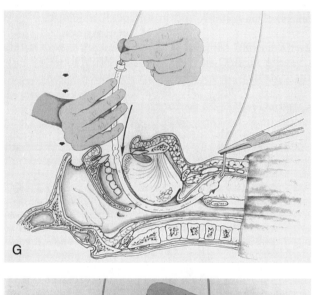

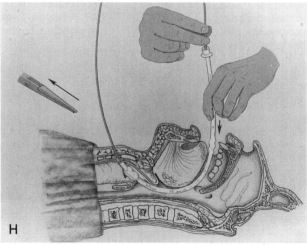

Figure 6–2 *Continued.* *G*, When the ET reaches the CTM, it is important to maintain pressure *(small arrows)*, forcing the ET into the oropharynx *(large arrow)* to cause continuing pressure against the CTM with the tip of the ET. (Note: You are still maintaining moderate tension on the EC.) *H*, Have an assistant remove the hemostat *(large arrow)* while pressure is maintained *(small arrow)* to push the ET up against the CTM. (The EC may be cut flush with the hemostat before the hemostat is removed.)

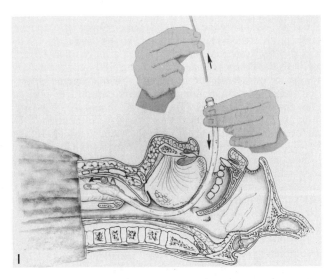

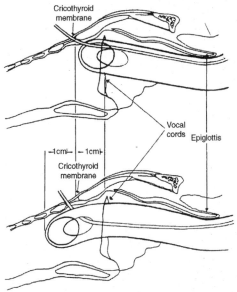

Figure 6–2 *Continued.* *I*, Simultaneously *(straight arrows)* remove the EC as you advance the ET. The tip of the ET will drop from its position up against the CTM to midtrachea *(curved arrow)*. Advance the ET to the desired depth. *J*, Cross-section of the larynx and trachea, with the ET and catheter guide passing through the CTM. *Top*, The catheter passes through the end of the ET, and 1 cm of the ET passes the cords. *Bottom*, The catheter exits the side hole, allowing 2 cm of the ET to pass beyond the vocal cords. (*A–I*, From University of California at Irvine, Department of Anesthesia, The Retrograde Cookbook. *J*, From Bourke D, Levesque PR: Modification of retrograde guide for endotracheal intubation. Anesth Analg 53:1014, 1974.)

tized, hold the scalpel blade in your dominant hand and make a small incision through the skin and the subcutaneous tissue.

Grasp the Tuohy needle (attached to a partially filled 10- to 20-mL syringe) with the dominant hand, like a pencil. Brace your hand on the patient's lower neck with the fifth digit and the medial aspect of the palm for better control; significant force is required to perforate the skin and the CTM with the Tuohy needle, and there is a risk of perforating the posterior tracheal wall as well.[34] Puncture the CTM, and aspirate for air to confirm placement in the tracheal lumen. If the needle is in the esophagus, it will be impossible to aspirate a large syringe full of air, since the esophagus will collapse under negative pressure.

Once the Tuohy needle is in place, advance the EC into the trachea. Pull the tongue anteriorly to prevent the EC from coiling up in the oropharynx. The EC usually exits on its own from either the oral or the nasal cavity. To assist in retrieving the EC from the oropharynx, we recommend using a nerve hook. Magill forceps, designed to grasp large objects like the ET, may not grip the EC securely, since the distal tips do not completely occlude and may also traumatize the pharynx.

Thread the EC in through the Murphy eye of the ET, then up and out the proximal lumen. (The EC was originally threaded through the main distal lumen [beveled portion] of the ET.) Threading the EC through the Murphy eye allows an additional 1 cm of ET to pass through the cords.[35] Using the cricotracheal ligament as the puncture site in combination with threading the EC through the Murphy eye enhances success over the original technique.[32, 33]

When advancing the ET over the EC, apply a moderate amount of tension.[36, 37] Excessive tension pulls the ET anteriorly, making it more likely to get caught up against the epiglottis, vallecula, or anterior commissure of the vocal cords. If there is difficulty in passing the opening of the glottis, first rotate the ET 90 degrees counterclockwise,[34, 38] then try using a smaller tube.[34]

Guide Wire Technique (Fig. 6–3)

Equipment
18-gauge angiocatheter
J-tip guide wire (0.038-inch outer diameter, 110 to 120 cm long)
Guide catheter (Cook Critical Care; Ellettsville, Ind.)
10- to 20-mL syringe partially filled with saline
Nerve hook (V. Mueller no. NL2490; Baxter, Deerfield, Ill.)
ET

The modified technique using a guide wire[18, 39] evolved because the flexible EC is prone to kinking and stretching.[40–42] The J-tip guide wire is relatively nontraumatic to the airway,[31, 43] is easy to retrieve from the oral or nasal cavity,[44, 45] is less prone to kinking and stretching, and can be used with the FB (see the section Fiberoptic Technique). The guide wire is easy to handle,[44, 46] and the technique takes less time to perform than the classic technique.[44]

Use the angiocatheter in place of the Tuohy needle. Place the catheter

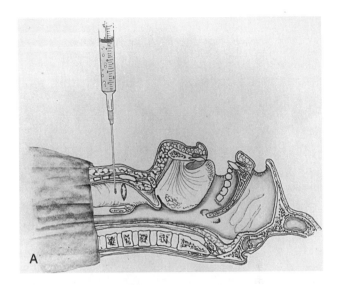

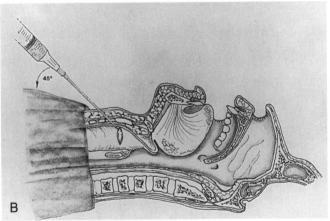

Figure 6–3   Guide wire technique. *A*, Place an 18-gauge angiocatheter 90 degrees to the CTM, aspirating for air to confirm the position. *B*, Change the angle to 45 degrees (again aspirating air to confirm the position).

Illustration continued on following page

over the needle and then remove the needle. Confirm the position by aspiration as in the classic technique. Advance the guide wire through the catheter into the trachea and out the mouth (or nose) in place of the EC as in the classic technique.

Discrepancy between the external diameter of the guide wire and the internal diameter of the ET allows a railroading (swaying side to side along the EC) effect to occur, with the tip of the ET catching

Text continued on page 132

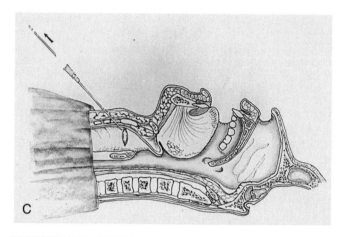

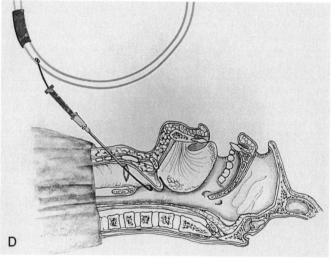

Figure 6–3 *Continued.*   *C,* Advance the sheath of the angiocatheter cephalad and remove the needle. *D,* Advance the J-tip guide wire through the angiocatheter sheath.

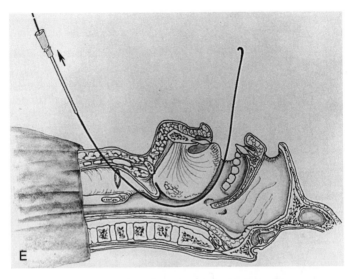

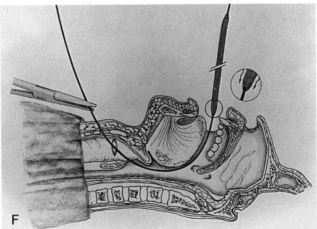

Figure 6–3 *Continued.* *E,* Retrieve the end of the guide wire from the mouth as in the classic technique. Remove the angiocatheter *(small arrow). F,* Clamp the hemostat flush with the skin, and advance the tapered tip of the guide catheter *(bullet)* over the guide wire into the mouth.

Illustration continued on following page

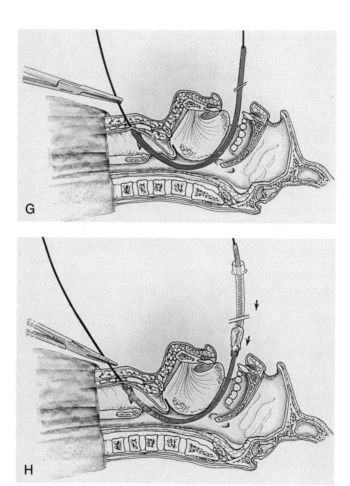

Figure 6–3 *Continued.* *G,* Advance the guide catheter to the CTM. *H,* Advance the ET over the entire structure *(arrows).* Use an ET that is 6- to 7-mm ID. The size of the ET is dictated by the external diameter of the guide catheter.

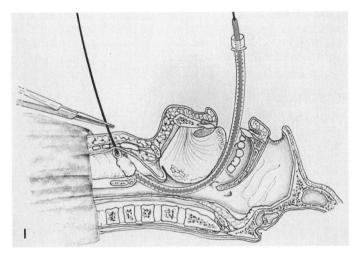

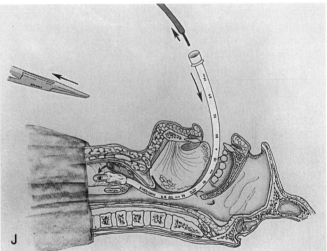

Figure 6–3 *Continued.* *I,* Advance the ET through the vocal cords and up against the CTM. *J,* Remove the hemostat, wire, and catheter as in the classic technique *(straight arrows),* except that the guide wire and guide catheter are removed simultaneously. (*A–J,* From University of California at Irvine, Department of Anesthesia, The Retrograde Cookbook.)

peripherally on the arytenoids or vocal cords instead of passing straight through the cords. Sliding the guide catheter (GC) down over the guide wire from above (antegrade) once it has exited the mouth or nose increases the external diameter of the guide apparatus.[38] The use of the GC in combination with a smaller-diameter ET allows the ET when passed over the GC to enter the glottis in a more centralized position with respect to the glottic opening.

Fiberoptic Technique (Fig. 6–4)

Equipment
18-gauge angiocatheter
J-tip GW (0.038-inch outer diameter, 110 to 120 cm long)
Guide catheter (Cook Critical Care; Ellettsville, Ind.)
10- to 20-mL syringe partially filled with saline
Nerve hook (V. Mueller no. NL2490; Baxter, Deerfield, Ill.)
ET
FB with light source

The FB is a versatile tool for the anesthesiologist,[10, 11] but the FB, like RI, has its limitations. In some cases, the combination of two techniques allows achievement of tracheal intubation after a single or serial techniques (e.g., blind nasal, direct laryngoscopy, fiberoptic intubation, retrograde intubation) have failed. For example, the combination of RI with direct laryngoscopy[20] and RI using the FB[25] can improve the chance of successful intubation.

Passing an FB antegrade over a guide wire placed by RI allows the outer diameter of the guide wire and the internal diameter of the suction port of the FB to form a tight fit, preventing railroading between both structures; thus, the FB follows a straight path through the vocal cords without getting caught on anatomic structures. The FB acts as a large GC (see the section Guide Wire Technique) and prevents railroading of the ET. Once the FB has passed over the guide wire through the vocal cords, it can be advanced freely beyond the puncture site to the carina, eliminating the problem of distance between cords and puncture site, and allowing placement of the ET under direct vision. The FB can be used by the less-experienced operator using this technique. It should be noted that oxygen can be delivered continuously through the FB with the guide wire still in place.

Prepare the FB before initiating RI. Remove the rubber casing from the proximal portion of the suction port (to allow the guide wire to exit from the handle) and place the appropriate ET over the FB. Perform RI using the guide wire technique, and then pass the FB antegrade over the guide wire like a GC. Once the tip of the FB abuts the CTM, there are three options:

1. Remove the guide wire distally or proximally (through the fiberoptic handle), and after advancing under direct vision to the carina, intubate. Removal distally is less likely to dislodge the FB from the trachea, but anecdotal evidence suggests that re-

Text continued on page 137

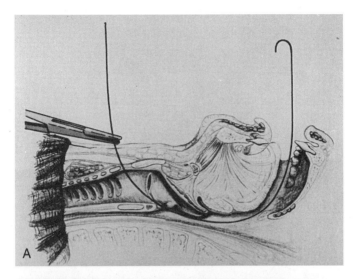

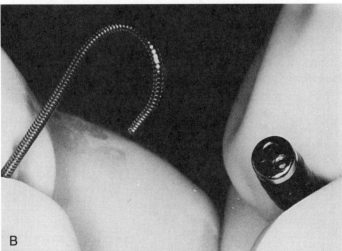

Figure 6–4 Fiberoptic technique. *A*, Place the guide wire as in the guide wire technique and pull it out to the appropriate length in order to accommodate the fiberoptic bronchoscope (FB) (hemostat in place). *B*, Closeup of the J-tip of the guide wire and distal tip of the FB.

Illustration continued on following page

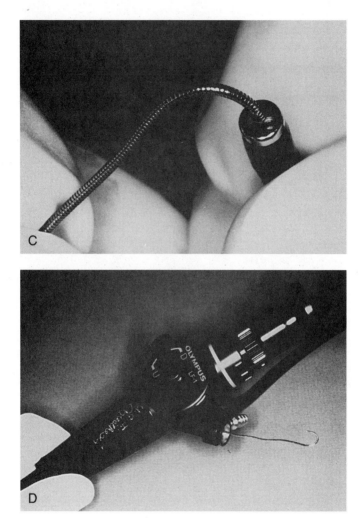

Figure 6–4 *Continued.* *C,* Closeup of the J-tip being fed into the suction port of the FB. *D,* Photograph of the J-tip exiting from the FB handle.

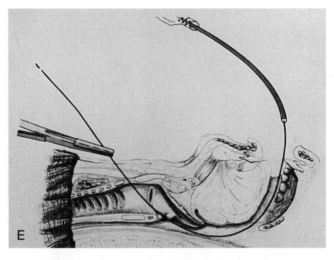

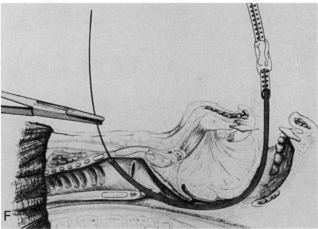

Figure 6–4 *Continued.* *E,* Begin advancing the FB (armed with the ET) over the guide wire. *F,* Advance the FB to the CTM.

Illustration continued on following page

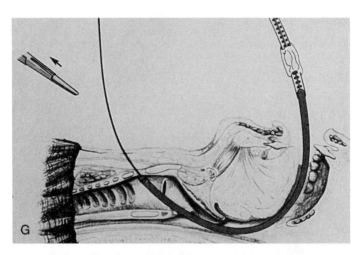

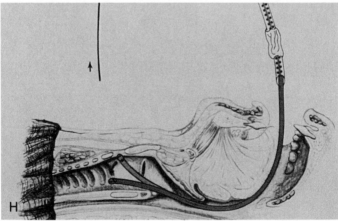

Figure 6–4 *Continued.* *G*, Have an assistant remove the hemostat. *H*, Remove the guide wire from the CTM *(straight arrow)*. The tip of the FB will then drop into midtracheal position *(curved arrow)*.

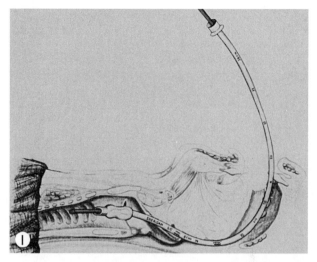

Figure 6–4 *Continued.* *I*, Continue as you would in a standard fiberoptic intubation. (*A–I*, From University of California at Irvine, Department of Anesthesia, The Retrograde Cookbook.)

moval proximally should decrease the incidence of infection from oral contaminants.[38]

2. Instead of removing the guide wire, allow it to relax caudad into the trachea, advance the FB below the cricoid cartilage, and then remove the guide wire. This allows a greater length of the FB in the trachea before the guide wire is removed.

3. Remove the guide wire proximally only until it is seen through the FB to have slipped out of the CTM and into the trachea, then advance the guide wire through the FB to the carina. Next, advance the FB over the guide wire to the carina. This option is probably preferable.

Silk Technique (Fig. 6–5)

Equipment
17-gauge Tuohy needle
EC with removable stylet
Scalpel blade (no. 11)
10- to 20-mL syringe partially filled with saline
Nerve hook (V. Mueller no. NL2490; Baxter, Deerfield, Ill.)
ET
30-inch length of silk suture (3–0) on a cutting needle (3–0 nylon monofilament may also be used)

This technique employs the principles and equipment of the classic technique, with the addition of the silk suture. All the equipment is readily available in the operating room.

Text continued on page 142

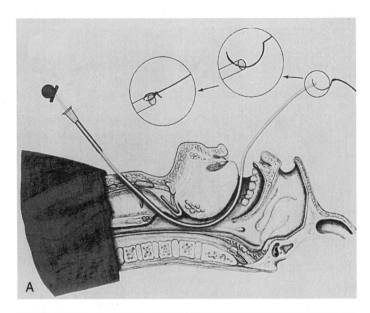

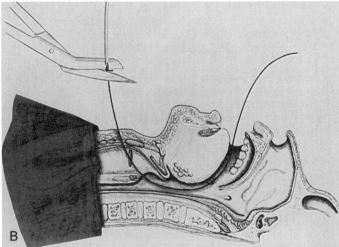

Figure 6–5 Silk technique. *A*, After proceeding as in the classic technique as the EC has exited the oral cavity, using a 3–0 noncutting silk suture (30-inch length), tie the suture to the EC as shown *(bullets)*. *B*, Pull the EC caudad until the silk suture exits the skin above the CTM, and then cut the EC off.

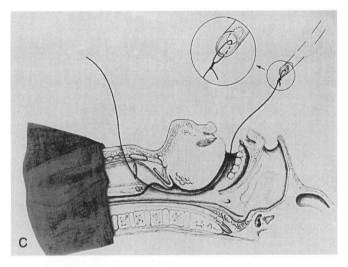

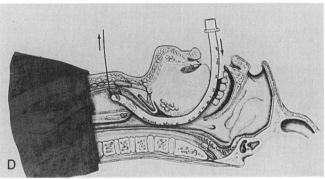

Figure 6–5 *Continued.* *C*, Tie the suture to the Murphy eye as shown *(bullets)*. Have an assistant pull the patient's tongue forward. Begin pulling the suture with one hand while the opposite hand holds the ET steady and in midline. At all times maintain tension on the suture while advancing the ET. *D*, Advance *(arrows)* the ET to the CTM.

Illustration continued on following page

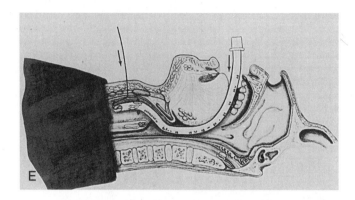

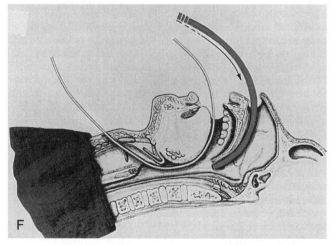

Figure 6–5 *Continued.* *E,* Release the suture and with the opposite hand advance the ET to the desired depth *(right arrow).* The suture will partially retract into the trachea *(left arrow)* as the ET is advanced past the CTM. Secure the remaining suture to the neck with Op-Site. On extubation leave the silk in place as a precaution should reintubation be required. Remove the suture in the recovery room on discharge by cutting it flush with the skin and pulling it out of the oral cavity. *F,* With the EC already in place, advance *(arrow)* a 16 Fr red rubber urologic catheter (UC) through the nose. *F,* Retrieve the tip of the UC from the oral cavity. *G,* Retrieve the tip of the UC from the oral cavity. *H,* Feed the EC into the UC *(bullet).* *I,* Remove the UC *(arrow),* with the EC now exiting the nose. (*A–I,* From University of California at Irvine, Department of Anesthesia, The Retrograde Cookbook.)

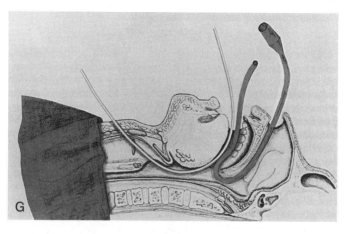

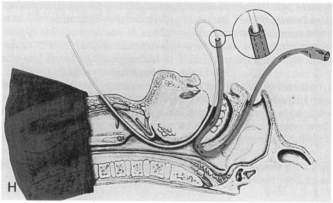

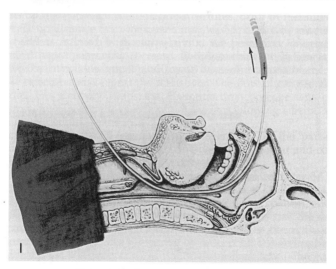

Figure 6–5 *See legend on opposite page*

This is a pull-through technique.[2, 34, 47] Various pull-through techniques have been described using ECs,[43, 48] central venous pressure (CVP) catheters,[27] monofilament sutures,[49] and Fogarty catheters.[50] The basic principle involves advancing the EC retrograde as in the classic technique, attaching it to the tip of the ET, and then using the EC to pull the ET into the trachea.

Once the EC (which is used only to place the silk) is out of the oral or nasal cavity, suture the silk to the cephalic end of the EC, cut off the needle and discard it, and then pull the silk antegrade through the CTM. Cut off and discard the EC, and tie the cephalic end of the silk to the Murphy eye of the ET. Use the silk suture to pull the ET into the trachea. If you attach the standard anesthesia circle system to the ET during placement, oxygen can be delivered via the ET, and in-line capnography can be used to verify the placement of the ET.

Because the silk is intimately attached to the ET, the railroading problem is eliminated, and multiple attempts at intubation are possible without repeating the puncture.

When a floppy epiglottis causes obstruction and the ET will not pass, you can deliberately intubate the esophagus. Gently withdraw the ET from the esophagus and apply tension simultaneously to the distal end of the silk, which will pop the tip of the ET anteriorly, lift the epiglottis, and allow the ET to enter the larynx.

If a nasal intubation is required, advance a urologic catheter (UC) through a naris into the posterior oropharynx. Attach the UC to the EC, which is exiting through the oral cavity. Withdraw the UC from the naris and the EC follows, now exiting the nasal rather than the oral cavity (Fig. 6–5).

The silk technique is easy, and because the silk can be left in place for the duration of the anesthesia, and in the recovery room after extubation with no discomfort, emergent reintubation can be accomplished. Sanchez has used this technique to reintubate two patients in the recovery room; both had suffered mandibular fractures, were initially intubated awake using a retrograde silk technique, and had arch bars placed in the operating room.

PEDIATRICS

The medical literature on the subject of RI in the pediatric population is not extensive.[17, 20, 30, 31, 34, 37, 45, 46, 51–56] RI has been used in the anticipated and the unanticipated difficult pediatric airway, primarily after failure of conventional intubating techniques (blind nasal intubation, direct laryngoscopy, fiberoptic intubation). The technique used is the same as that in the adult, but a higher incidence of difficulties has been reported, including problems in cannulating the ET and an inability to pass the ET through the glottic opening.[46]

In some cases, combined techniques have offered more success than blind RI. In one case report of a 16-year-old with acute epiglottitis, intubation was accomplished only by RI combined with rigid laryngoscopy: the retrograde catheter marked a path through an otherwise completely distorted anatomy.[20] The largest pediatric series with the highest success rate was reported by Audernaert;[46] in this series, RI was performed on 20 pediatric patients, aged 1 day to 17 years, with airway difficulties primarily due to congenital anomalies. The preferred approach, a combination of fiberoptic with retrograde guide wire, offered a higher success rate, faster intubation, the ability to insufflate oxygen through the suction port of the FB with the guide wire in place, easy passage of the ET through the glottis, minimal reliance on anatomic landmarks to guide the FB into the trachea, and less experience required to manage the FB. No major complications were reported, and the technique was considered a valuable addition to pediatric airway management.

COMPLICATIONS AND CAUTIONS

Although it has been demonstrated that transtracheal needle puncture is safe and associated with only minor complications,[57] numerous potential complications of RI have been suggested in the literature (Table 6–4). Actual documented complications are relatively few, and most were self-limited (Table 6–5). The most common complications cited are bleeding[24, 37, 42, 43, 58–61] and subcutaneous emphysema.[42, 54, 59]

Bleeding

Insignificant bleeding (4 to 5 drops) is associated with CTM puncture[37, 42] during RI. Even a patient who was heparinized intraoperatively and had postoperative disseminated intravascular coagulation had only a small, self-limited hematoma.[24] Controversy exists with respect to making the puncture below the cricoid cartilage because of a greater potential for bleeding.[33, 43, 51] Three studies with a total of 57 patients who underwent RI with punctures at the cricotracheal ligament or between the second and third tracheal rings showed no evidence of major bleeding.[43, 54, 59] There are, however, scattered reports of severe hemoptysis following transtracheal needle puncture with resultant hypoxia, cardiorespiratory arrest, dysrhythmias, and death.[62–66] Two patients suffered epistaxis[37, 67] after nasal intubation (with no vasoconstricting agent used).[37, 67] In order to decrease the potential for bleeding, avoid performing RI in patients with bleeding diatheses. When per-

---

Table 6–4   Potential Complications of Retrograde Intubation

Esophageal perforation
Hemoptysis
Intratracheal submucosal hematoma with distal obstruction
Laryngeal edema
Laryngospasm
Pretracheal infection
Tracheal fistula
Tracheitis
Vocal cord damage

From University of California at Irvine, Department of Anesthesia Teaching Aids.

Table 6–5   Reported Complications of Retrograde Intubation*

Self-limited
    Bleeding
        Puncture site (8)
        Peritracheal hematoma (1)
        Epistaxis (2)
    Subcutaneous emphysema (4)
        Pneumomediastinum (1)
        Breath holding (1)
        Catheter traveling caudad† (2)

Not self-limited
    Trigeminal nerve trauma (1)
    Pneumothorax (1)
    Loss of hook‡ (2)

*Numbers in parentheses indicate the number of reported complications.
†Refers to catheter traveling in a caudad direction toward the lungs instead of cephalad toward the oral cavity.
‡Refers to Waters' technique of retrieving catheter from nasopharynx using a self-made hook. From Waters DJ: Guided blind endotracheal intubation: For patients with deformities of the upper airway. Anaesthesia 18:158, 1963, and University of California at Irvine, Department of Anesthesia Teaching Aids.

forming RI, apply digital pressure to the puncture site for 5 minutes, apply a pressure dressing to the puncture site for 24 hours, and maintain the patient in the supine position for 3 to 4 hours after the puncture.

Subcutaneous Emphysema

Subcutaneous emphysema localized to the area of a transtracheal needle puncture site is common but self-limited. In severe cases, air may track through the fascial planes of the neck, leading to tracheal compression with airway compromise, pneumomediastinum, and pneumothorax.[54, 62, 68–72] Accumulation of air occurs gradually over 1 to 6 hours after a transtracheal puncture.[68, 70] Severe subcutaneous emphysema has been attributed to the use of a large-bore needle and exposure of the puncture site to persistent elevated intratracheal pressure (coughing, grunting, sneezing).

Other Complications

Other reported self-limited complications are breath holding[37] and caudad travel of the catheter (a straight, flexible guide wire)[54] (this is also possible when the catheter is inserted through a tracheostomy stoma).

Complications that were not self-limited include trigeminal nerve trauma,[73] which the author suspects was due to multiple laryngoscopies; guide wire fracture, in which the wire had to be surgically removed;[23] loss of the hook of a type that is no longer used;[37, 51, 56] and pneumothorax, requiring a chest tube.[68]

CONCLUSION

RI has been a particularly useful alternative in difficult intubations after multiple manipulations have caused bleeding, in facial injuries where bleeding is already present, and in patients with limited neck movement. The technique is easy to learn, requires little equipment, and in practiced hands is a rapid, safe, and effective method for intubating the trachea.

In the vast majority of cases, the airway can be secured using conventional techniques, but in a small number of cases these techniques cannot be successfully applied to the clinical problem at hand. No method offers 100% success rate, and therefore, it is wise to have multiple available options and to be facile with alternative techniques for intubation. Techniques allowing access to the airway via the CTM should be included as part of the armamentarium of clinicians involved in the care of seriously injured or ill patients.

ACKNOWLEDGMENT

With special thanks to Tay McClellan for her outstanding medical illustrations.

REFERENCES

1. American Society of Anesthesiologists Task Force: Practice guidelines for management of the difficult airway. Anesthesiology 78:597, 1993.
2. Sanchez AS: Cricothyroid Membrane [videotape]. ASA Airway safety video, part II, 1992.
3. Clemente CD: Gray's Anatomy, 13th ed. Philadelphia, Lea & Febiger, 1985, pp 1366–1368.
4. Caparosa RJ, Zavatsky AR: Practical aspects of the cricothyroid space. Laryngoscope 67:577, 1957.
5. Shantha TR: Retrograde intubation using the subcricoid region. Br J Anaesth 68:109, 1992.
6. Naumann H (ed): Head and Neck Surgery, vol 4. Philadelphia, WB Saunders, 1984, pp 162–181.
7. Bergman R, Thompson S (eds): Compendium of Human Anatomic Variation: Text, Atlas, and World Literature. Baltimore-Munich, Urban & Schwartzenberg, 1988, pp 65–116, 175–190.
8. Anson BJ (ed): Morris Human Anatomy: A Complete System Treatise, 12th ed. New York, McGraw-Hill, 1966, pp 674–702, 1545–51.
9. Sanchez A, Pallares V: Retrograde intubation technique. In Benumof JL (ed): Airway Management: Principles and Practice. St Louis, Mosby–Year Book, 1996, p 320.
10. Ovassapian A: Topical anesthesia. In Fiberoptic Airway Endoscopy in Anesthesia and Critical Care, 3rd ed. New York, Raven, 1990, pp 45–56.
11. Ovassapian A: Fiberoptic tracheal intubation. In Fiberoptic Airway Endoscopy in Anesthesia and Critical Care, 3rd ed. New York, Raven, 1990, pp 57–79.
12. Stone DJ, Gal TJ: Airway management. In Miller RD (ed): Anesthesia, 3rd ed. New York, Churchill Livingstone, 1990, p 1265.
13. Wedel DJ, Brown DL: Nerve blocks. In Miller RD (ed): Anesthesia, 3rd ed. New York, Churchill Livingstone, 1990, p 1407.
14. Shapiro HM, Drummond JC: Neurosurgical anesthesia and intracranial hypertension. In Miller RD (ed): Anesthesia, 3rd ed. Churchill Livingstone, New York, 1990, p 1737.
15. Cucchiara RF, Black S, Steinkeler JA: Anesthesia for intracranial procedures. In

Barash PG, Cullen BF, Stoelting RK (eds): Clinical anesthesia. Philadelphia, JB Lippincott, 1989, p 849.

16. Stehling SC: Management of the airway. *In* Barash PG, Cullen BF, Stoelting RK (eds): Clinical Anesthesia. Philadelphia, JB Lippincott, 1989, p 543.

17. Cooper CM, Murray-Wilson A: Retrograde intubation: Management of a 4.8 kg 5-month infant. Anaesthesia 42:1197, 1987.

18. Lechman MJ, Donahoo JS, Macvaugh H: Endotracheal intubation using percutaneous retrograde guidewire insertion followed by antegrade fiberoptic bronchoscopy. Crit Care Med 14:589, 1986.

19. Pintanel T, Font M, Aguilar JL, et al: Retrograde orotracheal intubation. Rev Esp Anestesiol Reanim 35:344, 1988.

20. Heslet L, Christensen KS, Sanchez R, et al: Facilitated blind intubation using a transtracheal guide wire. Dan Med Bull 32:275, 1985.

21. Lee YW, Lee YS, Kim JR: Retrograde tracheal intubation. Yonsei Med J 28:3, 1987.

22. Schmidt SI, Hasewinkel JV: Retrograde catheter-guided direct laryngoscopy. Anesthesiol Rev 16:49, 1989.

23. Contrucci RB, Gottlieb JS: A complication of retrograde endotracheal intubation. Ear Nose Throat J 69:776, 1989.

24. Casthely PA, Landesman S, Fynaman PN: Retrograde intubation in patients undergoing open heart surgery. Can Anaesth Soc J 32:661, 1985.

25. Carlson CA, Perkins HM: Solving a difficult intubation. Anesthesiology 64:537, 1986.

26. Maestro CM, Andujar MJJ, Sancho CJ, et al: Intubacion retrograda en un paciente con una malformacion epiglotica (cartas al director). Rev Esp Anestesiol Reanim 35:344, 1988.

27. Raza S, Levinsky L, Lajos TZ: Transtracheal intubation: Useful adjunct in cardiac surgical anesthesia. J Thorac Cardiovasc Surg 76:721, 1978.

28. Gupta B, McDonald JS, Brooks HJ, et al: Oral fiberoptic intubation over a retrograde guidewire. Anesth Analg 68:517, 1989.

29. Amanor-Boadu SD: Translaryngeal guided intubation in a patient with raised intracranial pressure. Afr J Med Sci 21:66, 1992.

30. France NK, Beste DJ: Anesthesia for pediatric ear, nose and throat surgery. *In* Gregory GA: Pediatric Anesthesia, 2nd ed. New York, Churchill Livingstone, 1989, p 1127.

31. Gregory GA: Induction of anesthesia. *In* Gregory GA: Pediatric Anesthesia, 2nd ed. New York, Churchill Livingstone, 1989, p 557.

32. Lleu JC, Forrler M, Forrler C, et al: L'intubation oro-tracheale par void retrograde. Ann Fr Anesth Reanim 8:632, 1989.

33. Lleu JC, Forrler M, Pottecher T, et al: Retrograde intubation using the subcricoid region [letter]. Br J Anaesth 55:855, 1983.

34. Sanchez AS: The retrograde cookbook. Presented at the First International Symposium on the Difficult Airway, Newport Beach, Calif, 1993.

35. Bourke D, Levesque PR: Modification of retrograde guide for endotracheal intubation. Anesth Analg 53:1013, 1974.

36. Freund PR, Rooke A, Schwid H: Retrograde intubation with a modified Eschmann stylet [letter]. Anesth Analg 67:596, 1988.

37. Akinyemi OO: Complications of guided blind endotracheal intubation. Anaesthesia 34:590, 1979.

38. Benumof JL: Management of the difficult adult airway. Anesthesiology 75:1087, 1991.

39. King HK, Wang LF, Wooten DJ: Endotracheal intubation using translaryngeal guided intubation vs percutaneous retrograde guidewire insertion [letter]. Crit Care Med 15:183, 1987.

40. Heller EM, Schneider K, Saven B: Percutaneous retrograde intubation. Laryngoscope 99:555, 1989.

41. Hines MH, Meredith JW: Modified retrograde intubation technique for rapid airway access. Am J Surg 159:597, 1990.

42. Powell WF, Ozdil T: A translaryngeal guide for tracheal intubation. Anesth Analg 46:231, 1967.

43. Abou-Madi MN, Trop D: Pulling versus guiding: A modification of retrograde guided intubation. Can J Anaesth 36:3:336, 1989.
44. Stern Y, Spitzer T: Retrograde intubation of the trachea. J Laryngol Otol 105:746, 1991.
45. Thomas P: Retrograde intubation. *In* Dailey RD, Simon B et al (eds): The Airway: Emergency Management. St Louis, Mosby–Year Book, 1992, p 107.
46. Audenaert SM, Montgomery CL, Stone B, et al: Retrograde-assisted fiberoptic tracheal intubation in children with difficult airways. Anesth Analg 73:660, 1991.
47. Sanchez AS: Preventing the difficult airway from becoming the impossible airway: Retrograde intubation. Presented at the Annual Meeting of the American Society of Anesthesiologists, Las Vegas, Oct 16, 1990.
48. Kubo K, Takahashi S, Oka M: A modified technique of guided blind intubation in oral surgery. J Maxillofac Surg 8:135, 1980.
49. Harrison CA, Wise CC: Retrograde intubation [letter]. Anaesthesia 43:609, 1988.
50. Carlson RC, Sadove MS: Guided non-visualized nasal endotracheal intubation using a transtracheal Fogarty catheter. Illinois Med J 143:364, 1973.
51. Waters DJ: Guided blind endotracheal intubation using translaryngeal guided intubation vs percutaneous retrograde guidewire insertion [letter]. Crit Care Med 15:183, 1987.
52. Borland LM, Swan DM, Leff S: Difficult pediatric endotracheal intubation: A new approach to the retrograde technique. Anesthesiology 55:577, 1981.
53. Manchester GH, Mani MM, Master FW: A simple method for emergency orotracheal intubation. Plast Reconstr Surg 49:312, 1972.
54. VanNiekerk JV, Smalhout B: Retrograde endotracheal intubation using a catheter. Ned Tijdschr Geneeskd 131:1663, 1987.
55. Levin RM: Anesthesia for cleft lip and cleft palate. Anesthesiol Rev 6:25, 1979.
56. Akinyemi OO, John A: A complication of guided blind intubation. Anesthesia 29:733, 1974.
57. Gold MI, Buechel DR: Translaryngeal anesthesia: A review. Anesthesiology 20:181, 1959.
58. Barriot P, Bruno R: Retrograde technique for tracheal intubation in trauma patients. Crit Care Med 16:712, 1988.
59. Mahiou, Bouvet FR, Korach JM: Intubation retrograde [abstract R26]. *In* Proceedings of the Thirty-First Congress de Intubacion Tracheal, Paris, July 14, 1983.
60. Guggenberger H, Lenz G: Training in retrograde intubation [letter]. Anesthesiology 69:292, 1988.
61. Guggenberger H, Lenz G, Heumann H: Success rate and complications of a modified guided blind technique for intubation in 36 patients. Anaesthesist 36:703, 1987.
62. Ries K, Levison ME, Kaye D: Transtracheal aspiration in pulmonary infection. Arch Intern Med 133:453, 1974.
63. Unger KM, Moser KM: Fatal complication of transtracheal aspiration: A report of two cases. Arch Intern Med 132:437, 1973.
64. Spencer CD, Beaty HN: Complications of transtracheal aspiration. N Engl J Med 286:304, 1972.
65. Schillaci RF, Iacovoni VE, Conte RS: Transtracheal aspiration complicated by fatal endotracheal hemorrhage. N Engl J Med 295:4884, 1976.
66. Hemley SD, Arida EJ, Diggs AM, et al: Percutaneous cricothyroid membrane bronchography. Radiology 76:763, 1961.
67. Corleta O, Habazettl H, Kreimeier U, et al: Modified retrograde orotracheal intubation technique for airway access in rabbits. Eur Surg Res 24:129, 1992.
68. Poon YK: Case history number 89: A life-threatening complication of cricothyroid membrane puncture. Anesth Analg 55:298, 1976.
69. Kalinske RW, Parker RH, Brandt D, et al: Diagnostic usefulness and safety of transtracheal aspiration. N Engl J Med 276:604, 1967.
70. Massey JY: Complications of transtracheal aspiration: A case report. J Ark Med Soc 67:254, 1971.
71. Won KH, Rowland DW, et al: Massive subcutaneous emphysema complicating

transcricothyroid bronchography. Am J Roentgenol Radium Ther Nucl Med 101:953, 1967.
72. Wilson JKV: Cricothyroid bronchography with a polyethylene catheter: Description of a new technique. Am J Roentgenol 81:305, 1959.
73. Faithfull NS: Injury to terminal branches of the trigeminal nerve following tracheal intubation. Br J Anaesth 57:535, 1985.

Chapter 7

Airway Gadgets

Harold S. Minkowitz

"Accessories for endotracheal anesthesia are without end. There is no living Anaesthetist who holds the distinction of not having designed one or more devices."[1] This statement, although written almost 40 years ago, is equally true today and indicates that we have not yet designed the perfect intubation device. Normally, the limiting factor in choosing a particular intubating technique is the anesthesia practitioner's familiarity and skill. Therefore, everybody involved in airway management should be familiar with several different devices or techniques so that when a difficult airway management problem arises, it can be safely managed.

LIGHTED STYLETS

In 1957, MacIntosh and Richards first described intubation of the trachea under direct vision, using a lighted introducer to guide the endotracheal tube (ET) through the cords.[2] The first transillumination technique to guide nasotracheal intubation was described 2 years later.[3]

Transillumination techniques rely on the transillumination of the tissues of the anterior neck to demonstrate the location of the tip of the ET. A well-circumscribed glow visible in the anterior neck indicates tracheal location, whereas a diffuse glow is seen with esophageal intubation.[4]

In the last several years, a number of commercial transillumination products have been developed, including the disposable Flexilum (Concept Corp., Clearwater, Fla.) and TubeStat Lighted Stylet (Concept Corp., Clearwater, Fla.); the partially disposable Trachlight (Laerdal Medical Corp., Long Beach, Calif.) (Fig. 7–1), Imagica Fiberoptic Lighted Stylet (Fiberoptic Medical Products, Allentown, Pa.), and Vital Light (Vital Signs, Totowa, N.J.); and the nondisposable versions, the Fiberoptic Lighted Intubation Stilette and "The Shuttle," Fiberlightview Lighted Stilette (Anesthesia Medical Specialties, Santa Fe Springs, Calif.), the latter of which is available in both adult and pediatric sizes, allowing its use in ETs as small as 4.0-mm inner diameter (ID). These products have been used effectively and safely for both orotracheal and nasotracheal intubations.[5–8]

A number of reports have described successful intubation using lightwands.[5–9] However, the following problems were noted:[4]

1. Under ambient light, the beam intensity was insufficient to produce adequate transillumination. This requirement for a darkened environment limited its use in certain situations.

2. The light source projected only forward; thus, the transilluminated beam would be visible only if the tip of the stylet

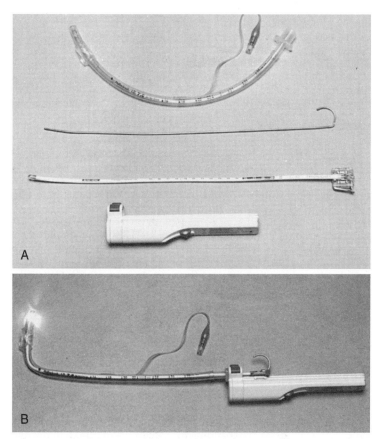

Figure 7–1 *A,* The Trachlight consists of three parts: a removable handle, a flexible wand, and a stiff retractable stylet. *B,* The Trachlight assembled.

pointed toward the skin surface. This may be a problem if the tip of the stylet points posteriorly or caudad in the trachea.

3. Inadequate stylet length limited the length of the ETs that could be used.
4. Some devices did not have a tube clamp to secure the ET.
5. The rigid wand portion occasionally resulted in dislodging the ET from the trachea when withdrawing the lightwand after intubation. After withdrawal of the stylet, detection of the location of the tip of the ET is not possible.
6. Disposable units resulted in increased costs.

Trachlight

In view of these problems, a new lighted stylet, the Trachlight (Laerdal Medical), was designed. The Trachlight comprises three parts: a reusable handle, a disposable flexible wand, and a stylet. The stylet attaches to the handle by a ratchet-like mechanism, and its position on the handle may be adjusted; thus, ETs of varied lengths can be accommodated. The stylets are now available in three sizes: infant, child, and adult. A clamp on the distal end of the handle locks the ET into place. A bright light source, powered by three AAA batteries held within the handle, emits light both anteriorly and distally into the airway. After 30 seconds, the light begins to flash, as a reminder to ventilate the patient and also to minimize heat production.[9] The tip of the light bulb is encased within the ET, and therefore burn injury is unlikely during intubation. Within the wand is a stiff malleable stylet, which is bent into a "field hockey stick" shape on order to facilitate placement of the ET into the glottic opening.

Lightwand techniques have been shown to safely intubate a large number of surgical patients. However, trauma may result if lightwands are used for the intubation of patients with pharyngeal masses or with anatomic abnormalities of the upper airway. Thus, they should not be used in these circumstances. Although a similar technique may be employed for all lightwand devices, particular reference is made to the Trachlight, as the author has had the most experience with this device.

■ Technique

With this device, initial attempts on an airway mannequin make the intubation of human patients easier, because the technique is so different from that of standard endotracheal intubation. Once you are comfortable with the technique, you should intubate patients with normal airway anatomy in order to gain experience with this device.

Lubricating the rigid metal internal stylet with silicone fluid facilitates its retraction during intubation. Before securing the wand to the handle, secure the internal stylet into place in the wand connector. Then slide the wand onto the handle from below, and through the tube clamp. Secure an ET to the handle, and then insert the wand into the ET, with the light bulb just proximal to the bevel of the ET. Note and match the distance markings located on both the ET and the light wand. Next bend the ET-trachlight (ET-TL) over the area marked "bend here." It is important to measure each patient's thyromental distance in order to accurately estimate the arc the stylet must make around the tongue to enter the trachea. If the patient's head and neck are in the neutral position, the angle should approximate 90 degrees. With head flexion, an angle less than 90 degrees is required, and with head extension greater than 90 degrees is required.[10] Position the patient in such a manner that the anterior neck is clearly visible. In the absence of any contraindications, both the head and the neck of the patient should be extended, unlike the sniffing position used for conventional laryngoscopy. In patients with a short neck, a shoulder roll increases the exposure of the anterior neck. Most patients may be intubated in ambient light, and a dimmed environment is recommended only in patients in whom transillumination of the anterior neck would be difficult, such as obese patients.

Following standard preparation for intubation, lift the supine patient's jaw upward using the thumb and index finger of the nondominant hand. This lifts the epiglottis and tongue off the posterior pharyngeal wall, facilitating intubation. Turn the Trachlight on and insert it into the patient's oropharynx. Rotate it around the patient's tongue, maintaining a midline position, and gently rock the ET-TL combination forward and backward until the tip is directed into the trachea. If a faint glow is seen above the thyroid prominence, the tip is located in the vallecula. If a dim glow appears, or no glow is visualized, the tip is probably in the esophagus. When the tip enters the glottic opening, a well-defined glow is visualized in the anterior neck, just below the thyroid prominence. Withdrawing the inner stylet about 10 cm increases the flexibility of the distal tip, and the trachea can then be intubated. Advance the ET-TL until the glow begins to disappear at the sternal notch, indicating that the tip of the ET is located approximately midway between the carina and the vocal cords.[11] Release the locking clamp and remove the Trachlight from the ET. If it is difficult to advance the ET once the stylet has been retracted, rotate the ET 90 degrees counterclockwise and attempt reinsertion. Never apply force in order to intubate, as trauma, and possible loss of the airway, may result.

The Trachlight may also be used to facilitate nasal intubation. Perform standard preparation for nasal intubation and remove the internal stylet before inserting the Trachlight into the ET. If a directional tip (e.g., Endotrol) ET is used, exert traction on the loop in order to direct the tip anteriorly. Pass the ET-TL combination through the nose, lift the jaw upward, and turn the Trachlight on. Gently advance the ET-TL using the glow as a guide, redirecting the tip toward the thyroid prominence should resistance be encountered. Flexing the patient's neck may aid in nasotracheal intubation. Finally, the Trachlight with its internal stylet removed may also be used to confirm the proper location of any ET.

ENDOTRACHEAL TUBE GUIDES

A number of stylets have been used to aid in intubation. Four of these devices are discussed.

Eschmann Tracheal Tube Introducer

The Eschmann introducer (Eschmann Health Care, Kent, England), also known as a gum elastic bougie, is a 60-cm-long, 15 Fr–gauge stylet that is angled 40 degrees approximately 3.5 cm from the distal end and is made from a woven polyester base.[12] It has been popular in Europe for many years and its use was first described in 1949. This introducer can be used in one of two ways. It can be advanced through the ET until the tip protrudes from the ET. The tip can then be guided through the vocal cords and the ET advanced over it. Alternatively, the introducer can itself be guided into the trachea and an ET railroaded over it.

It is very helpful in patients with an "anterior larynx." If only the epiglottis is visualized, the Eschmann introducer can be guided under the epiglottis and into the trachea. It may prove lifesaving in an unexpected difficult intubation in which only a portion of recognizable laryngeal structures are visualized. In addition, it may be used as a tube changer, over which ETs are exchanged.[13] However, it is not marketed for use as such because of its limited length. Concord, Portex also manufactures two tracheal tube guides that are 70 cm long, although the diameters differ (10 versus 15 Fr) and allow both adult and pediatric tube exchange. These guides are made of the same material as the introducer, but they do not have any distal angulation. Correct placement in the trachea is indicated by feeling a "clicking" as the tip slides over the tracheal cartilages, the bougie gets "held up" as it reaches the small bronchi, or the patient coughs.[14, 15] If difficulty occurs when attempting to advance the ET, one should rotate the ET 90 degrees counterclockwise so that the bevel faces posteriorly and advance the ET, therefore avoiding the right arytenoid. If this is not successful, a smaller ET may pass through the cords.

It is very easy to use, with a steep learning curve. Difficult airway anatomy may be simulated by performing laryngoscopy in the regular manner. Once the vocal cords and epiglottis are visualized, withdraw the laryngoscope blade until only the tip of the epiglottis is visualized. The difficult airway may now be simulated and the bougie used as a guide.

Patil Two-Part Intubation Catheter

The Patil two-part intubation catheter, manufactured by Cook Critical Care, is made of polyvinyl chloride, with a radiopaque stripe down its length. It is 63 cm long with a 6-mm outer diameter (OD) and a 3.4-mm inner diameter and may be used with ETs with an ID greater than 7 mm. Two parts of the device are attached by a threaded connector. The first part, with a malleable stylet in situ, facilitates intubation. There are eight side ports on the distal end of this part.

The second part can be connected to the first and the extended device used as a tube changer.[16] Two Rapi-Fit connectors are included in the package. These adapters are easily engaged or disengaged from the stylet in order to allow jet ventilation. Should difficulty arise in passing the ET over the extended catheter, ventilation can be accomplished by attaching either Rapi-Fit adaptor and ventilating the patient until a permanent airway has been established.

Augustine Guide

The Augustine guide (Augustine Medical, Eden Prairie, Minn.) has been developed for performing blind intubation in adults. It is composed of two pieces, a guide handle and a stylet. The stylet has an S-shaped distal tip with three aspiration holes on each side. A 35-mL syringe serves as an esophageal detection system and is attached to the proximal end. A positioning blade resembling a short MacIntosh laryngoscope blade is connected to a handle that contains a guide channel to hold an ET.[17]

The device was designed for prehospital airway management in patients with difficult airways. No cervical spine movement is needed; hence it is an appropriate device for use in patients with cervical spine injuries. It may also be used to intubate patients in a variety of positions and settings, including the operating room and the intensive care unit. Although this device has not been commercially available, it is going to be reintroduced as an instrument to assist fiberoptic tracheal intubation rather than blind tracheal intubation.

■ Technique

Before intubation, insert the stylet into a 7- to 8-mm ID ET and advance it to the distal tip of the ET. Then insert the stylet-ET combination into the guide channel with the ET and stylet tip at the opening under the positioning blade.[18] Advance the device around the tongue and into the vallecula. The handle should be at 90 degrees to the plane of the face. Confirm correct placement by moving the device from side to side in the vallecula and palpating hyoid bone movement in the neck.[18]

Advance the syringe-stylet unit until the syringe meets the ET connector. Confirm the tracheal location by encountering no resistance to the passage of the stylet, easy aspiration of air into the syringe, and no recoil of the syringe plunger. Resistance to aspiration of the syringe and recoil of the plunger indicate esophageal placement. It is important always to aspirate a full 30 to 35 mL of air to check for lack of recoil of the plunger of the syringe.

With tracheal placement of the stylet confirmed, hold the handle firmly and advance the ET over the stylet into the trachea. If any resistance to passage of the ET occurs, rotate the ET 90 degrees counterclockwise.[19] This changes the orientation of the bevel of the ET from a lateral to a downward position, facilitating advancement of the ET over the right arytenoid into the trachea. Confirm correct ET placement by the standard techniques.

The Augustine guide uses a blind intubation technique, so patients with blood, vomitus, or secretions in the oropharynx and those with limited direct airway visualization can be managed with this device. The handle can be used as a guide for oral fiberoptic bronchoscopy.

Airguide Tube

The "bubble-tip" (Airguide) tracheal tube system (Linder nasotracheal tube with Airguide inflatable introducer; Polamedco, Inglewood, Calif.) was developed to minimize mucosal and soft tissue injuries. This system consists of a nonbeveled tracheal tube with a Murphy eye, and a soft stylet, called the Airguide inflatable introducer, that is 30 to 45 cm long and has an OD of 3 mm. There is an air-inflatable balloon on one end and a self-closing valve on the other. When the balloon is inflated for use, it is called a "bubble-tip" or an obturator. Before insertion into the naris, the Airguide inflatable introducer is inserted into an ET and the balloon is inflated. Once intubation is successful, the Airguide is deflated and the introducer is removed. Watanabe and colleagues studied the use of this device in 66 elective surgical patients who underwent nasotracheal intubation and found that the Airguide minimized the incidence of epistaxis and increased navigability in the subglottic region during nasotracheal intubation.[20]

RIGID LARYNGOSCOPES

Various laryngoscopes have been described since MacEwan, a distinguished surgeon of the Glasgow Royal Infirmary, first used his fingers to guide an ET into the trachea in 1878.[21] More than 80 laryngoscope blades have since been described. It is beyond the scope of this chapter to discuss them all; rather, a number have been selected and important differences are highlighted.

A laryngoscope consists of a handle, a blade, and a light source. The main shaft of the blade is called the *spatula*. The *web* or *step* is the upward projection on the blade toward the roof of the mouth. The lateral projection from the web is called the *flange*. The *beak* is the tip of the blade, and near the beak is a light source.

Jackson Laryngoscope Blade

In 1908, Jackson developed a straight-bladed laryngoscope with an O-shaped flange and a U-type handle that resembled three sides of a square with the lifting handgrip parallel to the blade. This laryngoscope facilitated the exposure of the larynx without applying direct pressure to the upper teeth and became the standard instrument for performing laryngeal examinations and for directly inspecting the vocal cords before intubation.

Miller Laryngoscope Blade

In 1941, Miller designed a laryngoscope blade to decrease the risk of tooth trauma and lift the epiglottis. This laryngoscope was longer than the Jackson blade, smaller at the tip with a shallower base, and rounded at the bottom and had an extra curve beginning about 5 cm from the distal tip.[22] This new design required less mouth opening for intubation, as well as freer anterior movement of the mandible, so that when the small round end of the blade pressed against the tongue and the distal tip entrapped the epiglottis, a channel was created to expose the larynx. The Miller blade has become a standard against which other laryngoscope blades are compared.

MacIntosh Laryngoscope Blade

In 1943, MacIntosh designed a curved blade in order *not* to entrap the epiglottis. The MacIntosh blade is advanced until the distal tip is placed in the vallecula, and then upward traction is applied to the tongue base, facilitating exposure of the larynx.

Modifications

Since the invention of these three primary laryngoscope blades, many modifications have been proposed. These modifications were primarily designed to overcome certain difficult airway problems.

■ Limited Mouth Opening

There are various reasons why a patient may have limited mouth opening, such as trauma, congenital abnormalities, or medical disease. In order to facilitate the passage of the laryngoscope to accomplish intubation, a reduction or abolition in the step will help fit the blade between the teeth,[23, 24] although this sacrifices its role of separating the upper and lower teeth once the blade has been positioned appropriately.

A retromolar approach, which is an oblique approach to the vocal cords through the corner of the mouth, reduces the distance to the vocal cords and renders them more accessible in patients with restricted mouth opening.[25] A number of laryngoscopes for people with limited mouth opening have been designed. These include the Soper, Parrott, Gould, Bowen-Jackson, Gabuya-Orkin, Bizzarri-Giuffrida, Onkst, Orr, and Schapira laryngoscope blades, the improved-vision MacIntosh laryngoscope blade, and the double-angled laryngoscope blade. The double-angled blade was designed to combine the advantageous features of the Miller and MacIntosh laryngoscope blades and eliminate their disadvantages.[26] The blade has two incremental curves (20 and 30 degrees) that allow visualization of an anteriorly located larynx without the need to look through the laryngoscope posteriorly. In order to decrease the risk of tooth damage and provide more room for intubation, the vertical flange was eliminated. Additionally, a wider and flatter tip was designed for ease of manipulation of a large tongue or floppy epiglottis. The double-angled laryngoscope blade is a simple blade but requires further testing before widespread use.

The Levering laryngoscope blade was designed to elevate the epiglottis in certain clinical situations, such as in patients with a recessive mandible and decreased mouth opening. The laryngoscope was designed to decrease the risk of tooth damage caused by the clinicians levering back with the laryngoscope on the teeth in an attempt to lift the epiglottis. This laryngoscope is a modification of the MacIntosh laryngoscope but has a hinged tip controlled by a lever at the proximal end. It is inserted into the mouth, and the distal tip is placed into the vallecula. Compression of the lever results in elevation of the hinged tip approximately 70 degrees upward, which elevates the epiglottis. Tracheal intubation is then followed in the standard technique. The lever is then released and the blade is removed. A number of case reports have shown its use in difficult airways.[27, 28] Tuckey and associates evaluated the effect of the levering laryngoscope on the view obtained at laryngoscopy in 210 consecutive patients who required tracheal intubation.[29] They found that elevation of the levered tip of the blade significantly improved laryngeal visualization in patients with a grade III view of the larynx, whereas the neutral position of the blade was most beneficial in those with grades I or II.

■ Anterior Larynx

A number of laryngoscopes, including the Siker laryngoscope, have been designed to overcome the problem of the operator's not being able to visualize the vocal cords in patients with an "anterior larynx." This blade was designed to manage patients with prominent or overriding upper incisors, recessed mandibles, and an anterior larynx.[30] The Siker blade incorporates a mirror in the laryngoscope blade located 3 inches from the distal tip.

Two laryngoscope blades have been designed with prisms in the blade. The Huffman blade has a prism fitted on a standard MacIntosh no. 3 laryngoscope. The other laryngoscope using a prism is the Belscope angulated laryngoscope. This is a straight-bladed laryngoscope bent 45 degrees at its midpoint and is available in three sizes. The angled blade requires less compression and anterior displacement of the tongue to obtain a view of the larynx, and the epiglottis is lifted forward as with a Miller blade. It is similar conceptually to the Siker blade. The Belscope can be used as a regular laryngoscope, or in difficult cases, the prism can be used to "see" around the corner and provide an indirect view of the glottic opening.[25] The Belscope is recommended when poor neck extension, a large tongue, or a short mandible hinders optimal positioning of a MacIntosh laryngoscope blade, causing the curvature of the MacIntosh blade to obscure vision of the larynx. Concerns regarding the use of these blades include the paucity of extensive clinical evaluation, the amount of practice necessary to achieve proficiency, and fogging of the prisms.[31]

■ Sternal Space Restriction

A number of laryngoscopes have been designed in order to manage patients with sternal space restriction, which may be caused by thoracic cage abnormalities, flexion deformity of the neck, skull traction, obesity, large breasts, and cricoid pressure. In order to perform intubations in these patients, the laryngoscope blade may be inserted laterally and then rotated 90 degrees. Alternatively, the handle and blade can be detached, the laryngoscope inserted into the mouth, and the handle reattached. A number of laryngoscopes have been designed to address this clinical problem. Solutions include fixed-angle modified blades,[32] adjustable multiangle adapters,[33] single-position adapters, and hinge blocks.[34, 35] The problem with all these blades is that the angle between the handle and the blade results in a different pattern of intubation from that which the practitioner has become accustomed, which may result in unsuccessful intubation. Also, the mechanical advantage of the 90-degree-or-less angle is sacrificed, and the simplest solution to most of the situations may be a shortened laryngoscope handle.[36]

■ Small Intraoral Cavity

A small oral cavity reduces the space available for and the maneuverability of a laryngoscope blade and ET. In order to optimize compression of the tongue into the mandibular space compartment, a blade with an ample flange and step is required.[37] The Wisconsin, Flagg, and Guedel laryngoscopes are examples of these blades. The Macintosh blade, by stretching the hyoepiglottic ligament, may also increase the intraoral space.[1]

The Bainton pharyngolaryngoscope (Pilling Instruments, Fort Washington, Pa.) was designed specifically for patients with pharyngeal obstructions.[38] It resembles a standard straight blade while incorporating a 7-cm tube into the distal portion. Within its lumen, a dual fiberoptic light source is recessed, thus protected from secretions and obstruction by the surrounding oropharyngeal tissue. An oral opening is created at the distal tip of the blade by its 60-degree bevel. The tip of the blade elevates the epiglottis to permit a view of the larynx. Using a tubular design, this laryngoscope creates pharyngeal space and facilitates the passage of an 8-mm ID or smaller ET without an adapter through or around the laryngoscope blade. The right hand should stabilize the ET as the blade is removed over the proximal end of the ET.

■ Immobile or Unstable Cervical Spines

For immobile or unstable cervical spines (see also the section Indirect Fiberoptic Laryngoscopes), the redesign of laryngoscope blades involves remodeling not only the blade but also the handle and light source. Mercury Medical developed the 2001 Fiberlight, which is a fiberoptic laryngoscope blade that fits onto standard laryngoscope handles. This modification involves both pediatric- and adult-sized MacIntosh, Miller, and Phillips laryngoscopes.

INDIRECT FIBEROPTIC LARYNGOSCOPES

Conventional direct laryngoscopy requires wide mouth opening, flexion of the cervical spine, and extension of the atlantooccipital joint in order to create a direct line of vision from the mouth to the vocal cords. In certain conditions, positioning in this fashion is not possible and may even be contraindicated. Also, it may be impossible to visualize the larynx using direct laryngoscopy because the curve between the front teeth and the larynx cannot be straightened. New fiberoptic laryngoscopes have been designed for use in such circumstances. Four of these laryngoscopes are discussed: the Bullard and Upsher fiberoptic laryngoscopes, the WuScope system, and the Augustine scope. They have several features in common, including an anatomically shaped blade, fiberoptic bundles, and a light source. They do, however, have a number of important differences, which are discussed.

Bullard Laryngoscope

The Bullard laryngoscope (Circon, ACMI, Stamford, Conn.) (Fig. 7–2) is an indirect fiberoptic laryngoscope with a rigid anatomically shaped

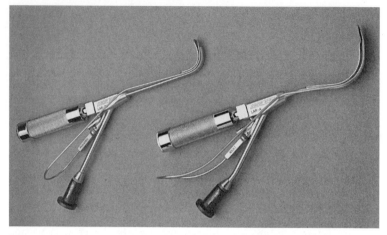

Figure 7–2 Bullard laryngoscope. An adult scope is next to a pediatric scope with introducing stylets and battery handles. (Courtesy of Circon Corporation.)

blade with fiberoptic bundles.[9] Indirect laryngoscopy is performed without aligning the oral, pharyngeal, and laryngeal axes, making the device ideal for patients with cervical spine abnormality. Both adult and pediatric sizes are available. Few studies have been performed to evaluate the advantages of the Bullard over conventional laryngoscopy and flexible fiberoptic bronchoscopy, but many reports have detailed the use of the Bullard laryngoscope in patients with difficult airways.[39, 40] Also, it can be used in conjunction with new instruments and intubation modalities, which may provide an easy approach and effective anesthesia in these patients.

The larynx is well visualized because the fiberoptic bundle, located on the posterior aspect of the blade, comes to within 26 mm of the distal tip of the blade. At the level of the larynx, the field of view is 55 ± 5 degrees. Two light sources are available, a battery-powered handle or a flexible fiberoptic cable connected to a high-intensity light source (e.g., halogen or xenon). This latter option provides superior visibility. The eyepiece has an attachable diopter for correction of visual acuity. A video camera may be attached to the eyepiece.

A 3.7-mm channel with a Luer-Lok connection can be used for suction, oxygen insufflation, or the administration of local anesthetics during laryngoscopy. A three-way stopcock allows accommodation of more than one option. A second port accepts a nonmalleable intubating stylet, designed to follow the contour of the laryngoscope blade. Older versions of the Bullard laryngoscope incorporated intubating forceps, which have been abandoned in favor of the newer stylets. Another intubating stylet with a hollow core has been developed. This lumen allows the passage of a 4-mm flexible fiberoptic bronchoscope or other guide device to facilitate intubation. This new stylet is attached to the body of the Bullard laryngoscope with a finger screw. The thin laryngoscope blade allows the insertion of the device into the mouth of a patient with a minimal (0.64 cm) mouth opening. The greatest limitation to the insertion of the device is the OD of the ET, since the entire unit is inserted simultaneously.

The Bullard laryngoscope may be used in awake (after proper topicalization) or anesthetized patients. Six methods of intubation have been described using the Bullard laryngoscope.[41, 42] These include an ET with a malleable stylet, an ET exchanger, an ET with a movable tip, the Bullard intubating forceps, and the two intubating stylets. The most commonly employed techniques involve the use of the intubating stylets. Either stylet must be lubricated and attached to the Bullard laryngoscope in the appropriate fashion. If the older, solid stylet is used, the ET adapter should be removed and the ET should be positioned properly over the stylet so that the distal end of the stylet projects through the Murphy eye of the ET. If the newer, hollow-core stylet is used, the ET is simply passed over it and not threaded through the Murphy eye.

■ Technique

Once the patient's mouth is open, the use of a tongue blade to elevate the tongue facilitates its passage. Hold the device in the left hand and insert it into the oropharynx in the horizontal plane. Once the blade clears the tongue, rotate the handle 90 degrees in the vertical plane, sliding the blade around the tongue, remaining in the midline position. Then gently lift the laryngoscope in order to view the rima glottis. The device may be used with the blade tip posterior to the epiglottis, or it may be placed into the vallecula. If the epiglottis is large or difficult to trap, a plastic blade extender is available for use. Once the larynx is visualized, place the stylet tip to the left centrally between the vocal cords. Next advance the ET under direct vision until the cuff passes distal to the vocal cords. Then remove the device in the reverse manner in which it was inserted. Confirm the correct placement of the tube in the standard fashion. Occasionally, it may be difficult to pass an ET into the trachea despite good vocal cord visualization. The most common difficulty is that the ET is unable to pass over the right arytenoid. It may be necessary to displace the blade posteriorly and then lift vertically to optimize conditions. Other options include a flexible guide through the forceps channel of the Bullard laryngoscope into the trachea,[43, 44] withdrawing the Bullard and then passing the ET over the guide into the trachea. In order to become proficient with the device, training and commitment are necessary.[42] The intubating stylet has been shown to require less time to intubate and also requires fewer attempts than the original three mechanisms.[45] It was also found that the ease of intubation was not influenced by the laryngoscopic grade. When the Bullard is used for intubation, some neck movement does occur, although it is minimal.[46] It is not known whether this movement is clinically significant.

UpsherScope

The UpsherScope (Mercury Medical, Clearwater, Fla.) (Fig. 7–3) is also an anatomically designed fiberoptic laryngoscope. Only an adult size is available, but a pediatric size is being developed.[47] It is constructed of three pieces of stainless steel, the largest of which is the "tubeguide," approximately C-shaped in cross-section. Along the right side of the instrument is the "delivery slot," which runs the length of the tube guide. The open part of the C slot allows the ET to be removed from the device after intubation. The C-shaped section ends about 2 cm from the distal end of the blade. As with the Bullard laryngoscope, two light sources are available, a battery-powered handle or a flexible fiberoptic cable that is connected to a high-intensity light source. The eyepiece is focusable and immersible. The device does not have any extra ports, and therefore any suctioning, insufflation of oxygen, or local anesthetic instillation is performed through the lumen of the ET. Secretions interfere with the view, and therefore an antisialagogue should be administered in a timely fashion and the oropharynx should be suctioned before the insertion of the device.

■ Technique

In order to intubate using the UpsherScope, place the device in the left hand. Gently lift the tongue forward using a tongue blade, and carefully insert the instrument behind the tip of the tongue blade, always remaining midline. Remove the tongue blade and advance the device,

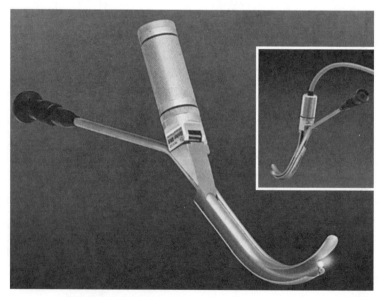

Figure 7–3   UpsherScope. (Courtesy of Mercury Medical.)

following the oropharyngeal curve. Once the epiglottis has been identified, place the tip of the device into the vallecula or under the epiglottis. The vocal cords will be exposed by gently lifting the device vertically. Because the angle of the tip of the blade and the emergence of the ET are different, intubation is facilitated by localizing the vocal cords in the lower half of the viewfinder. The ET can then be advanced through the vocal cords under vision.

Should any doubt be present as to the ET's location, the ET position can be confirmed using conventional means, with the device in situ. To remove the device, grasp the ET firmly and slide the device from the ET, using a motion that is a reverse of that used to enter the pharynx.

Should difficulty arise in intubation while the cords are visualized, a number of options are available. A control-tip ET or a Schroeder stylet may be used to guide the tip through the vocal cords. Similarly, a bougie can be passed through the ET in order to guide the ET through the cords. If a very difficult airway is encountered, a fiberoptic bronchoscope may be passed through the ET to guide the ET through the cords. This technique is especially useful in those patients with an anterior larynx.

The UpsherScope was evaluated in 200 patients with normal airways and was successful in 191, with a median intubation time of 38 seconds.[47] Difficulties were encountered in elevation of the epiglottis, passage of the ET through the vocal cords, and secretions' interference with the view.

WuScope System

The WuScope (Pentax) (Fig. 7–4) is conceptually similar to both the Bullard laryngoscope and the UpsherScope. It has a handle, an anatomi-

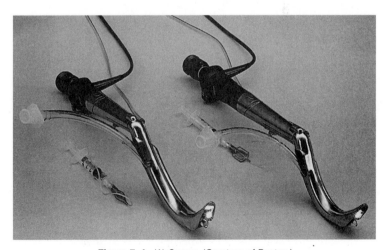

Figure 7–4 WuScope. (Courtesy of Pentax.)

cally designed blade, a fiberoptic view port, and a port for oxygen insufflation. There are, however, a number of differences. The fiberoptic mechanism consists of a Pentax fiberoptic rhinolaryngoscope Achi LA-S1 and thus cannot be used with a battery handle. This custom fiberscope is equivalent to the Pentax FNL-10RP2, the Olympus ENF-P3, or the Machida ENF-3L flexible fiberscopes. The blade portion has three detachable stainless steel parts including a cone-shaped tube that receives the fiberscope superiorly and connects to the main blades at the base. The main blade and the bivalve element are arc shaped, each having corresponding grooves that form a larger passageway for the ET and a smaller passageway for the fiberscope insertion cord. An opening to insert the ET is created when the three parts are positioned together. The tubular aspect of the blade helps create a viewing space when tumors, trauma, edema, or inflammation obscure the posterior pharynx.[10] The oxygen channel is positioned along the fibercord passageway.

The axes of the handle and the blade lie at an angle of 110 degrees. By separate interlocking mechanisms, the bivalve element can be attached or released easily at the main blade and the handle. Using the rigid bivalved blade is difficult initially but is soon mastered. It is recommended that assembling the rigid blade portion be practiced until familiarity is gained with all the parts and interlocking mechanisms before attempting to assemble the entire device together. Two adult sizes are available, large adult and adult.[10] The regular adult-sized blade is adequate for intubation in most cases (85%). The best way to gauge the appropriate size is to hold it next to the patient's profile so that the distal end of the blade reaches the hyoid. When the adult-sized scope blade is used, the extender should always be attached to the handle. Once the device is assembled, certain rules must be followed: (1) always hold the device at the metal handle portion, not the extender portion, and (2) *do not* touch the angulation control lever (a piece of tape may be placed over the lever for a reminder).

■ Technique

The ET is encased within the device. Using the same technique as for the UpsherScope and Bullard laryngoscopes, insert the device into the mouth, remaining midline. When the vocal cords are visualized, align a suction catheter that was passed through an ET with the glottis and advance the ET through the vocal cords.[48] Disassemble the WuScope after intubation and gently remove it from the mouth. Remove the bivalve element from the patient's mouth first; the handle, main blade, and fiberscope are then removed as one unit, leaving the ET in place. In order to use the WuScope for nasal intubation, the bivalve element is not attached. After the ET is passed into the oropharynx through the naris, insert the device into the oral cavity, as previously described. Allow the concave undersurface of the distal main blade to straddle the ET and guide it toward the larynx and into the trachea.

The inventor evaluated the WuScope in more than 350 tracheal intubations over a 15-month period, including intubations in 56 patients with Mallampati classification III and IV without any complications. Visualization of the larynx was easy in all cases, with an average intubation time (from insertion of the blade into the patient's mouth to the removal of the device) of 47 seconds (range 25 to 75). A longer average intubation time (72 seconds) was found in patients with acute pathologic changes to the upper oral airway.

Augustine Scope

The Augustine scope also has an anatomically designed blade with an ET channel (which holds the ET in place), a battery power source, and a fiberoptic scope. A number of differences exist between it and the other rigid fiberoptic laryngoscopes. The leading edge has a midline indentation and two lateral bulbous protrusions. When seated in the vallecula, the midline indentation straddles the hyoepiglottic ligament, and the two bulbous protrusions lock into the recesses of the vallecula and engage beneath the hyoid bone. The vocal cords are exposed by lifting the device anteriorly. An improved view of the vocal cords is attained with an epiglottis lifter that is activated by sliding the ET through the tube channel.[48] The ET channel positions the ET at the opening between the vocal cords, and the ET is inserted under direct vision. This device also does not have any suction ports, and any suctioning, oxygen insufflation, and local anesthetic instillation are performed through the lumen of the ET.

Although the Augustine scope has yet to be manufactured, researchers have found it to be an effective device. One clinical study has been published that compared the Augustine scope to direct laryngoscopy[49] and found that the mean time to perform intubation was 19 ± 10 seconds compared with 21 ± 13 seconds in the direct-laryngoscopy group. In the Augustine group, 102 of 104 patients were successfully intubated. Three patients who could not be intubated in the direct-laryngoscopy group were successfully intubated with the Augustine scope. Unlike the situation with the Bullard laryngoscope, once the vocal cords are in view, directing the ET into the trachea is fairly simple.

All of the fiberoptic laryngoscopes described have a number of features in common. All should be inserted in the midline, have the potential to traumatize the airway, and should be used with caution. Also, they all have an anatomically shaped blade that does not require head motion for insertion. With the exception of the Augustine scope, all can be used to facilitate nasotracheal intubation. An ET is passed through one of the nares while the device is passed into the oropharynx in the usual fashion. The ET is then guided into place under vision. A video camera can be attached to the eyepiece of any of the scopes for teaching purposes. Finally, all can be used in anesthetized or awake patients, provided topical anesthetic has been applied to the airway. The anesthesia practitioner should become familiarized with the use of these devices and gain proficiency in routine intubations before using them in difficult intubations. The most common mistakes made with the use of the fiberoptic laryngoscopes, compared with other methods of intubation, include the tendency of the practitioner to

1. Move the head and neck, which is unnecessary and contraindicated in certain clinical situations
2. Use force, which often distorts the patient's natural anatomy
3. Move too quickly, loosing proper orientation
4. Approach the glottic opening too closely, causing difficult alignment of the device with the ET

CUFFED OROPHARYNGEAL AIRWAY

In 1992, Greenberg and Toung were the first to describe the cuffed oropharyngeal airway (COPA) (Mallinckrodt Medical, Athlone, Ireland) as a potential airway during administration of anesthesia in spontaneously breathing patients.[50] The device is a modified Guedel airway with an inflatable distal cuff and a proximal 15-mm connector for attachment to the anesthetic breathing system (Fig. 7–5). The cuff was designed such that when inflated it would displace the base of the patient's tongue, form a seal with the pharynx, and elevate the epiglottis from the posterior pharyngeal wall in order to provide a clear airway. It is

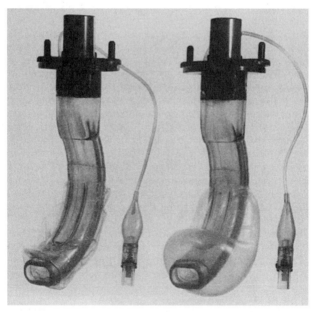

Figure 7–5 The cuffed oropharyngeal airway with the cuff inflated and deflated. (From Greenberg RS, Brimacombe J, Berry A, et al: A randomized controlled trial comparing the cuffed oropharyngeal airway and the laryngeal mask airway in spontaneously breathing anesthetized adults. Anesthesiology 88:970–977, 1998.

inflated through a one-way valve and pilot balloon that emerges from the COPA tube at the flange. The flange at the proximal end is fitted with two posts in order to secure the strap, which stabilizes the COPA at the mouth against the upper teeth or gums. The COPA is disposable, made from polyvinyl chloride, and available in four sizes—80, 90, 100, and 110—which refer to the distance measured in millimeters between the flange and the distal tip.

Recently, Greenberg and colleagues showed that the COPA and the laryngeal mask airway (LMA) are similar in establishing a safe and effective airway for spontaneously breathing anesthetized adults. They found that there were fewer manipulations required for insertion of the LMA and that it was faster to insert as compared to the COPA, whereas the use of the COPA was associated with fewer complications such as bleeding and sore throat.[51]

CONCLUSION

The devices discussed in this chapter all have limitations for their clinical use, but a knowledge of these devices can help facilitate particular specific airway problems.

REFERENCES

1. Ellis RH: The Cheerful Centenarian, or the Founder of Laryngoscopy. *In* Sykes WS (ed): Essays on the First Hundred Years of Anesthesia. Vol 2. Huntington, NY, Robert E Kreiger, 1972, pp 95–111.
2. MacIntosh R, Richards H: Illumination introducer for endotracheal tubes. Anesthesia 12:223, 1957.
3. Yamamura H, Yamamoto T, Kamiyama M: Device for blind nasal intubation. Anesthesiology 20:21, 1959.
4. Hung OR, Murphy M: Lightwands, lighted stylets and blind techniques of intubation. Anesthesiol Clin North Am 13:2, 1995.
5. Vollmer TP, Stewart RD, Paris PM, et al: Use of a lighted stylet for guided orotracheal intubation in the prehospital setting. Ann Emerg Med 14:324–328, 1985.
6. Ellis GE et al: Guided orotracheal intubation in the operating room using a lighted stylet: A comparison with direct laryngoscopic technique. Anesthesiology 64:823, 1986.
7. Ainsworth QP, Howells TH: Transilluminated tracheal intubation. Br J Anaesth 62:494, 1989.
8. Weis FR, Hatton MN: Intubation by use of the lightwand: Experience in 253 patients. J Oral Maxillofac Surg 47:577, 1989.
9. Trachlight™ Stylet and Tracheal Lightwand Instruction Manual. Armonk, N.Y., Laerdal Medical, Revised 1994.
10. Cooper SD: The evolution of upper airway retraction: New and old laryngoscope blades. *In* Benumof JL (ed): Airway Management Principles and Practice. St Louis, Mosby–Year Book, 1996, pp 374–411.
11. Stewart RD, La Rosee A, Kaplan RH, Ilkanipour K: Correct positioning of an endotracheal tube using a flexible lighted stylet. Crit Care Med 18:97–99, 1990.
12. Good ML: Airway Gadgets. ASA Refresher Course Lectures 531, San Francisco, Calif., Oct. 15–19, 1994.
13. Desai SP, Fenci V: A safe technique for changing endotracheal tubes. Anesthesiology 53:67, 1980.
14. Sellers WFS, Jones GW: Difficult tracheal intubation [letter]. Anaesthesia 41:93, 1986.

15. McCarroll SM, Lamont BJ, Buckland MR, Yates AP: The gum elastic bougie: Old but still useful [letter]. Anesthesiology 643–644, 1988.
16. Cooper RM: The difficult airway. II. Anesthesiol Clin North Am 13:3, 1995.
17. Kovac AL: The Augustine guide: A new device for blind orotracheal intubation. Anesthesiol Rev 20(1):25–29, 1993.
18. Instructions for Intubation Using the Augustine Guide. Eden Prairie, Minn, Augustine Medical, 1991.
19. Schwartz D, Johnson C, Roberts J: A maneuver to facilitate flexible fiberoptic intubation. Anesthesiology 71:470–471, 1989.
20. Watanabe S, Yaguchi Y, Suga A, Asakura N: A "Bubble-Tip" (Airguide) tracheal tube system: Its effects on incidence of epistaxis and ease of tube advancement in the subglottic region during nasotracheal intubation. Anesth Analg 78:1140–1143, 1994.
21. MacEwan W: Clinical observations on the introduction of tracheal tubes by mouth instead of performing tracheotomy or laryngoscopy. BMJ 2:122–124, 1880.
22. Miller RA: A new laryngoscope. Anesthesiology 2:317, 1941.
23. Choi JJ: A new double angled-blade for direct laryngoscopy. Anesthesiology 72:516, 1990.
24. Bizarri BV, Guffrida JG: Improved laryngoscope blade designed for ease of manipulation and reduction of trauma. Anesth Analg 37:231, 1958.
25. Cooper SD: Evolution of upper airway retraction: New and old laryngoscopy blades. In Benumof JL: Difficult Airway Management. Philadelphia, Mosby, 1996.
26. Choi JJ: A new double-angle blade for direct laryngoscopy. Anesthesiology 72:576, 1990.
27. Farling PA: The McCoy levering laryngoscope blade [letter]. Anaesthesia 49:358, 1994.
28. Johnston HM, Rao U: The McCoy levering laryngoscope blade [letter]. Anaesthesia 49:358, 1994.
29. Tuckey JP, Cook TM, Render CA: Forum. An evaluation of the levering laryngoscope. Anaesthesia 51:71–73, 1996.
30. Siker ES: A mirror laryngoscope. Anesthesiology 17:38, 1956.
31. Benumof JL: Management of the difficult adult airway: With special emphasis on awake tracheal intubation. Anesthesiology 75:1087–1110, 1991.
32. Kessell J: A laryngoscope for obstetrical use. Anaesth Intensive Care 5:265, 1977.
33. Patil VU, Stehling LC, Cander HL: An adjustable laryngoscope handle for difficult intubations. Anesthesiology 60:609, 1984.
34. Jellicoe JA, Harris NR: A modification of a standard laryngoscope for difficult tracheal intubations in obstetric cases. Anaesthesia 39:800, 1984.
35. Yentis SM: A laryngoscope adapter for difficult intubation. Anaesthesia 42:764, 1987.
36. Datta S, Briwa J: A modified laryngoscope for endotracheal intubation of obese patients. Anesth Analg 60:120, 1981.
37. McIntyre JWR: Airway equipment. Laryngoscopes, prisms, fiberoptic devices, and other adjuncts. Anesthesiol Clin North Am 13:309–324, 1995.
38. Bainton CR: A new laryngoscope blade to overcome pharyngeal obstruction, Anesthesiology 67, 767, 1987.
39. Abrams KJ: The Bullard Laryngoscope. Anesthesiol News Oct:66, 1995.
40. Abrams KJ, Desai N, Katsnelson T: Bullard laryngoscopy for trauma airway management in suspected cervical spine injuries. Anesth Analg 72;623: 1992.
41. Gorback MS: Management of the challenging airway with the Bullard laryngoscope. J Clin Anesth 3:473:1991.
42. Bjopraker DG: The Bullard intubating laryngoscopes. Anesth Rev 17(5):64, 1990.
43. Dyson A, Harris J, Bhatia K, et al: Rapidity and accuracy of tracheal intubation in a mannequin: Complications of the fiberoptic with the Bullard laryngoscope. Br J Anaesth 65:268–270, 1990.
44. Baraka A, Muallem M, Sibai AN: Facilitation of difficult tracheal intubation by the fiberoptic Bullard laryngoscope. Middle East J Anaesthiol 11:73–77, 1991.
45. Cooper SD, Benumof JL, Ozki GT: Evaluation of the Bullard laryngoscope using

the new intubating stylet: Comparison with conventional laryngoscopy. Anesth Analg 79:965, 1994.

46. Hastings RH, Vigil AC, Hanna R, et al: Cervical spine movement during laryngoscopy with the Bullard, Macintosk and Miller laryngoscopes. Anesthesiology 82:859–869, 1995.

47. Pearce AC, Shaw S, Macklin S: Evaluation of the UpsherScope. A new rigid fiberscope. Anaesthesia 51:561–564, 1996.

48. Wu T, Chou H: A new laryngoscope: The combination intubating device. Anesthesiology 81:1085, 1994.

49. Krafft P, Krenn CG, et al: Clinical trial of a new device for fiberoptic orotracheal intubation (Augustine scope) Anesth Analg 84:606–610, 1997.

50. Greenberg RS, Toung T: The cuffed oro-pharyngeal airway—a pilot study. Anesthesiology 77:A558, 1992.

51. Greenberg RS, Brimacombe J, Berry A, et al: A randomized controlled trial comparing the cuffed oropharyngeal airway and the laryngeal mask airway in spontaneously breathing anesthetized adults. Anesthesiology 88:970–977, 1998.

Chapter 8

Laryngeal Mask Airway

and Esophageal Tracheal

Combitube

Harold S. Minkowitz

The laryngeal mask airway (LMA) was first introduced in 1983 as an adjunct to airway management during anesthesia[1] and received FDA approval in 1991. This device is designed to seal the patient's larynx and direct inspired and expired gases to and from the trachea. The device consists of an oval inflatable cuff (which seals the larynx) in continuity with a wide-bore tube (Fig. 8–1). The anesthesia circuit or Ambu bag can be connected to the wide-bore tube by means of a standard 15-mm endotracheal tube (ET) connector. A number of sizes

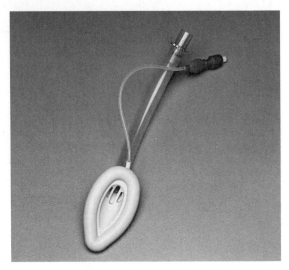

Figure 8–1 Laryngeal mask airway. (Courtesy of Kendall Healthcare Products Company.)

of LMA are available, each specifically designed to fit the larynx of patients of different weights (Table 8–1).

The LMA is a reusable device that must be sterilized before each use. The integrity of the cuff is determined by maximal inflation (checking for leaks) followed by maximal deflation (checking valve patency). The LMA should not be used if there is a herniation or thinning of the

Table 8–1   Description of Different Sizes of Laryngeal Mask Airway

Mask Size	Patient Size	LMA Tube (ID, mm)	LMA Tube Length (cm)	Maximum Cuff Volume (mL)	Largest ET (ID, mm)	FB Size (mm)
1	Neonates/infants up to 5 kg	5.25	11.5	4	3.5	2.7
1½	Infants 5–10 kg	6.1	13.5	7	4.0	3.0
2	Infants/children 10–20 kg	7.0	15.5	10	4.5	3.5
2½	Children 20–30 kg	8.4	17.5	14	5.0	4.0
3	Children over 30 kg and small adults	10	22	20	6.0 cuffed	5.0
4	Normal and large adults	10	22	30	6.0 cuffed	5.0
5	Large adults	11.5	23.5	40	7.0 cuffed	5.0

LMA, laryngeal mask airway; ET, endotracheal tube; FB, fiberoptic bronchoscope; ID, internal diameter.
Modified from Brain AIJ, Denman WT, Goudsouzian NG: *Laryngeal Mask Airway LMA-Classic™/LMA-Flexible™ Instruction Manual.* The Laryngeal Mask Company Ltd., LMA North America, Inc., San Diego, CA 92121, February 1999.

cuff when inflated with a volume of air greater than 50% of the maximal volume recommended.[2] Once examined in this fashion, the device can be prepared for use. The cuff should be maximally deflated, with its rim pointing away from the mask aperture forming a canoe-shaped cuff.[3] The posterior surface of the cuff is lubricated.

LARYNGEAL MASK AIRWAY INSERTION TECHNIQUE

After induction of anesthesia, the patient should be placed in the sniffing position and the LMA inserted into the oropharynx. Neither a laryngoscope nor muscle relaxation is necessary for its insertion. Using the correct insertion technique greatly facilitates its placement and optimal positioning. The LMA should be held between the thumb and index finger as close to the junction of the cuff and the tube as possible. The tip of the cuff is placed midline against the patient's hard palate, maintaining upward pressure. The device is advanced using the index finger and pushed as far as possible into the hypopharynx until resistance is met (usually at the location of the upper esophageal sphincter). The cuff is then filled with the correct volume of air for that particular size LMA (see Table 8–1). Additional inflation may result in suboptimal placement of the device, and no more air than recommended should be inserted. The tube should not be held or connected to the circuit during inflation. Once the cuff is inflated, the anesthesia circuit is attached and the ability to adequately ventilate is assessed.

Various other insertion techniques and aids to insertion have been described, although this technique provides superior results in terms of function and final anatomic position.[2] Optimal positioning is crucial when using the LMA as an intubation aid. The LMA should be removed only after the patient's protective airway reflexes have returned and the patient is able to open the mouth on command.[3] Removing the LMA under deep levels of anesthesia has been described[4] and may be useful in certain circumstances.

For most patients, spontaneous ventilation through the LMA is satisfactory. Positive-pressure ventilation can also be used with the LMA, but a leak between the larynx and the LMA may occur at higher inflation pressures. As ventilatory pressures increase, the leak fraction (leak as a fraction of inspired volume) increases. At 15 cm H_2O, the leak fraction was 13%, increasing to 25% at 25 cm H_2O.[5] A decrease in compliance may also increase the leak fraction. Composite data from three studies have shown that the esophagus lies within the LMA bowl in zero of 170 patients with the standard insertion technique, 8 of 140 when insertion was with the cuff inflated, and 3 of 30 when insertion was as a Guedel airway. Thus gastric distention may occur with prolonged positive-pressure ventilation. Research has not shown a clinically significant difference in gastric distention using positive-pressure ventilation with an LMA or an ET, provided inflation pressures remain below 20 cm H_2O.[6]

LARYNGEAL MASK AIRWAY AND THE DIFFICULT AIRWAY

The LMA is useful as an aid to oral intubation because of the anatomic alignment of the LMA aperture with the glottic opening when the LMA is properly placed. The clinician may use the LMA as the primary airway or as a conduit to facilitate endotracheal intubation. The LMA has been used to successfully intubate adults with a history of difficult tracheal intubation, limited mouth opening, or restricted neck movement, as well as children with Treacher Collins syndrome, Apert's syndrome, cleft palate, and juvenile chronic arthritis. It has also been used in patients in whom intubation or ventilation with a face mask proved to be impossible. The LMA fits into the American Society of Anesthesiologists (ASA) Difficult Airway Algorithm in four different places as either an airway (ventilatory device) or a conduit for endotracheal intubation (see Fig. 8–1).

Elective Use in Known Difficult Intubation

Patients with a history of difficult intubation should not be paralyzed, even if use of an LMA is intended, because placement may fail (up to 6%). There are a number of reports of failed ventilation through the LMA in patients with difficult airways,[7–9] as well as in patients whose tracheae were initially predicted to be easy to intubate. In certain circumstances, the LMA should be placed while the patient remains awake.[10] With good topical anesthesia, the LMA is very well tolerated. Once awake ventilation is confirmed, anesthesia may be induced or awake endotracheal intubation through the LMA may be performed.

Failed Intubation, Ability to Mask Ventilate

In the scenario of failed intubation with adequate face mask ventilation, LMA insertion may not be necessary and may even compromise the airway (i.e., if difficulty in LMA placement arises, or if coughing, aspiration, or laryngospasm occur because of light anesthesia). The LMA may even be placed if positive-pressure ventilation is desired or if subsequent tracheal intubation is required.

Failed Intubation, Inability to Mask Ventilate

In the scenario of failed intubation with inadequate face mask ventilation, the decision to use an LMA should be made early. While attempts are made to secure the airway with the LMA, preparation for a surgical airway or percutaneous transtracheal airway should be initiated, in the event that ventilation through the LMA is not successful. Once the airway has been secured with an LMA, decisions should be made as to further airway management. The patient may be awakened, and depending on the necessity of the operation and the condition of the airway, (1) the surgery can be canceled, (2) the patient can be intubated awake, or (3) regional anesthesia can be administered. If indicated, a surgical airway can be created. The decision for each technique must be individualized and tailored to the patient's specific situation.

Laryngeal Mask Airway as a Conduit for Endotracheal Intubation

The trachea may be intubated using the LMA as a conduit in patients known to be difficult to intubate.[11, 12] Also, in one study in which 96% of adult patients were thought to be easy to intubate by conventional means, successful endotracheal intubation was achieved by blindly passing an ET through the LMA.[13] In patients with difficult airway anatomy and limited neck movement, this technique may be associated with a lower success rate since the sniffing position cannot be used. The ET should be well lubricated. Rotating the ET 90 degrees counterclockwise can prevent the bevel from catching the bars of the LMA.[14] If the airway management plan is to intubate the trachea using the LMA as a guide, the tip of an ET may be passed through the aperture bars of the LMA before placement of the LMA in the airway.

One of the disadvantages of using the LMA as a conduit is that the ET diameter is limited by the size of the LMA (see Table 8–1). If a large ET is desired, a commercial tube changer or bougie may be used through the ET within the LMA in order to reintubate with the larger-sized ET. It must be remembered that after removal of the LMA, difficulty in placing the larger ET may arise, possibly resulting in the loss of the airway. A prototype intubating LMA has been described that allows the passage of larger-sized ETs (8 or above), thus eliminating this problem.[15] When intubating through the LMA, one should use the largest ET available (i.e., the nasal ET or Mallinckrodt microlaryngeal tube) to ensure an adequate distance beyond the vocal cords. Several other airway devices may be used in order to facilitate endotracheal intubation through the LMA.

The most reliable technique of endotracheal intubation using the LMA as a conduit involves using the fiberoptic bronchoscope as a guide. The fiberoptic bronchoscope, preloaded with an ET, can be guided into the trachea. The carina is visualized and the ETs railroaded over the fiberoptic bronchoscope into the trachea. This technique has a high success rate in patients with difficult airways.[11] Also, one may pass a bougie through the LMA with the angulated tip pointing anteriorly, rotating it 180 degrees once it passes through the grille of the LMA.[16] Once the bougie has passed through the vocal cords, an ET can be railroaded over it either with the LMA in place or with the LMA removed.

Cricoid Pressure with the Laryngeal Mask Airway

The application of cricoid pressure may reduce the ease of placement of the LMA. The combined results from five studies suggest that LMA insertion has a higher success rate without than with the application of cricoid pressure (94% versus 79%).[17–21] However, these studies used different techniques to apply cricoid pressure along with different neck positioning. Cricoid pressure may be temporarily released during LMA placement to obtain a higher success rate, although there is an increased risk of pulmonary aspiration during this period.[2] Cricoid pressure applied after placement of the LMA is effective[22] and does not usually dislodge the mask.[23] An algorithm has been developed for the use of cricoid pressure with the LMA (see Fig. 13–2).

LARYNGEAL MASK AIRWAY IN RESUSCITATION

Securing the airway with an ET is an essential part of all resuscitation protocols. However, the LMA may provide better airway management than a face mask or attempts at intubation made by inadequately trained personnel. With inexperienced personnel, the LMA can be correctly placed more often than an ET.[24] Having more personnel trained in sufficient airway management skills may prevent hypoxia until more experienced personnel are available to provide definitive care.[25] Most patients being resuscitated are considered to be at risk for aspiration, and therefore cricoid pressure should be maintained, if possible.

Contraindications

The LMA may be unsuitable under the following conditions (Table 8–2):[26]

1. *Risk of aspiration.* The LMA does not protect the tracheobronchial tree from the contents of the gastrointestinal tract. The LMA may actively reduce lower esophageal sphincter tone by reflex relaxation,[27, 28] but this may not be clinically significant.

2. *Residual upper airway reflexes.* Full mouth and pharyngeal relaxation are required to insert the LMA. Thus, patients need to be adequately anesthetized: otherwise, patients may gag, cough, vomit, develop laryngospasm, or bite down on the tube.

3. *Poor pulmonary status.* The LMA is unsuitable for positive-pressure ventilation of patients with either high airway resistance or low pulmonary compliance. At high inspiratory pressures, an air leak around the cuff may occur.

4. *Laryngeal problems.* The LMA cannot overcome obstruction at the level of the larynx. It is a supraglottic method of intubation. In the patient with laryngospasm, attempting to ventilate the lungs may force air into the stomach and increase the risk of aspiration.

5. *Local pharyngeal abnormality.* The device is generally unsuitable in patients with local pharyngeal abnormality, including

Table 8–2 Contraindications to the Use of the Laryngeal Mask Airway

Risk of aspiration
Residual upper airway reflexes
Poor pulmonary status
Laryngeal problems
Local pharyngeal abnormality

parapharyngeal or pharyngeal abscesses, edema, and hematomas.

Special Indications

The LMA may be used for airway management for patients anesthetized for fiberoptic bronchoscopy. As discussed earlier, the LMA provides an excellent conduit for flexible fiberoptic bronchoscopy, with the patient either under general anesthesia or awake with adequate topicalization. The LMA may be used in patients with tracheal stenosis when general anesthesia is required, or when a face mask cannot be used because of limited access or poor fit. Also, the LMA may be advantageous for professional voice users requiring general anesthesia, since it has been reported to produce fewer voice changes than endotracheal intubation.

In 1997, a modification that enhances the use of the LMA as an intubation guide was introduced into the clinical setting. This device, referred to as the intubating laryngeal mask (ILM), can be used for elective or emergency ventilation and serves as an excellent conduit for intubation.

The ILM (Fig. 8–2) consists of a mask attached to a rigid stainless steel tube curved to align the barrel aperture to the glottic vestibule. The ILM has a 13-mm internal diameter that can accommodate an 8.0-mm cuffed tracheal tube, which can be inserted into the larynx either

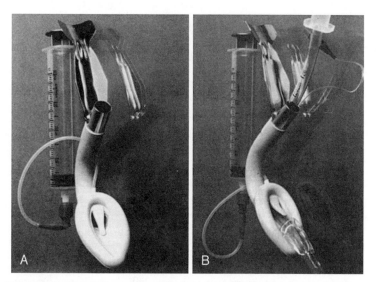

Figure 8–2 *A*, Intubating laryngeal mask. *B*, Intubating laryngeal mask with the tracheal tube. (From Rosenblatt WH, Murphy M: The intubating laryngeal mask; use of a new ventilating-intubating device in the emergency department. Ann Emerg Med 33:234–238, 1999.)

blindly or fiberoptically. The device is short enough to ensure that the tracheal tube cuff extends beyond the vocal cords. The mask of the ILM is similar to that of the standard LMA, but with two important differences: lying vertically across the mask aperture is a single, stiff bar designed to lift the epiglottis away from the path of the tracheal tube, and within the barrel mask junction is a ramp designed to direct the tube centrally. A handle incorporated into the ILM facilitates its insertion, manipulation, and removal, especially in patients whose head and neck cannot be manipulated (e.g., because of cervical spine injury). The ILM is produced in adult sizes with cuffs equivalent to size 3, 4, and 5 LMAs.[29–31]

The ILM offers a method of rescue ventilation and oxygenation in any failed intubation when there is anticipated difficulty with direct laryngoscopy, or when awake blind nasal intubation is contraindicated or impossible. As with any new airway device, practice is required in order to become proficient and is encouraged during treatment of nonemergent cases.[32]

ESOPHAGEAL OBTURATOR AIRWAY

The esophageal obturator airway was designed as an alternative means to secure the airway in an emergency. The device is 34 cm long, with a balloon at its distal tip. It has one lumen and one balloon. The distal end is closed. Sixteen holes lie proximal to the balloon. When correctly positioned, these holes lie in the region of the hypopharynx. Proximally, a face mask is connected, sealing the mouth and nose during ventilation. The esophageal obturator airway is placed in the esophagus and the balloon is inflated. The face mask is placed against the patient's face. Air then enters through the holes in the hypopharynx and ventilates the trachea since the mouth and nose are sealed by the mask and the esophagus is sealed by the balloon. In the controlled environment of the operating room, technical difficulties were associated with the device.[33] There were a number of problems with the esophageal obturator airway, including significant difficulties in obtaining a tight mask seal[33, 34] and unrecognized tracheal intubation resulting in total airway obstruction.[35] With these disadvantages in mind, the esophageal tracheal Combitube was designed.

ESOPHAGEAL TRACHEAL COMBITUBE

The Combitube (Kendall Sheridan Catheter Corp., Argyle, N.Y.) (Fig. 8–3) combines the features of a conventional ET and that of an esophageal obturator airway. It is a double-lumen tube with an esophageal lumen and a tracheal lumen. The esophageal lumen has an open upper end and a closed distal end. There are perforations at the pharyngeal level. The tracheal lumen has an open distal end with no perforations down its length. An oropharyngeal latex balloon seals the oral and nasal cavities, and after inflation the balloon presses against the base of the tongue and closes the soft palate. A smaller distal cuff seals the esophagus or the trachea depending on the position of the Combitube.

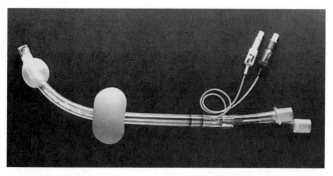

Figure 8–3 Combitube. (Courtesy of Gensia Automedics, Inc.)

The proximal end of the esophageal lumen is blue and marked as number 1. It is 2 cm longer than the tracheal lumen, which is clear and marked number 2.

Physical Features

The Combitube is a disposable double-lumen tube that comes in two sizes, the large adult size (for individuals greater than 5½ feet tall) and small adult size (for individuals 4 to 5½ feet tall). The longer lumen resembles a cuffed ET. The shorter lumen resembles an esophageal obturator airway since its distal end is occluded. It has eight oval side openings, each approximately 4 mm in diameter. A large proximal balloon seals the upper airway and anchors the device in place. Lung ventilation is possible with either tracheal or esophageal intubation. Unlike the LMA, the Combitube should protect against aspiration and was designed for emergency ventilation. It was approved by the FDA for use as an airway device in 1988.

Insertion Technique

The Combitube is inserted blindly into the mouth with the thumb of the nondominant hand after pulling the tongue and lower jaw upward. After the device is inserted into the mouth, it is advanced in a downward and curved movement until the printed rings are aligned with the teeth. The esophagus is usually entered with blind placement, and if difficulty is experienced, a rigid laryngoscope may be used to aid placement. The distal balloon is then filled with 5 to 15 mL of air in order to seal the esophagus. In order to seal the oral and nasal passages and to secure the tube in position, the proximal balloon is filled with approximately 100 mL of air in the large-adult–sized Combitube or approximately 85 mL in the small-adult–sized Combitube using the large syringe provided. This balloon should actually be inflated until an adequate seal has been obtained.

With blind insertion, there is a high probability that esophageal placement will result; therefore, one should ventilate through the esophageal lumen (blue, marked number 1) first. Ventilation forces air through the perforations in the esophageal lumen into the pharynx and out into the trachea. Esophageal placement is confirmed by breath sounds in the absence of gastric insufflation, and ventilation is continued through this lumen. If breath sounds are absent when ventilating through lumen number 1, the device has entered the trachea. The tube position is not changed, and ventilation through the clear, shorter tracheal tube number 2 is commenced. Correct position is confirmed by auscultation.

If ventilation is unsatisfactory through both lumens, then the Combitube was probably advanced too far, resulting in obstruction of the airway by the proximal balloon. The device should then be withdrawn about 1 inch, with both cuffs deflated. Ventilation is then confirmed in the standard manner as described earlier.[36] Confirmation of correct placement has also been accomplished using the Easy Cap in the dog model.

The major indication is as a backup device for airway management.[37] Indications for placement of a Combitube include emergency use both in and out of the hospital environment. It can be used in situations of difficult or failed intubation or for resuscitation by individuals not skilled in endotracheal intubation;[38] in situations of limited access to the patient's head; and in patients in whom neck movement is contraindicated (e.g., cervical spine injury). Uses in elective surgery include patients with known difficult airways or professional voice users concerned about vocal cord damage with endotracheal intubation. Contraindications to the use of the Combitube are listed in Table 8–3.

There are a number of differences between Combitube insertion and endotracheal intubation. For Combitube insertion, the patient does not have to be in the "sniffing" position, and the operator may stand behind the patient, to the side of the patient, or face to face with the patient.[37]

To replace a Combitube (Table 8–4) located in the esophagus with an ET, one should first deflate the proximal balloon and attempt endotracheal intubation with the Combitube in place. If the endotracheal intubation is successful, the lower balloon may be deflated and the device removed. If intubation of the trachea with an ET is unsuccessful, one should keep the lower balloon inflated, thus preventing aspiration, reinflate the proximal balloon, and recommence ventilation until either another attempt at intubation is begun or a surgical airway is estab-

Table 8–3   Contraindications to the Use of the Combitube

Height <4 ft
Intact gag reflexes
Esophageal abnormality
Ingestion of caustic substances
Upper airway obstruction
Latex allergy

Table 8–4   Exchanging Esophageal Tracheal Combitube for Endotracheal Tube

ESOPHAGEAL POSITION

1. Deflate oropharyngeal balloon
2. Move ETC to left side
3. Perform direct laryngoscopy or use FB
4. Place ET and confirm placement
5. Deflate small distal cuff and remove ETC

TRACHEAL POSITION

1. Use airway exchange device in lumen no. 2 (tracheal lumen)
2. Deflate both oropharyngeal balloon and distal cuff
3. Remove ETC
4. Railroad ET over AEC

ETC, esophageal tracheal Combitube; FB, fiberoptic bronchoscope; ET, endotracheal tube; AEC, airway exchange catheter.

lished. To replace a Combitube with an ET in the trachea, one can simply use an appropriately sized tube exchange catheter through the tracheal lumen, deflate both cuffs, and remove it over the exchange catheter.

Advantages of the Combitube include rapid control of the airway, protection against aspiration, no requirement for head movement, and potential use by relatively inexperienced personnel. Disadvantages include possible esophageal damage and an inability to suction the trachea in the esophageal position.

In patients undergoing elective general anesthesia, ventilation with the Combitube results in a higher Pao_2 than ventilation with an ET. This was found to be caused by a small degree of positive end-expiratory pressure with the Combitube caused by an increased resistance to expiratory flow with this device. Additionally, the vocal cords were not bypassed with the Combitube, in contrast to the situation when an ET was used.[39] The Combitube has been used successfully in obstetric anesthesia, using a laryngoscope to guide the tube into the esophagus.[40] The Combitube inserted by intensive care unit nurses under medical supervision was found to be as effective as an ET inserted by intensive care unit physicians during cardiopulmonary resuscitation.[41] In the prehospital setting, the Combitube was successfully inserted by paramedics in 71% of patients when inserted as a first-line device to control the airway. It was successfully inserted in 64% of patients who could not be intubated using direct laryngoscopy.[42] The ASA Task Force on Management of the Difficult Airway has recommended use of the Combitube when an anesthetized patient cannot be intubated or mask ventilated.[43] When compared with the LMA, the Combitube provides some protection against regurgitation and allows positive-pressure ventilation at inflation pressures greater than 20 cm H_2O. The Combitube may be used in patients in whom direct visualization of the vocal cords is not possible, as in patients with massive airway bleeding or regurgitation.[44]

CONCLUSION

The LMA and Combitube have revolutionized modern airway management in both the emergent and nonemergent securing of the airway.

REFERENCES

1. Brain AIJ: The laryngeal mask airway—A new concept in airway management. Br J Anesth 55:801–805, 1983.
2. Brimacombe J, Berry A: Insertion of the laryngeal mask airway—A prospective study of four techniques. Anaesth Intensive Care 21:89–92, 1993.
3. Asai T, Morris S: The laryngeal mask airway: Its features, effects and role. Can J Anaesth 41:10, 930–60, 1994.
4. Erskine RJ, Rabey PG: The laryngeal mask airway in recovery [Letter]. Anaesthesia 47:531–532, 1992.
5. Devitt JH, Wenstone R, Noel AG, O'Donnell MP: The laryngeal mask airway and positive pressure ventilation. Anesthesiology 80:550–555, 1994.
6. Brain AIJ: Risk of aspiration with the laryngeal mask [Letter]. Br J Anaesth 73:278, 1994.
7. Collier C: A hazard with the laryngeal mask airway [letter]. Anaesth Intensive Care 19:301, 1991.
8. Christian AS. Failed obstetric intubation [letter]. Anaesthesia 45:995, 1990.
9. Russsell SH, Hirsch NP: Simultaneous use of two laryngoscopes [letter]. Anaesthesia 48:918, 1993.
10. McCirrick A, Pracillio JA. Awake intubation: A new technique. Anaesthesia 46:661–663, 1991.
11. Silk JM, Hill HM, Calder I: Difficult intubation and the laryngeal mask. Eur J Anesthesiol 4:47–51, 1991.
12. Asai T: Fiberoptic intubation through the laryngeal mask in an awake patient with a cervical spine injury [letter]. Anesth Analg 77:404, 1993.
13. Heath ML, Allagain J: Intubation through the laryngeal mask. A technique for unexpected difficult intubation. Anaesthesia 46:545–548, 1991.
14. Heath ML: Endotracheal intubation through the laryngeal mask: Helpful when laryngoscopy is difficult or dangerous. Eur J Anaesthesiol 4:41, 1991.
15. Brain AIJ: Three cases of difficult intubation overcome by the laryngeal mask airway. Anaesthesia 40:353, 1985.
16. Chadd GD, Ackers JWL, Bailey PM: Difficult intubation aided by the laryngeal mask airway [letter]. Anaesthesia 44:1015, 1989.
17. Ansermino JM, Blogg CE: Cricoid pressure may prevent insertion of he laryngeal mask airway. Br J Anaesth 69:465–467, 1992.
18. Asai T, Barclay K, Power I, Vaughan RS: Cricoid pressure impedes placement of the laryngeal mask airway. Br J Anaesth 74:521–525, 1995.
19. Brimacombe J: Cricoid pressure and the laryngeal mask airway. Anaesthesia 46:986–987, 1991.
20. Brimacombe J, White A, Berry A: Effect of cricoid pressure on ease of insertion of the laryngeal mask airway. Br J Anaesth 71:800–802, 1993.
21. Heath ML, Allagain J: Intubation through the laryngeal mask—A technique for unexpected difficult intubation. Anaesthesia 46:366–367, 1991.
22. Strang TI: Does the laryngeal mask airway compromise cricoid pressure? Anaesthesia, 47:829–831, 1992.
23. Asai T: Use of the laryngeal mask for tracheal intubation in patients at increased risk for aspiration of gastric contents. Anesthesiology 77:1029–1030, 1992.
24. Pennant JH, Walker MB: Comparison of the endotracheal tube and laryngeal mask in airway management by paramedical personnel. Anesth Analges 74:531, 1992.
25. Joshi GP, Smith I, White PF: Laryngeal mask airway. In Benumof JL (ed): Airway Management: Principles and Practice. St Louis, Mosby–Year Book, 1996, pp 353–373.
26. Fisher JA: Role of the laryngeal mask in airway management. Can J Anaesth 39:1–3, 1992.

27. Owens T, Robertson P, Twomey K, et al: Incidence of gastroesophageal reflux with the laryngeal mask. Anesthesiology 79:A1053, 1993.
28. Rabey PG, Murphy PJ, Langton JA, et al: The effect of the laryngeal mask airway on lower esophageal sphincter pressure in patients during general anesthesia. Br J Anaesth 69:346–348, 1992.
29. Kapila A, Addy EV, Verghese C, et al: The intubating laryngeal mask airway: An initial assessment of performance. Br J Anaesth 79:710–713, 1997.
30. Brain AI, Verghese C, Addy EV, et al: The intubating laryngeal mask: II. A preliminary clinical report of a new means for intubating the trachea. Br J Anaesth 79:704–709, 1997.
31. Brain AI, Verghese C, Addy EV, et al: The intubating laryngeal mask: I. Development of a new device for intubation of the trachea. Br J Anaesth 79:703, 1997.
32. Rosenblatt WH, Murphy M: The intubating laryngeal mask: Use of a new ventilating-intubating device in the emergency department. Ann Emerg Med 33(2):234–238, 1999.
33. Bryson TK, Benumof JL, Ward CF: The esophageal obturator airway: A clinical comparison of ventilation with a mask and oropharyngeal airway. Chest 74:537, 1978.
34. Hammargren Y, Clinton JE, Ruiz E: A standard comparison of the esophageal obturator airway and endotracheal tube intubation in cardiac arrest. Ann Emerg Med 14:953, 1985.
35. Gertler JP, Cameron DE, Shea K, Baker CC: The esophageal obturator airway: Obturator or obtundator? J Trauma 25:424–426, 1985.
36. Frass M, Johnson JC, Atherton GL, et al: Esophageal tracheal Combitube (ETC) for emergency intubation: Anatomical evaluation of ETC placement by radiography. Resuscitation 18:95–102, 1989.
37. Frass M: The Combitube: Esophageal/tracheal double lumen airway. *In* Benumof JL (ed): Airway Management: Principles and Practice. St Louis, Mosby–Year Book, 1996.
38. Johnson JC, Atherton GL: The esophageal tracheal Combitube: An alternative route to airway management. JEMS 29, May 1991.
39. Frass M, Rodler S, Frenzer R, et al: Esophageal tracheal Combitube, endotracheal airway and mask: Comparison of ventilatory pressure curves. J Trauma 29:1476–1479, 1989.
40. Wissler RN: The esophageal-tracheal Combitube. Anesth Rev 20:147, 1993.
41. Staudinger T, Brugger S, Watschinger B, et al: Emergency intubation with the Combitube: comparison with endotracheal airway. Ann Emerg Med 22:1572–1575, 1993.
42. Atherton GL, Johnson JC: Ability of paramedics to use the Combitube in prehospital cardiac arrest. Ann Emerg Med 22:1263, 1993.
43. The American Society of Anesthesiologists Task Force on Management of the Difficult Airway: Practice guidelines for management of the difficult airway. Anesthesiology 78:597, 1993.
44. Cozine K, Stone G: The take back patient in ear, nose and throat surgery. Anesthesiol Clin North Am 11(3):651–679, 1993.

Chapter 9

Surgical Approaches to
Airway Management for
Anesthesia Practitioners

Mark E. K. Wong and Jon P. Bradrick

SURGICAL AIRWAYS: PERSPECTIVE OF AN ANESTHESIA PRACTITIONER

A surgical airway may be defined as an airway established transcutaneously as an alternative to traditional transoral or transnasal intubation. Most discussions of this topic adopt the perspective of the surgeon, which is different from that of the anesthesia practitioner in several important respects. Professional expertise notwithstanding, the surgeon may require a surgical airway under conditions different from those required by the anesthesia practitioner. Although surgeons may be called on to perform an emergent cricothyroidotomy or tracheostomy, most surgical airways are established under controlled conditions. The patient is already intubated or sufficient time permits careful dissection under local anesthesia. The emphasis in this chapter is therefore on providing guidance to individuals who do not routinely establish surgical airways and who, when faced with this requirement, find themselves confronted with a true medical emergency. Anticipation, preparation, simplicity, speed, and verification form the fundamental characteristics of the primary procedures advocated. More sophisticated and time-consuming maneuvers are included for completeness, but these techniques are often not feasible during emergency airway management.

ANTICIPATION OF POTENTIAL AIRWAY PROBLEMS

A surgical airway becomes necessary when impending airway loss cannot be averted with mask-supported oxygenation and ventilation or traditional transnasal or transoral intubation. Situations in which this might occur include patients with airway compromise from maxillofacial trauma or from pharyngeal or laryngeal trauma or abnormality; and patients who lack oral access because of intermaxillary fixation, or masticatory space infection limitation of temporomandibular joint motion. Early identification of these patients allows anesthesia practitioners an opportunity to prepare for potential airway loss while attempting intubation in this potentially problematic group of patients.

Maxillofacial Trauma

Severe injury to the maxillofacial skeleton may complicate oral or nasal intubation for several reasons. Active bleeding into the nasopharynx and oropharynx can obscure the field or cause laryngospasm. Continuous suctioning through a large-diameter suction tip (e.g., Yankauer) and a strong light are used to improve visualization of the upper airway. Facial fractures can also distort the anatomy, causing airway embarrassment. During emergencies, the exact location and extent of facial fractures are less important than the following features, which can be determined rapidly:

- *Narrowing of the upper airway through displacement of bony structures.* Fracture and displacement of the nasal bones may reduce the size of the posterior nares, although a decrease on one side may be accompanied by an increase in diameter of the contralateral nostril. Bilateral fractures of the mandible may compromise the airway if anterior support to the tongue is lost. Obstruction results from the tongue falling back and may not be corrected with the classic chin-lift or jaw-thrust maneuver. However, direct laryngoscopy is still possible, and successful intubation will protect the upper airway.

- *Communication of the nasal airway with the anterior cranial fossa.* Much is made of the potential for inadvertently introducing an endotracheal tube into the anterior cranial fossa through a fractured cribriform plate. According to the *Advanced Trauma Life Support Provider Manual,*[1] nasal intubations are strictly contraindicated in the presence of cribriform plate or basilar skull fractures.[2] The problem lies in accurately identifying the presence of such a fracture during emergencies. Cerebrospinal fluid leakage, which appears as a thin, yellow discharge from the nose, is a sign of disruption of the cribriform plate *with* an associated dural tear. However, this sign is often obscured by nasal bleeding and may be absent in the presence of a cribriform plate fracture if the dura remains intact. If a nasal intubation is contemplated, deliberately directing the endotracheal tube in a caudal direction will avoid insertion of the tube intracranially. Alternatively, a flexible guide may be introduced first through the nose and visualized in the nasopharynx before an endotracheal tube is passed over the guide.[3, 4] If excessive bleeding or mobility of the facial skeleton prevents oral or nasal intubation, a surgical airway remains the only alternative. This should be established without undue delay or multiple attempts at intubation, which often provokes more bleeding and increases soft tissue edema.

Pharyngeal Trauma or Abnormality

Pharyngeal trauma affects soft tissue and results in bleeding and edema that may prevent visualization of the vocal cords. Abnormalities that may affect this region include harmatomas, neoplasms, or peritonsillar abscesses (quinsy) that occupy the pharyngeal space, reducing patency. These conditions are identified through a quick examination of the oropharynx with direct laryngoscopy or rigid bronchoscopy. Even if sufficient space adjacent to a pathologic lesion is available for tube passage, the possibility of violating the lesion during intubation should still be considered. Such an event may result in excessive bleeding or rupture of an abscess into the airway. If the upper airway has been sufficiently narrowed, a surgical airway should be considered.

Laryngeal Trauma or Abnormality

Suspicions should be raised concerning the possibility of a laryngeal fracture in patients who sustain blunt or penetrating trauma to the neck and present with ecchymosis over the larynx, hoarseness, stridor, or cervical subcutaneous emphysema.[1] These patients are candidates for a cricothyroidotomy or tracheostomy, which ideally should be performed under local anesthesia before acute airway distress occurs.[5] High-pressure insufflation techniques should be avoided because of the likelihood of introducing additional air into the paralaryngeal soft tissue.[6] If the patient is sufficiently stable for a computed tomographic examination of the neck, essential information concerning the level and characteristics of the laryngeal injury can be obtained. Neoplasms of the larynx or enlarged cervical lymph nodes can distort or displace the larynx, and this should be taken into consideration if a surgical airway is required. Once again, preoperative computed tomography is invaluable for characterizing the size and position of space-occupying masses.[7]

Restricted Oral Access from Intermaxillary Fixation

Patients with fractures of the maxilla or mandible or those who have undergone elective osteotomies (e.g., orthognathic surgery) are often placed into intermaxillary fixation to facilitate healing in the correct position. Fixation may be achieved with stainless steel wires or elastic bands. If a patient in intermaxillary fixation experiences airway compromise, the fixation may be removed by cutting the wires or elastic bands with wire cutters or a pair of scissors. Direct laryngoscopy can then be performed in the standard fashion. When the fixation cannot be released because of a lack of instrumentation or patient compliance, blind or fiberoptic-guided intubations or a surgical airway remain the only alternatives.

Restricted Oral Access from Masticatory Space Infection

Infections of the head and neck, regardless of the source, may become disseminated and involve the various fascial spaces surrounding the different muscles of mastication: the temporalis, masseter, and medial pterygoid. In the early stages, a reflex myospasm restricts the mandible's range of motion, producing trismus.[8] This condition may be relieved by administering muscle relaxants or inducing a deep plane of anesthesia. Chronic infections, on the other hand, limit mouth opening, because of muscle fibrosis. Muscle relaxants or oversedation will not improve the situation and if administered with the expectation of relieving trismus, hasten the need for an emergent surgical airway if mask ventilation fails.[9] Distinguishing between an early or chronic infection is difficult, although the patient's history may be helpful. Alternatively, regional local anesthetic blocks of the affected muscles may be used to differentiate between myospasm or fibrosis as causes of trismus.

Infections adjacent to facial muscles not involved with mandibular motion complicate intubation through different mechanisms. Sublingual space abscesses located between the floor of the mouth and the mylohyoid muscle can elevate the tongue, preventing anterior retraction during laryngoscopy. Bilateral infections of the submandibular spaces in association with bilateral sublingual abscesses and submental space involvement represent a particularly dangerous condition known as *Ludwig's angina*. When this occurs, significant swelling around the neck can displace and narrow the airway while producing edema of the pharyngeal and laryngeal soft tissue and vocal cords. Cervical involvement can be demonstrated through the use of computed tomographic studies.[10] Patients also experience difficulty controlling their secretions, which makes intubation even more difficult. A potentially lethal variation of Ludwig's angina is associated with direct extension of the infection from the cervical region through the paralaryngeal spaces into the mediastinum.[11] Erythema over the neck and chest and signs of gross septicemia are signs of mediastinal involvement.[12] Immunocompromised patients should be considered at significant risk for developing this condition. Infection involving the paralaryngeal spaces complicates surgical airways by altering the tissue planes of the neck as a result of muscle necrosis and accumulation of purulent material. If at all possible, this situation should be avoided by early and aggressive incision and drainage of orofacial infections.

Restricted Access from Temporomandibular Joint Abnormality

There are essentially two categories of temporomandibular joint abnormality that may restrict mandibular mobility. Internal derangements of the joint comprise a number of conditions in which distortion of intraarticular or periarticular structures limits joint motion through either physical obstruction or pain.[13] The obstruction, however, is seldom so significant as to prevent direct laryngoscopy, and standard induction techniques can be used. If there is an element of doubt, diagnostic injections of local anesthetic into the affected joint should establish the mandible's range of motion. The second group of temporomandibular joint abnormalities encompasses conditions in which the joint is ankylosed to the cranial base with bone *(bony ankylosis)* or tight scar bands *(fibrous ankylosis)*.[14] When either is present, the restriction of mandibular motion is absolute and intubation invariably involves a fiberoptic-guided technique, blind intubation, or surgical airway.

DEVELOPMENT OF AN APPROACH TO AIRWAY PROBLEMS

The different conditions that commonly affect airway access have been described. Recognizing their potential impact on the airway alerts anesthesia practitioners to critically evaluate their attempts with traditional intubation. The number of attempts at intubation is ultimately determined by the patient's ability to maintain a satisfactory level of oxygenation, either spontaneously or through mask ventilation. Prolonged attempts are also influenced to a large degree by the willingness of the anesthesia practitioner to establish a surgical airway. The decision to abandon traditional intubation methods in favor of a surgical airway is difficult, especially for those unaccustomed to these techniques. This difficulty is compounded by the emergent circumstances and the lack of time for deliberation or consultation with colleagues. Prior psychologic preparation is therefore stressed repeatedly in numerous publications including the Anesthesia Safety Foundation's monograph on difficult airway management.[15]

After assessing the patient's condition, anesthesia practitioners should determine a priori a cutoff point when a surgical airway becomes the procedure of choice. They should also survey their environment and identify the appropriate individual with the necessary skills and experience to assume responsibility for airway decisions. A reasonable basis for developing a systematic approach to surgical airways begins with an appreciation of several fundamental concepts:

1. Multiple attempts at intubating a patient who has already lost the airway prolong the duration of tissue hypoxia.

2. Multiple attempts at intubating a patient with airway compromise traumatize the upper airway, producing more soft tissue edema, possibly more bleeding, an increase in local secretions, and, depending on the degree of pharmacologic sedation employed, either an obtunded state or heightened agitation. All these conditions predispose to airway loss.

3. A patient cannot be "overoxygenated," that is, a patient who is capable of maintaining the airway will not be hurt with additional support through a surgical airway. In contrast, a patient who has lost the airway will be endangered if oxygenation is not restored rapidly.

4. Familiarity with surgical airway techniques reduces the natural hesitation to consider alternatives to traditional intubation.

The anatomy of the pediatric airway differs sufficiently from that of adults so that different surgical airway techniques are required.[16]

With these concepts in mind, all anesthesia practitioners should be prepared to establish surgical airways, and their repertoire should include techniques for both adults and children. If the airway has already been lost, a limited number of attempts at transoral or transnasal intubation can be attempted before establishing a surgical airway. This is especially true when the period of hypoxia is unknown.

When a fragile but intact airway exists, initial assessment of the patient should be directed at determining how best to improve the chances for successful intubation while not further endangering the airway.[17] A review of radiologic images, if available, will provide valuable information concerning the patency of the upper airway. Axial computed tomography soft tissue windows of the pharynx and larynx provide the most information.[10] However, underpenetrated (soft tissue views), lateral plain films of the neck are also useful and can demonstrate stenosis of the airway shadow in an anteroposterior dimension.[18] Ultrasonography and magnetic resonance imaging are also effective in demonstrating the presence, size, and location of cervical soft tissue abnormalities that may compromise the airway.[19, 20] Pharmacologic measures to reduce secretions, soft tissue edema, and vascularity as well as regional anesthesia to promote the comfort of the patient should be employed if time permits. Oversedation of the patient or placement in a recumbent position, in which secretions are more difficult to control, must be strenuously avoided. After optimization of the airway, inspection with direct laryngoscopy or endoscopy will reveal the feasibility of intubation. Fortunately, in most cases in which the airway is not lost, sufficient space is present for intubation. This initial maneuver also provides information regarding the ease of transnasal or transoral access in patients with limited mandibular or tongue mobility. If mobility or upper airway patency are significantly compromised, early consideration should be given to a surgical airway.

SELECTION OF A SURGICAL AIRWAY

There are essentially two environments in which anesthesia practitioners confronted with the need for a surgical airway may find themselves. The first is an environment, such as the operating room or emergency center, that is well equipped with good light, suction, and the ability to produce pressurized ventilation and with the necessary instruments and personnel to perform a surgical procedure. The second is less suitable for sophisticated techniques and includes locations outside these areas in the hospital, such as the operating room recovery area, or wards. The selection of an appropriate technique will be governed by the available facilities and the age of the patient.

Three procedures qualify for consideration in the emergency setting: needle cricothyroidotomy, surgical cricothyroidotomy, and emergency tracheostomy. The emergency tracheostomy is included because it is the only procedure indicated for surgical airway access in the newborn, where there is insufficient space between the cricoid and thyroid cartilages, both of which are positioned high in the neck. Percutaneous dilatational cricothyroidotomy or tracheostomy are not considered primary techniques during emergencies, even though they may be performed relatively quickly by experienced operators. The rapid introduction of an airway using dilatational methods relies on familiarity with the technique and the tactile requirements of the procedures.

Unequipped Environment

In the absence of proper instrumentation or facilities, a needle cricothyroidotomy is the primary procedure for rapidly gaining surgical access to the airway in adults and children (nonneonates).[21] Because highly pressurized oxygen delivery systems are usually not available, the catheter is connected to any low-flow oxygen source as a temporary measure. Although oxygenation is possible with this technique, adequate ventilation cannot be supported, even with a resuscitation bag.[22] Supplemental oxygen should be maintained through a face mask or nasal cannula even after the placement of a needle cricothyroidotomy. The low-flow system should be replaced as soon as possible with a formal cricothyroidotomy, tracheostomy, or high-pressure insufflation system.

Equipped Environment

When acute airway distress occurs in an equipped environment, the procedure of choice for securing an airway is a surgical cricothyroidotomy with the insertion of either an endotracheal tube or the components of a cricothyroidotomy kit.[23, 24] Introduction of a regular tracheostomy tube, for example, Shiley or Portex types, may not be possible because of the fixed angulation of the tube. Even though a needle cricothyroidotomy with high-pressure jet insufflation is capable of providing oxygenation and ventilation, this system is limited by a number of significant factors including

- An inability to protect the airway from aspiration
- An inability to suction the airway
- Problems associated with a blind procedure such as the potential for introducing air into the cervical soft tissues (subcutaneous emphysema) if the catheter tip is misplaced during introduction or as a result of dislodging
- Kinking, to which the thin-walled catheter is prone
- Time limitations: jet insufflation cannot be continued for more than 30 to 40 minutes, because hypoventilation (hypercarbic acidosis) and barotrauma will result

A surgical cricothyroidotomy is also preferred over tracheostomy in patients with suspected or confirmed cervical spine trauma. The superficial position of the airway below the cricothyroid membrane reduces the need to hyperextend the neck, a maneuver necessary to raise the level of the trachea closer to the skin.[25]

Needle cricothyroidotomy may be considered in pediatric patients younger than 10 years with a palpable cricothyroid membrane. Surgical cricothyroidotomy is contraindicated in this population because the cricoid constitutes the only complete circumferential cartilaginous support to the airway and may be damaged during a more extensive procedure.[26] Needle cricothyroidotomy is also an acceptable alternative for individuals who are uncomfortable with the prospect of surgical cricothyroidotomy. This is an important concession, especially considering the limitations of this procedure outlined earlier. However, as stated previously, the greatest obstacle to a timely establishment of a surgical airway is operator apprehension. If an individual is more comfortable with a needle cricothyroidotomy, this technique should be attempted first. Surgical cricothyroidotomy can always follow the insertion of a needle.

Emergency tracheostomy is rarely performed in the presence of acute airway loss, because it is a slower procedure involving a greater degree of dissection with the potential for encountering more anatomic obstacles such as vessels and the thyroid gland. However, in neonates or other individuals with altered airway anatomy, such as those with laryngeal fractures, a surgical or needle tracheostomy may be the only alternative. In these cases, access to the trachea is gained just below the level of the cricoid cartilage in the region of tracheal rings 1 and 2.[27]

SURGICAL AIRWAY TECHNIQUES

Cricothyroidotomy

The term *cricothyroidotomy* encompasses a number of different procedures that have in common the insertion of a tube or catheter through the cricothyroid membrane. Alternative terms synonymous with cricothyroidotomy include *cricothyrotomy, coniotomy,* and *minitracheostomy.* There are essentially three ways to provide an airway through the cricothyroid membrane, differentiated by the size of the opening through the membrane, how the opening is created, or the rigidity of the cannula. The smallest access, and therefore the least efficient mechanism for oxygenation and ventilation, employs a needle and thin-walled intravenous catheter assembly. The lack of rigidity of the catheter makes the system difficult to advance into the airway, and it is also prone to kinking. The largest opening is provided by an incision made through the membrane using a scalpel, after which an endotracheal tube is inserted. This is also the most rapid technique. Between these two methods is a group of procedures that use specially designed devices for the rapid insertion of a precontoured, relatively rigid tube after a trochar-cannula assembly is used to puncture the membrane. The most refined variation of this last group of procedures employs dilators of increasing diameter to serially increase the size of the initial opening through the skin, subcutaneous tissue, and cricothyroid membrane. The operator's preference and the surroundings affect the choice of procedure.

■ Indications and Contraindications

The indications for a cricothyroidotomy have already been discussed at length. In short, this procedure is performed to gain emergent airway access when attempts at mask ventilation or transnasal or transoral intubations have failed.[28] Cricothyroidotomy is also the procedure of choice when a tracheostomy cannot be performed, for example, in patients with cervical injuries that preclude hyperextension of the neck. Contraindications to the procedure may be divided into absolute and relative categories.

Absolute contraindications include

1. Neonates or infants younger than 6 years
2. Patients with laryngeal fractures

Relative contraindications require an element of operator judgment and include conditions such as

1. Patients with laryngeal abnormality (e.g., neoplasms and inflammatory states)
2. Patients who have been intubated translaryngeally for more than 3 days who may be at increased risk for subglottic stenosis

■ General Preparations

Unless a surgical airway is completely unexpected, preparations should begin with the initial anesthesia preoperative assessment and include three major components:

1. The anesthesia practitioner determines ahead of time the cutoff point at which to switch from conventional oral or nasal routes to a transcutaneous approach.

2. The necessary equipment for a needle or surgical cricothyroidotomy is assembled.

3. The individual patient's laryngeal anatomy is examined and the position of the cricothyroid membrane, thyroid cartilage, cricoid cartilage, and possible puncture points and incision lines marked on the skin.

■ Surgical Anatomy

The cricothyroid membrane extends from the inferior border of the thyroid cartilage (superiorly) to the superior border of the cricoid cartilage (inferiorly). It is composed of a thick, triangular, centrally located web of tissue continuous with thin lateral membranes. Anteriorly, the cricothyroid membrane is approximately 9 mm in height and 22 mm in width (Fig. 9–1). In comparison, the width of an average index finger measures approximately 15 mm. The cricothyroid membrane lies close to the skin in the midline of the neck. It is approximately 1 to 1½ fingerbreadths below the laryngeal prominence of the thyroid cartilage.[29] Vascular structures adjacent to the membrane pose the major surgical risk to a cricothyroidotomy.[30] The superior cricoid vessels may traverse the superior one third of the membrane horizontally and may be transected. Laterally, the vertically oriented anterior jugular veins and branches of the inferior thyroid vein are usually avoided by the midline dissection. The vocal cords are protected by the thyroid cartilage and are found between 5 and 11 mm above the inferior border of the thyroid cartilage. In consideration of these relationships, a cricothyroidotomy should be performed in the midline of the neck in the lower third of the membrane just above the cricoid cartilage.[31]

■ Surgical Technique

Needle Insufflation (Intravenous Catheter Technique)

Despite its name, this technique employs a soft catheter for ventilation while the needle is used as an introducer.[21] In its most basic form, a 12-, 14-, or 16-gauge intravenous catheter is used to enter the airway. An interface between the cannula hub and the standard 15-mm connector of an oxygen delivery system such as a resuscitation bag or anesthesia circuit is required. This may be fashioned out of a 5- or 10-mL Luer-Lok syringe with the plunger removed and the connector from a 7.5-mm endotracheal tube. The Luer end of the syringe is inserted into the

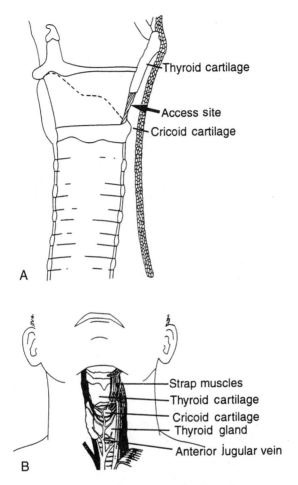

Figure 9–1 *A*, Lateral view of laryngeal cartilages and cricothyroid member. *B*, Anterior view of cricothyroid membrane and adjacent structures.

cannula while the connector is attached to the opposite end of the syringe. Alternatively, a 15-mm connector from a 3-mm pediatric endotracheal tube may be directly inserted into the cannula hub as an interface.[32]

Two types of oxygen delivery systems can be used once access has been achieved.[33] A *low-flow* system, such as that provided by a resuscitation bag or anesthesia circuit, offers as its chief advantage common accessibility. Although oxygenation is possible, ventilation is seriously impeded, and this technique is regarded as a temporary measure until more efficient forms of oxygenation or ventilation become available. *High-pressure* systems utilizing pressures of 50 psi, insufflation rates of 12 L/min, and inspiratory durations of 1 to 1.5 seconds are capable of delivering tidal volumes of between 400 and 750 mL through a 16-gauge cannula. This pressure is provided most conveniently by a jet injector connected to a regulated wall or tank oxygen source (Mercury Medical Inc.). Alternatively, the flush valve on an anesthesia machine may be used, although these systems produce less than 10 psi of pressure and cannot be relied on for adequate ventilation. True high-pressure systems can sustain oxygenation and ventilation for periods up to 40 minutes and offer a significant advantage over low-flow systems.

The technique for inserting a needle-catheter assembly is as follows.[21] The patient is ideally placed in a supine position with extension of the neck (provided that cervical injury is absent); however, a 45-degree semirecumbent position may be necessary if the patient is unable to control secretions or experiences air hunger. Continuous oxygenation with 100% oxygen by face mask is maintained throughout the procedure. The anesthesia practitioner's position is to the right of the patient if right-handed or to the left if left-handed. With adequate preparation, the puncture site is already marked and the necessary equipment assembled. The patient's head and neck are aligned centrally and maintained in this position with the help of an assistant or stabilizing tape. If time permits, the skin overlying the cricothyroid membrane is prepared with povidone-iodine (Betadine). Local anesthesia, even in the conscious patient, is usually not employed, because it may obscure the position of the membrane by raising a skin wheal. The nondominant hand is used to stabilize the thyroid cartilage from above while the index finger of the dominant hand is used to confirm the position of the cricothyroid membrane. An appropriately sized (e.g., 16-gauge) intravenous needle-catheter with syringe attached is inserted through the skin at the level of the inferior third of the membrane. A slight caudal direction is taken to reduce the chance of posterior wall puncture. The syringe is aspirated continuously as the needle-catheter is advanced. Perforation through the cricothyroid membrane into the tracheal lumen is confirmed by a free flow of air into the syringe. If the syringe is filled with a small amount of saline, the appearance of air bubbles provides visual confirmation of entry (Fig. 9–2). Once the needle has been inserted through the membrane and advanced for a short distance to ensure that the cannula tip also sits within the lumen of the airway, the needle is withdrawn and the necessary interface between the cannula and the oxygen delivery system connected (Fig. 9–3).

Oxygenation and ventilation through an intravenous catheter requires specific measures to counteract some of the limitations of this technique.[34] Low-pressure oxygenation should be performed with high flow rates of 15 L/min. The mouth and nose are sealed if air escape reduces ventilatory efficiency. If the patient is unable to expire because of glottic obstruction, insertion of a second catheter into the airway is indicated. Diminished expiration is also a concern when high-pressure systems are employed, and patients ventilated with this modality

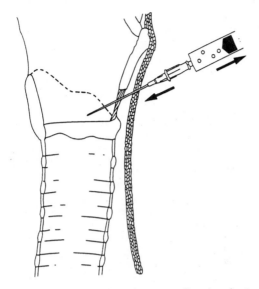

Figure 9–2 Needle cricothyrotomy: confirmation of entry.

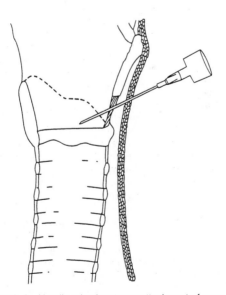

Figure 9–3 Needle cricothyrotomy: attachment of connector.

should be closely observed for carbon dioxide retention. Jet insufflation is performed at rates of 8 to 10 breaths per minute with inspiratory durations of 1 second. An alternative technique uses high-frequency jet insufflation with rates of 150 breaths per minute. Relief of airway pressure is accomplished by including a stopcock in the circuit and not a second cannula, which decreases inspiratory pressure through air escape. Alternatively, cutting a hole in the side wall of the oxygen tubing and occluding it with a finger in a pattern of 1 second "on" and 4 seconds "off" also permits passive exhalation.

Insufflation Through Rigid or Semirigid Cricothyroidotomy Cannulas

Efforts to improve ventilation through the cricothyroid membrane have resulted in the development of special cricothyroidotomy devices such as the Melker Emergency Cricothyrotomy Catheter Set (Cook Critical Care) or Nu-Trake Weiss Emergency Airway System (International Medical Devices, Inc.). These sets overcome the difficulties encountered with the use of small-diameter, thin-walled intravenous catheters by introducing larger (3.5- to 7.2-mm ID) cannulas into the airway. Tissue resistance to cannula advancement is reduced by a skin incision and the use of a dilator before insertion of the cannula. The principal differences between the sets lie in their method of insertion and rigidity of the cannula walls. The Melker cricothyrotomy set uses a Seldinger guide wire technique to position a semirigid cannula into the cricothyroid space. The Nu-Trake device employs a rigid metal cannula and is inserted over a needle. The QuickTrach Transtracheal Catheter (VBM Medizintechnik GMBH) uses a plastic cannula housed over a curved needle for a single-puncture technique. Anesthesia practitioners should become familiar with whichever system is available in their practicing environment.

Melker Emergency Cricothyrotomy Catheter Set

Advocates of this system point to the familiarity of anesthesia practitioners with the Seldinger guide wire technique and the relatively low amount of force required to insert the cannula into the airway. Three cannula sizes are available with internal diameters of 3.5, 4, and 6 mm. Insertion of this device begins with essentially the same initial steps taken for placement of an intravenous catheter through the cricothyroid membrane. The patient is ideally positioned supine with slight extension of the neck if the cervical spine is clear of injury. Once again, the head and neck should be aligned along the long axis of the body. Before the procedure is begun, the lubricated dilator is inserted into the airway cannula to reduce the number of steps once the membrane is punctured. After the skin is prepared, a 1- to 1.5-cm vertical incision is made in the midline of the neck overlying the inferior third of the cricothyroid membrane (Fig. 9–4). An 18-gauge needle-catheter assembly is passed through the incision in a caudad direction (45 degrees to the frontal plane) while continuous aspiration is done with the attached syringe. Once the tip of the needle and catheter enter the cricothyroid space and free air is aspirated, the syringe and needle are detached, leaving

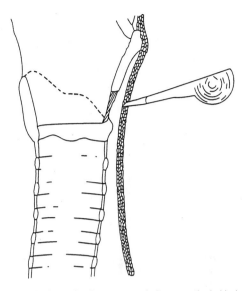

Figure 9–4 Melker cricothyrotomy technique: vertical skin incision.

the catheter in place. A flexible guide wire is inserted through the catheter for 2 to 3 cm, maintaining a caudal bias (Fig. 9–5). The catheter is then removed and the curved dilator with airway cannula is threaded over the guide wire (Figs. 9–6 and 9–7). Stabilization of the guide wire against the skin is necessary during this maneuver to prevent displacing the wire farther into the trachea. The tip of the dilator extends beyond the end of the cannula. This design allows the skin incision and soft tissue overlying the criocothyroid membrane to be gradually enlarged by an in-out motion of the dilator alone. Before the skin is dilated, one should ensure that the guide wire protrudes from the handle end of the dilator to maintain proximal control. Once the soft tissue has been sufficiently stretched to accommodate the diameter of the cannula, both the cannula and the dilator are advanced through the membrane into the airway. The dilator and guide wire are withdrawn together, leaving the cannula in place (Fig. 9–8). After confirmation of cannula position with standard techniques, cloth tapes are used to secure the cannula in place.[33]

Nu-Trake (Weiss Emergency Airway System)

This device differs from the Melker system in the cannula design and method of insertion. Whereas other preformed cannulas are curved, the Nu-Trake employs a straight cannula. The cannula housing is also different and uses tapered metal flanges protruding from a plastic stem to hold the margins of the cricothyroid fenestration open as cannulas of different diameters are inserted (Fig. 9–9). The preparation and positioning of the patient are similar to the previously described tech-

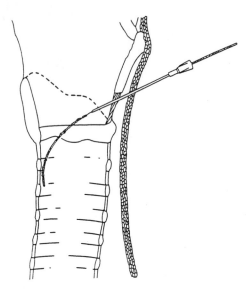

Figure 9–5   Melker cricothyrotomy technique: insertion of guide wire.

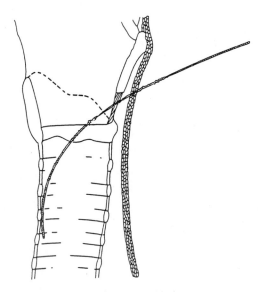

Figure 9–6   Melker cricothyrotomy technique: guide wire in place.

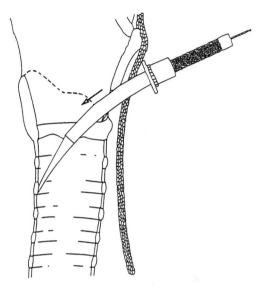

Figure 9–7   Melker cricothyrotomy technique: dilator and cannula assembly threaded over wire.

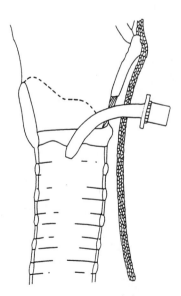

Figure 9–8   Melker cricothyrotomy technique: cannula in place.

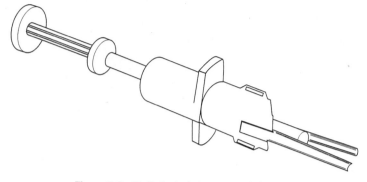

Figure 9–9 Nu-Trake technique: cannula housing.

niques. The internal diameter of cannulas available for this system measure 4.5, 6, and 7.2 mm. At the start of the procedure, the cannula housing, 13-gauge needle stylet, and syringe are assembled as a single unit (Fig. 9–10). The needle stylet attaches to the cannula housing with a simple twist lock, whereas the syringe and needle are connected with a Luer fitting. A vertical 1- to 2-cm skin incision is made in the midline of the neck at the level of the lower third of the cricothyroid membrane. The stylet-housing-syringe assembly is inserted through the incision in a slightly caudal direction with the application of controlled force to push the stylet and tips of the metal flanges through the membrane. Confirmation of entry into the cricothyroid space is made by aspirating free air into the syringe (Fig. 9–11). At this point, the stylet is unlocked from the cannula housing and removed with the syringe. The smallest cannula-obturator assembly (B1; ID 4.5 mm) is used first and inserted through the housing. The cannula housing position is controlled by locking the second and third fingers under the stabilizing flanges while pushing on the cannula-obturator assembly with the thenar eminence of the hand (Fig. 9–12). As the cannula advances into the cricothyroid space, the metal flanges of the housing separate to accommodate the dimensions of the cannula. Larger-diameter cannulas are inserted through the housing in a serial fashion to introduce the largest airway

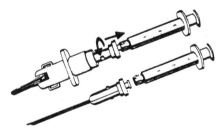

Figure 9–10 Nu-Trake technique: assembly of needle stylet to cannula housing.

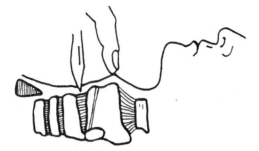

Figure 9–11   Nu-Trake technique: skin incision.

possible for a particular trachea. Once correct positioning of the airway has been achieved, the housing is secured with cloth tape (Fig. 9–13).[33]

Although this device employs a rigid cannula that is not likely to kink, critics of this technique describe difficulties dissecting through the soft tissue with the stylet and cannula assembly. Significant forces were therefore required to insert the assembly, resulting in lacerations or perforations of the posterior tracheal wall. Also, the length and direction of the straight cannula made it prone to occlusion from the posterior tracheal wall.[35]

QuickTrach Transtracheal Catheter

The simplest cricothyroidotomy device is represented by the QuickTrach, which uses a single step to puncture through the membrane with a sharp, curved needle and advance a curved plastic cannula over the needle into the trachea. Two cannula sizes are available, a 4-

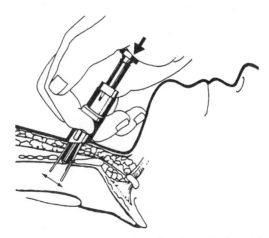

Figure 9–12   Nu-Trake technique: insertion of cannula through housing.

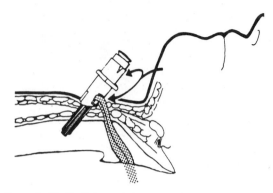

Figure 9–13 Nu-Trake technique: securing cannula with tape.

mm-ID cannula for adults and a 2-mm-ID cannula for children older than 6 years. The same difficulties encountered with the Nu-Trake also apply to this device. Sufficient force must be applied to the stylet-cannula assembly to dissect through the skin and soft tissue overlying the cricothyroid membrane. Unfortunately, if this force is not properly moderated, inadvertent trauma to the posterior laryngeal wall can occur.

The patient is positioned in a manner similar to that for the other procedures. The QuickTrach is first assembled by attaching the syringe to the stylet. The stylet and cannula are slightly curved to facilitate

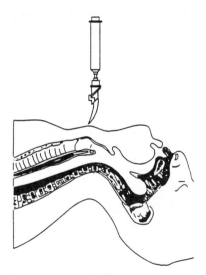

Figure 9–14 QuickTrach technique: orientation of stylet-cannula-syringe before insertion.

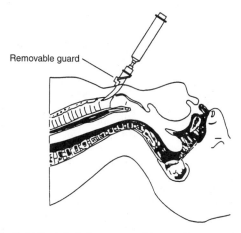

Figure 9–15   QuickTrach technique: removable guard to prevent overinsertion.

entry into the trachea. Penetration of the skin in the midline of the cricothyroid membrane is performed with the stylet-cannula-syringe assembly oriented 90 degrees to the skin surface (Fig. 9–14). As the stylet and cannula are advanced through the soft tissue, a slight caudal bias is adopted. Penetration into the cricothyroid space is confirmed by the aspiration of free air into the syringe. The stylet is advanced farther into the trachea by approximately 5 mm. Overinsertion is prevented by a removable guard that clips onto the cannula (Fig. 9–15). When the stylet and cannula have been inserted to the proper depth, the depth guard is removed before the plastic cannula is slid over the stylet so that the flange rests against the skin. The syringe and stylet are removed and the cannula is secured in place (Fig. 9–16).[36]

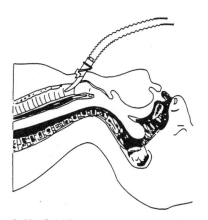

Figure 9–16   QuickTrach technique: cannula in position.

Surgical Cricothyroidotomy

During emergencies, speed is of the essence. Establishing a successful airway rapidly, however, is more dependent on an operator's familiarity with a particular technique than on the technique itself. A surgical cricothyroidotomy represents a quick method for accessing the airway. Its place in the algorithm of difficult airway management should be determined by the individual anesthesia practitioner and not by claims made by operators experienced with open approaches to the airway.

Although the instrumentation required for a surgical cricothyroidotomy is fairly basic, an important requirement is the provision of adequate light and a good suction device. The patient is placed in a supine position with hyperextension of the neck if possible. However, if airway compromise is significant, the procedure may be performed in a semirecumbent position. Maintaining the head and neck in a straight line with the long axis of the body minimizes distortion of the laryngeal anatomy, and this can be accomplished either with the patient's cooperation or through assisted restraints. A particularly challenging situation is created by patients who become combative as a result of hypoxia. If attempts at securing an airway are compromised by motion of the patient, consideration should be given to the exceptional step of paralyzing the patient.

A right-handed operator should stand to the right of the patient. Three surgical landmarks are defined and marked on the patient's skin: the inferior border of the thyroid cartilage, the superior border of the cricoid cartilage, and the midline of the cricothyroid membrane (Fig. 9–17). A significant and not unusual error is to mistake the thyrohyoid membrane for the cricothyroid membrane. If time permits, a small amount of local anesthesia can be infiltrated into the skin overlying the membrane. Too much anesthetic agent obscures the surgical field and makes it more difficult to dissect.

Two approaches to the cricothyroid airway may be adopted de-

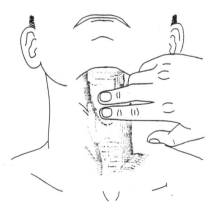

Figure 9–17 Surgical cricothyroidotomy: palpation of landmarks.

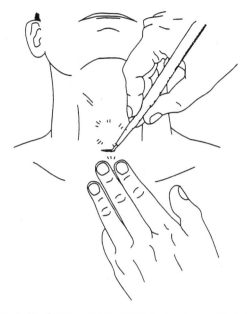

Figure 9–18 Surgical cricothyroidotomy: transverse skin incision.

pending on the circumstances. The so-called slash cricothyroidotomy implies a supreme effort to access the airway in the most rapid fashion possible.[1] In this procedure, the thyroid cartilage is stabilized between the thumb and forefinger of the nondominant hand while a full-thickness, 3-cm transverse incision is made through the middle of the crico-thyroid space with a no. 11 scalpel blade (Fig. 9–18). Vertical midline incisions are also acceptable, although care must be taken to avoid incising the thyroid or cricoid cartilages. After retraction of the skin and overlying soft tissue with a small rake retractor, the airway should become immediately apparent. Dilation of the incision is performed by inserting the blade handle into the airway and rotating it through a 90-degree arc. Alternatively, a Trousseau tracheal dilator is inserted and spread while an endotracheal tube is inserted (Fig. 9–19). Tracheostomy tubes are often unsuitable for cricothyroidotomy sites, because the angulation of the tube is incorrect and does not correspond with the more superficial position of the trachea. When a patient's cricothyroid space is too small to accommodate an endotracheal tube, a suction catheter may be substituted as a temporary measure until an alternative cannula is found. A more controlled form of surgical cricothyroidotomy incises through the tissues superficial to the cricothyroid membrane in layers.[37] After the thyroid cartilage is stabilized, a partial-thickness 3-cm incision is made through the skin alone. Blunt dissection with the tips of a curved hemostat or Mayo scissors is performed to the level of the cricothyroid membrane while avoiding vessels present in the region.

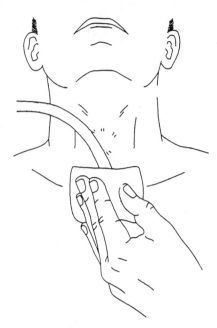

Figure 9–19 Surgical cricothyroidotomy: insertion of endotracheal tube and dressing.

A transverse incision is made through the inferior third of the membrane and a Trousseau dilator inserted. Additional stabilization of the trachea can be achieved by inserting a tracheal hook through the opening and engaging the inferior surface of the thyroid cartilage. Anterior and superior retraction applied to the hook raises the trachea superficially and facilitates insertion of an endotracheal tube. If tracheal control is a concern because of motion of the patient or a deeply located trachea, placement of the tracheal hook before incising through the membrane is often helpful.

■ Complications

The complication rate for nonemergent cricothyroidotomy ranges from 6% to 8%. This incidence increases markedly to 10% to 40% when a cricothyroidotomy is performed as an emergency.[28] Complications stem from a variety of causes, which may be divided into those arising from the procedure itself and those that develop later as a result of cannulation through the cricothyroid membrane. Problems that may occur during a cricothyroidotomy include voice changes (hoarseness, weakness, or decreases in pitch) resulting from superior laryngeal nerve damage; an inability to cannulate the airway; hemorrhage; aspiration; perforation through the tracheal wall producing subcutaneous or mediastinal emphysema; pneumothorax; laryngeal damage; and esophageal or mediastinal perforation. In the adult population, voice changes represent the most common complication and can occur in up to 50% of all cases, whereas in the pediatric population, pneumothorax occurs with the greatest frequency. Complications associated with cannulation include the development of subglottic stenosis; problems with swallowing; infection; erosion through adjacent vessels; persistent stomas; and tracheomalacia.[38] It should be noted that these complication rates apply to surgical cricothyroidotomies and not to needle or dilatational techniques.

■ Verification of Tube Placement

It is essential to confirm that adequate oxygenation and ventilation are taking place. The tube's position should also be checked and the pateint examined to rule out the presence of complications resulting from the airway procedure. A rapid evaluation of these factors must be performed after cannulation, including an assessment of oxygenation levels with pulse oximetry; ventilation by observing the patient's expiration; the tube's position by auscultation; and subcutaneous emphysema by an examination of the neck and chest for signs of subcutaneous emphysema. A portable chest film should be requested as soon as possible to check the tube's position and rule out a pneumothorax. In the absence of adequate ventilation, end-tidal carbon dioxide measurements may be inaccurate, even if the cannula is properly placed within the airways.

Tracheostomy

A tracheostomy may be defined as establishing transcutaneous access to the trachea below the level of the cricoid cartilage. Unless an operator is very experienced, emergency tracheostomies are seldom performed, because of the depth of the trachea in the neck and the presence of significant overlying vascular structures such as the anterior cervical veins, inferior thyroid artery, or a high-riding innominate artery. An exception is made with children younger than 6 years whose cricothyroid space is inaccessible or too small for cannulation.

■ Indications and Contraindications

Tracheostomies performed under nonemergent conditions have a different set of indications from those done as emergencies. Emergency tracheostomies are usually performed when acute airway loss occurs in the following types of patients:

1. Children younger than 6 years or children whose cricothyroid space is considered too small for cannulation
2. Individuals whose laryngeal anatomy has been distorted by the presence of pathologic lesions or infection

Nonemergent tracheostomies are performed for a number of different reasons, including the following types of patients:

1. Patients with stable airways who cannot be intubated through a transoral or transnasal route

2. Patients in whom prolonged intubation (e.g., longer than 2 weeks) is anticipated

3. Patients who have been intubated translaryngeally for more than 3 days

Absolute contraindications to a tracheostomy do not exist since this is a lifesaving procedure. However, patients who might have an adverse outcome of a tracheostomy performed under both emergent and nonemergent circumstances include the following:

1. Patients with a coagulopathy

2. Patients with infections involving the fascial planes of the neck and paratracheal regions

3. Patients with cervical injuries or elderly patients who cannot fully extend their necks

■ General Preparations

As with cricothyroidotomies, preparations for a tracheostomy should begin with the initial anesthesia preoperative assessment and include three important components unless it is a true emergency:

1. The anesthesia practitioner determines ahead of time the cutoff point at which efforts to gain airway access switch from conventional oral or nasal routes to a transcutaneous approach.

2. A decision is made to perform a tracheostomy rather than a cricothyroidotomy.

3. The necessary equipment for a tracheostomy is assembled.

4. The individual patient's laryngeal and tracheal anatomy are examined, and the positions of the cricothyroid membrane, thyroid cartilage, cricoid cartilage, trachea, and possible puncture points or incision lines are marked on the skin.

■ Surgical Anatomy

The trachea extends from the inferior surface of the cricoid cartilage to the carina, where it bifurcates into the left and right main stem bronchi at the level of the fifth or sixth thoracic vertebra. The total length of an adult trachea is between 10 and 13 cm. Hyperextension of the neck positions approximately half the trachea in the neck, whereas flexion can push most of the trachea into the thorax. The trachea is supported by 16 to 20 incomplete "C-shaped" cartilaginous rings. The open end of the tracheal rings faces posteriorly. A tracheostomy incision is normally created approximately 2 fingers' breadth above the sternal notch. The structures below the skin at this level beginning with the most superficial plane are as follows (Fig. 9–20):

1. Subcutaneous tissue
2. Platysma muscle, which may be incomplete in the midline
3. Cervical fascia and anterior jugular veins (if present)
4. Strap muscles (sternohyoid and sternothyroid muscles)
5. Thyroid gland and isthmus, which normally overlie the second, third, and fourth tracheal rings
6. Inferior thyroid veins and thyroidea ima artery (if present), within a plane just deep to the gland
7. Pretracheal fascia

Lateral to the trachea are the internal jugular veins and carotid arteries. Within the tracheoesophageal groove lie the recurrent laryngeal nerves, and at the level of the sternal notch, the innominate artery may be found. In some patients, particularly children, the innominate may ride higher, interfering with the dissection.

■ Surgical Technique

Emergency Tracheostomy

A truly emergent tracheostomy is performed with a Bovie knife at a high setting (e.g., *cutting* and *coagulation* modes >20), a requirement

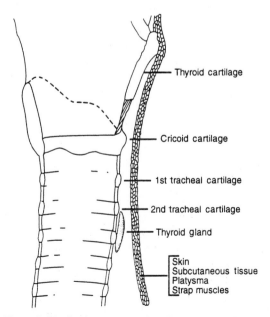

Figure 9–20 Tracheostomy sagittal view: anatomy of larynx.

that often limits this procedure to an operating room environment. The patient is placed supine with a roll under the shoulders to hyperextend the neck, unless cervical injuries preclude this position. Maintaining the head and neck in a central position helps prevent deviation of the trachea to one side. A midline vertical incision is made with the Bovie cautery using the *coagulation* mode. This incision extends from the inferior border of the cricoid cartilage to the sternal notch through the skin and subcutaneous tissue (Fig. 9–21). The position of the trachea is confirmed by palpation through the incision with the nondominant index finger before deepening the incision through the remaining soft tissue and anterior wall of the trachea. An attempt is made to incise the trachea below the level of the first tracheal ring, which helps to support the cricoid cartilage. After incision of the tracheal wall, an endotracheal tube is guided into the trachea with a finger, and oxygenation-ventilation is begun (Fig. 9–22). Vessels encountered by the dissection will hopefully be cauterized, but should bleeding continue, packing the area around the tube with gauze aids in tamponading the cut vessels. Standard tracheostomy tubes are not used in emergencies because the large flanges that extend from the tube base make it difficult to control bleeding once the tube is in place. With the use of endotracheal tubes, care must be taken not to intubate a bronchus. Emergency tracheostomies are usually accomplished in less than 1 minute.

Elective Tracheostomy

When an airway is not in imminent danger of being lost, a more careful dissection is performed with the patient under local anesthesia. After the skin is prepared and anesthetized, the surface landmarks indicating the cricoid cartilage, trachea, and sternal notch are marked on the skin. A 3-cm transverse incision 2 fingerbreadths above the sternal notch is made with a no. 15 scalpel blade. Vertical incisions have also been

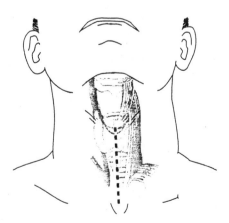

Figure 9–21   Tracheostomy anterior view: vertical skin incision for emergency tracheostomy.

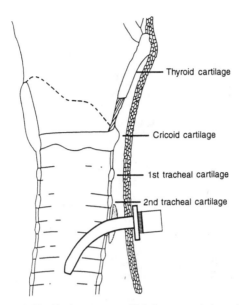

Figure 9–22 Tracheostomy sagittal view: cannula in position.

advocated because of esthetic concerns. However, the appearance of posttracheostomy stomas depends more on the duration and position of cannulation than the orientation of the incision.

Blunt dissection proceeds in the midline of the neck through the subcutaneous tissue, platysma muscle, and deep cervical fascia. Frequent palpation of the trachea and balanced retraction of the tissue on the left and right margins of the dissection help to keep the dissection centralized. Below or within the cervical fascia, the anterior jugular veins may be found and should be ligated and divided if they encroach on the field. The next plane is occupied by the strap muscles, which are vertically separated in the midline by further blunt dissection. The retractors should be continually repositioned at this time to pull the strap muscles laterally. Once the strap muscles have been separated, the thyroid isthmus is usually visualized at the superior extent of the dissection. The isthmus covers the second, third, and fourth tracheal rings unless it is small (Fig. 9–23).

Tracheal access is ideally gained through the second and third or third and fourth rings to avoid tube abutment against vessels that may cross the trachea at lower levels (Fig. 9–24). The first tracheal ring is spared to provide additional support to the cricoid cartilage. Exposure of the trachea at the level of the second and third tracheal ring requires division of the isthmus. A hemostat is used to separate the deep surface from the underlying pretracheal fascia, and the isthmus is freed sufficiently for the application of right-angled clamps on both sides. Division of the isthmus is then completed with a cautery. If a blade or

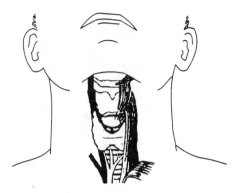

Figure 9–23 Tracheostomy anterior view: structures overlying the trachea.

scissors is used, the margins of the isthmus must be ligated with a nonresorbable suture, for example, 3–0 silk. The retractors are once again repositioned deeper into the field. Lateral stabilization of the trachea is aided by placing the blades of the retractor against the sides of the trachea. Care should be taken not to exert too much downward force with the retractors as this might force the blades into the tracheo-esophageal groove, traumatizing the recurrent laryngeal nerves. Removal of the pretracheal fascia is accomplished bluntly by wiping the fascia from the trachea with a peanut sponge. Before the trachea is

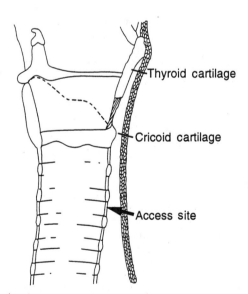

Figure 9–24 Tracheostomy sagittal view: access site.

entered, a transtracheal injection of local anesthetic should be given to prevent coughing.

After identification of the cricoid and first, second, third, and fourth tracheal rings, a tracheal hook is introduced through the anterior tracheal wall just below the ring superior to the level where the tracheal stoma will be created. For instance, if the stoma or flap will be created at the level of the third and fourth rings, the second ring is engaged by the hook. Gentle anterior retraction with the hook elevates the trachea into a more anterior position. There are several ways of creating a fenestration through the anterior wall. Some authors favor an inferiorly based U-shaped flap; others prefer an H-shaped flap or the removal of a circular window of trachea. Whichever design is used, nonresorbable stay sutures are usually passed through the flap or margin and secured to the skin to facilitate reintubation should accidental decannulation occur (Fig. 9–25). The incision through the tracheal wall is usually performed with a no. 11 scalpel blade and scissors. Precautions must be observed if a Bovie knife is used when a patient is receiving supplemental oxygen. An endotracheal tube or cuffed tracheostomy tube (with obturator) is inserted through the tracheal opening and secured to the neck with cloth tape (Fig. 9–26).[39]

Percutaneous Dilatational Tracheostomy

Despite the claims of some authors to the contrary, this technique is not advocated for emergent airway access. It is performed ideally on an intubated patient who requires a surgical airway for any number of reasons. Direct visualization of the procedure through an endoscope inserted translaryngeally is recommended to avoid accidental trauma to the posterior tracheal wall but is often omitted by experienced practitioners who rely on their tactile senses instead.[40]

This procedure is similar to that already described for the insertion of the Melker cricothyrotomy device. One difference is the level of cannulation that is in the interspace between the cricoid cartilage and the first tracheal ring or between the first and second rings. A 17-gauge needle-catheter assembly is used to access the trachea. When entrance

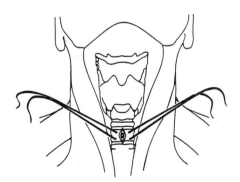

Figure 9–25 Tracheostomy: stay sutures through tracheal flaps.

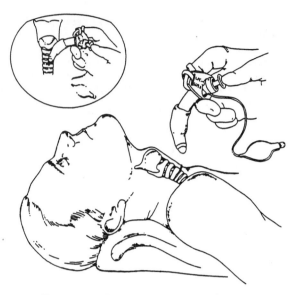

Figure 9–26   Tracheostomy: insertion of cannula.

to the trachea has been confirmed by the aspiration of free air, the catheter is advanced a few millimeters and the needle removed. A guide wire is threaded through the catheter and positioned several centimeters within the trachea before the catheter is removed. Proper guide wire depth is established through the alignment of a skin-level mark on the wire with the skin. Before the skin and soft tissue are dilated in preparation for cannula insertion, an 8 Fr guiding catheter is threaded over the guide wire and properly positioned by aligning the proximal end of the catheter with a corresponding mark on the guide wire. A safety ridge on the guiding catheter should also be at the skin surface. The first dilator is 12 Fr, and this is replaced with dilators of increasing diameter up to 36 Fr to accommodate different cannula sizes. A 24 Fr dilator corresponds to a 6-mm-ID endotracheal tube, whereas a 7-mm-ID tube should be preceded by a 28 Fr dilator. The dilator is passed over the guide wire–catheter assembly and the whole unit advanced until the skin-level indicator on the dilator reaches the skin. This prevents damage to the posterior tracheal wall. Overdilation of the skin is necessary for passage of the tracheostomy tube and balloon. When the appropriate amount of dilation has been completed, the tracheostomy tube is fed over the lubricated dilator into the trachea and secured in place.

■ Verification of Tube Placement

It is essential to confirm that adequate oxygenation and ventilation are taking place. The tube's position should also be checked and the patient examined to rule out the presence of complications resulting from the airway procedure. A rapid evaluation of these factors must be performed after cannulation, including an assessment of oxygenation levels with pulse oximetry; ventilation by observing the patient's expiration; the tube's position by auscultation; and subcutaneous emphysema by an examination of the neck and chest for signs of subcutaneous emphysema. A portable chest film should be requested as soon as possible to check the tube's position and rule out a pneumothorax. In the absence of adequate ventilation, end-tidal carbon dioxide measurements may be inaccurate, even if the cannula is properly placed within the airway.

REFERENCES

1. American College of Surgeons Committee on Trauma: Ventilatory management. *In* Advanced Trauma Life Support Program for Surgeons (Instructor Manual). 1993, First Impression, chapter 2.
2. Fremstad J, Martin S: Lethal complication from insertion of nasogastric tube after severe basilar skull fracture. J Trauma 18:820–822, 1978.
3. Bahr W. Stoll P: Nasotracheal intubation in the presence of frontobasal fractures: A retrospective study. J Oral Maxillofac Surg 50:445–447, 1992.
4. Smoot EC 3rd, Jernigan JR, Kinsley E, Rey RM Jr, et al: A survey of operative airway management practices for midface fractures. J Craniofac Surg 8:201–207, 1997.
5. Cohen A, Larson D: Laryngeal injury, a critical review. Arch Otolaryngol 102:166–170, 1976.
6. Turnball, AEA: High frequency jet ventilation in major airway or pulmonary disruption. Ann Thorac Surg 32:468, 1981.
7. Liebner E: Radiological studies of the lymphatic system of the head and neck. Otolaryngol Clin North Am 6:563, 1973.
8. Dierks E, Meyerhoff W, Schultz BEA: Fulminant infections of odontogenic origin. Laryngoscope 97:271, 1987.
9. Flynn T: Anesthetic and airway considerations in oral and maxillofacial infections. *In* Topazian R, Goldbert M (eds): Oral and Maxillofacial Infections, 2nd ed. Philadelphia, WB Saunders, 1987, p 352.
10. Hall M, Arteaga D, Mancuso A: Use of computed tomography in the localization of head and neck space infections. J Oral Maxillofac Surg 43:978, 1985.
11. Williams A, Guralnick W: The diagnosis and treatment of Ludwig's angina: A report of twenty cases. N Engl J Med 228:443, 1943.
12. Hendler B, Quinn P: Fatal mediastinitis secondary to odontogenic infections. J Oral Maxillofac Surg 36:308, 1978.
13. Wilkes C: Internal derangements of the temporomandibular joint: Pathological variations. Arch Otolaryngol Head Neck Surg 115:469, 1989.
14. Macintosh R, Henny F: A spectrum of application of autogenous costochondral grafts. J Maxillofac Surg 5:257, 1977.
15. American Society of Anesthesiologists Task Force on Management of the Difficult Airway: Practice Guidelines for Management of the Difficult Airway. Anesthesiology 78:597, 1993.
16. Hotaling A, Robbins W, Medgy DEA: Pediatric tracheotomy: A review of technique. Am J Otolaryngol 13:115, 1992.
17. Burtner D, Goodman M: Anesthetic and operative management of potential upper airway obstruction. Arch Otol 104:657, 1978.
18. Assael L, McCravy L: Use of soft tissue radiographs for assessing impending airway obstruction: Report of cases. J Oral Maxillofac Surg 44:398, 1986.
19. Ward-Booth R, Williams E, Faulkner T: Ultrasound: A simple noninvasive examination of cervical swellings. Plast Reconstr Surg 73:577, 1984.
20. Matt B, Lusk R: Delineation of a deep neck abscess with magnetic resonance imaging. Ann Otol Rhinol Laryngol 96:615, 1987.

21. Benumof J, Scheller M: The importance of transtracheal jet ventilation in the management of the difficult airway. Anesthesiology 71:769, 1989.
22. Frame S, Simon J, Kerstein M: Percutaneous transtracheal catheter ventilation (PTCV) in complete airway obstruction—A canine model. J Trauma 29:774–781, 1989.
23. Kress TEA: Cricothyroidotomy. Ann Emerg Med 11:197, 1982.
24. Mace S: Cricothyrotomy. J Emerg Med 6:309, 1988.
25. Aprahamian C, Thompson B, Finger WEA: Experimental cervical spine injury model: Evaluation of airway management and splinting techniques. Ann Emerg Med 13:584–587, 1984.
26. Gerson C, Tucker G: Infant tracheotomy. Ann Otol Rhinol Laryngol 91:413, 1982.
27. Gilmore B, Mickelson S: Pediatric tracheotomy: Controversies in management. Otolaryngol Clin North Am 19:141, 1986.
28. DeLaurier GA, Hawkins ML, Treat RC, Mansberger AR Jr, et al: Acute airway management: Role of cricothyroidotomy. Am Surg 56:12, 1990.
29. Caparosa R, Zavatsky A: Practical aspects of the cricothyroid space. Laryngoscope 67:577, 1957.
30. Little C, Parker M, Tarnopolsky R: The incidence of vasculature at risk during cricothyroidostomy. Ann Emerg Med 15:805, 1986.
31. Holst M, Hertegard S, Perrsson A: Vocal dysfunction following cricothyrotomy: A prospective study. Laryngoscope 100:749, 1990.
32. Finucane B, Santora A: Surgical approaches to airway management. *In* Principles of Airway Management, 2nd ed. St Louis, CV Mosby, 1996.
33. Melker R, Florete OJ: Percutaneous dilational cricothyrotomy and tracheostomy. *In* Benumof J (ed): Airway Management Principles and Practice. St Louis, CV Mosby, 1996, pp 484–512.
34. Ooi R, Sawcett N, Soni NEA: Extra inspiratory work of breathing imposed by cricothyrotomy devices. Br J Anaesth 70:17, 1993.
35. Abbrecht PEA: Insertion forces and risk of complications during cricothyroid cannulation. J Emerg Med 10:417, 1992.
36. Device package insert. Emergency Cricothyrotomy Device VBM Medizintechnik.
37. Van Hasselt E, Bruining H, Hoeve L: Elective cricothyroidotomy. Intensive Care Med 11:207, 1985.
38. Sise MJ, Shackford SR, Cruickshank JC, et al: Cricothyrotomy for long term tracheal access: A prospective analysis of morbidity and mortality in 76 patients. Ann Surg 200:13, 1984.
39. Davidson T, Magit A: Surgical airway. *In* Benumof J (ed): Airway Management Principles and Practice. St Louis, CV Mosby, 1996, pp 513–530.
40. Ciaglia P, Graniero K: Percutaneous dilatational tracheostomy—Results and long term follow-up. Chest 101:464, 1992.

Chapter 10

The Airway and Clinical

Postoperative Conditions*

D. John Doyle and Ramiro Arellano

A number of important postoperative conditions can present special clinical challenges to the anesthesia practitioner. This chapter summarizes some of the more common postoperative situations likely to require special attention from the perspective of airway management (Table 10–1).

AIRWAY COMPLICATIONS FOLLOWING TRACHEOTOMY

A number of airway-related problems may arise in the immediate postoperative period after a tracheotomy has been performed; these

*Note: This chapter is summarized from a presentation published in Doyle NJ, Arellano R: *Anesthesiology Clinics of North America* 13(3):615–633, 1995.

Table 10-1   Postoperative Surgical Conditions with Airway Implications

Thyroid or parathyroid surgery
Neck surgery (e.g., radical neck dissection)
Carotid artery surgery (e.g., endarterectomy)
Tonsil surgery (e.g., tonsillectomy)
Nasal surgery (e.g., septoplasty)
Transsphenoidal pituitary resection
Maxillofacial surgery
Fresh tracheotomy
Massive fluid resuscitation

include bleeding, subcutaneous emphysema, mediastinal emphysema, pneumothorax, airway obstruction, and hypoventilation. Late complications following tracheotomy include tracheal stenosis, tracheoesophageal fistula, tracheomalacia, and tracheal necrosis.

Bleeding, when it occurs after a tracheotomy, is usually minor, but even minor bleeding into the airway may lead to tracheal irritation and sometimes cause the patient to cough and buck vigorously. Major hemorrhage in the immediate postoperative period occasionally occurs as a result of bleeding from a large artery or vein (often the communicating branch of the superior thyroid artery). The latter situation requires immediate exploration of the surgical field. Major bleeding from the innominate artery may occur from erosion of this vessel by the distal end of the cannula in the presence of a mediastinal infection.[1] One hint that the tracheostomy could be applying pressure to the innominate artery is the finding of pulsations in the tracheotomy cannula after its initial insertion. If it is suspected that bleeding is from an innominate artery erosion, treatment includes inflating the tube cuff and pulling the tube assembly anteriorly to tamponade the bleeding. An oral tracheal tube should then be inserted for more definitive management of the airway, followed by repair in the operating room.[2]

Subcutaneous and mediastinal emphysema leading to hypoventilation and hypoxemia may occur as a result of partial obstruction of the tracheostomy cannula when the wound has been closed too tightly. Under these conditions, air may be forced down fascial planes.[3]

With long-term intubation, tracheomalacia, tracheal necrosis, and tracheal stenosis may occur, particularly when cuff pressures are chronically excessive. With tracheal necrosis or tracheomalacia, the airway may collapse with extubation or decannulation, and surgical management (tracheoplasty) is often necessary. Issues related to tracheal stenosis are discussed later in this chapter.

CHANGING FRESH TRACHEOTOMY TUBES

Changing a tracheotomy tube after a fresh tracheotomy is especially hazardous but may be required nonetheless because of a severe cuff leak or because of tube obstruction from the buildup of secretions. The main concern here is that the replaced tube may enter a false passage rather than the trachea. (This in itself is bad enough, but when the false passage is ventilated, the resulting subcutaneous emphysema soon removes all possibility of easily reestablishing the airway.) This problem eventually diminishes as the tracheal stoma matures to form a well-defined and self-supporting orifice. However, this rigidity and tissue support are lacking in a fresh tracheostomy; with removal of the tube, the tissue collapses on itself to obscure the passage. Accordingly, the clinician should be familiar with the precautions listed in Table 10–2 when dealing with a fresh tracheostomy tube.

HEAD AND NECK SURGERY

A number of head and neck surgical situations carry with them important airway implications. After thyroid surgery and parathyroid surgery, for example, hematomas may form and may compress the trachea and lead to suffocation. A similar situation can occur after carotid artery surgery. Specific management of hematomas of this kind depends on the clinical circumstances, but a number of important considerations exist. First, immediate intubation may be necessary should respiratory embarrassment occur. Second, intubation may be difficult if hematoma formation distorts airway anatomy (e.g., by causing deviation or compression of the trachea). Third, the use of muscle relaxants to facilitate intubation in this setting is especially hazardous; should intubation attempts fail, one cannot readily revert to spontaneous respiration. Fourth, reopening the surgical incision with manual evacuation of the hematoma may help reduce respiratory embarrassment and facilitate intubation.

Of interest in this context is the finding that based on preoperative and postoperative computed tomography, even in the absence of post-

---

Table 10–2 Clinical Precautions in Patients with a Fresh Tracheostomy

1. Before any tube change, the patient should be preoxygenated with 100% oxygen.
2. For the first week or so, all tube changes should be carried out in the operating room (OR) by an experienced surgeon, with good lighting and with a full set of surgical instruments (cricoid hooks, etc). An anesthesiologist should also be present in case intubation "from above" is necessary.
3. Once the tracheostomy site has begun to mature, it is no longer necessary to carry out tube changes in the OR, but a full set of tracheostomy instruments (especially cricoid hooks) should still be available. Changing the tube over a tube changer may also be useful, but some people find that it may complicate matters.
4. The fiberoptic bronchoscope may be potentially useful in confirming tracheal placement of a tracheostomy tube before attempting positive-pressure ventilation that could lead to subcutaneous emphysema if the tube is malpositioned.

operative hematoma formation, all patients undergoing carotid artery endarterectomy have some degree of reduction in airway diameter.[4] Carmichael et al note that in this setting emergency airway management is complicated by the reduced laryngeal lumen both for translaryngeal intubation and for cricothyroidotomy and suggest that the incidence of upper airway obstruction after carotid artery surgery may be reduced "by use of protamine, larger surgical drains, prophylactic steroids to prevent swelling or changes in surgical technique."

TONSILLECTOMY

Another postoperative bleeding problem with airway implications concerns the postoperative tonsillectomy patient who develops postoperative bleeding at the tonsillar bed. Considerations here include the following: first, the patient's stomach may contain blood (full-stomach situation); second, if the bleeding is extensive, the patient may be hypovolemic; third, the view at laryngoscopy may be obscured by fresh blood and clots, despite "apparently adequate" suction. In patients who have had nasal surgery (septoplasty, rhinoplasty, and so forth) or transsphenoidal pituitary resection, blood present in the oropharynx at the time of extubation may lead to coughing or laryngospasm, or both. Attempts at positive-pressure ventilation, should it be necessary, are complicated by concerns that the tight application of a face mask over the patient's nose may damage the surgeon's handiwork. The following methods can help make extubation uneventful. First, the use of a throat pack (e.g., saline-soaked gauze) intraoperatively or a laryngeal mask airway may reduce the amount of blood entering the glottis. Second, thorough suctioning of the oropharynx and nasopharynx before extubation is of value (blood clots are often present in the vicinity of the soft palate). Finally, it may be helpful to extubate the patient on his or her side while the patient is wide awake. In this context, special mention should be made of blood collections that may occur at the back of the soft palate during and after nasal and pituitary surgery. After extubation, clots may move from this site to fall into the glottis, leading to complete airway obstruction ("coroner's clot"). Thorough suctioning by both the nasal and the oral routes helps reduce the incidence of this problem.

MAXILLOFACIAL SURGERY

Maxillofacial surgery presents a number of potential airway challenges in the postoperative period.[5] Considerations are presented in Table 10–3.

MASSIVE FLUID RESUSCITATION

Surgical situations that require massive crystalloid resuscitation may lead to enormous head and neck edema such that reintubation becomes very difficult. Possible examples include liver transplantation surgery, thoracoabdominal aneurysm repair, and scoliosis surgery. The situation may be exacerbated when the surgery is carried out with the patient in

Table 10–3   Maxillofacial Surgery Considerations

1. Postoperative airway edema may be present.
2. The jaw may be wired shut postoperatively.
3. If the patient's jaw has been wired shut, a nasogastric tube should be in place and wire cutters should be readily available (e.g., one pair taped to the patient's chart and another taped to the wall above the patient's head.)
4. When possible, patients should be extubated awake with a leak present when the cuff is deflated (i.e., the patient should be able to breath around an occluded endotracheal tube when the cuff is deflated).
5. Extubation over a tube changer may facilitate reintubation should it become necessary.
6. Facilities to establish a surgical airway should be immediately nearby.

the prone position. Very often these patients are ventilated postoperatively; should a cuff leak occur in this setting, reintubation may be exceedingly difficult. Airway management principles are similar to those discussed earlier for maxillofacial surgery.

BURN PATIENTS

Burn patients present many potential airway problems.[6–8] Acutely, the findings of singed nasal hairs, facial burns, pharyngeal burns, or all of these may signify an inhalation injury and the need for early intubation before airway edema becomes problematic.[9–12] Hoarseness and stridor are especially ominous signs. Patients with very high carboxyhemoglobin levels and a depressed level of consciousness, patients who are unable to protect their airways, and patients with severe hypoxemia generally require intubation. Patients with very large burns who will require aggressive intensive care unit resuscitation often need intubation for respiratory support even in the absence of primary airway problems. Regrettably, long-term sequelae are common with prolonged intubation.[13] Fiberoptic bronchoscopy can be especially important when the airway has been involved in a burn patient.[14] Finally, as mentioned previously, fluid shifts associated with aggressive fluid resuscitation may result in such extensive tissue swelling that intubation becomes much more difficult.[15]

Surgery for wound débridement or escharotomy is frequently necessary in the first week. With time, severe scarring of the head and neck may limit neck movement and mouth opening to the extent that scar release under local anesthesia may be necessary before securing the airway.[16]

Although succinylcholine may be used safely in the immediate period following severe burn injuries (first 24 hours), after this period (and until healing is complete), a deadly hyperkalemic response may occur, leading to cardiac arrest. So deadly is this complication that many clinicians will not give succinylcholine immediately after or even within the first year of burn injury.

With facial burns it may be impossible to tape the endotracheal tube

(ET) to the face. Options include the use of a laryngeal mask airway, wiring of the ET to the teeth, and the use of special ET-securing devices. The laryngeal mask airway may be useful in this context as an alternative to tracheal intubation,[17] especially when repeated visits are made to the operating room for débridement and skin-grafting procedures.

POSTOPERATIVE SUBGLOTTIC STENOSIS AND TRACHEOBRONCHIAL STRICTURE

Stenotic airway lesions usually result from mucosal trauma produced by excessively pressurized ET cuffs.[18, 19] This excess pressure results in a circumferential area of necrosis leading to scarring and stricture. Similarly, laryngotracheitis in the presence of a preexisting ET may result in edema and inflammation, making a normally fitting tube too tight. Also, erosion at the site of the impingement of the cuff of an ET may result in inflammation of the trachea. Finally, a tracheotomy tube may result in erosion at the superior margin of the tracheal stoma, which may lead to granulation and stenosis, or alternatively, to tracheomalacia.

Stenotic lesions in the airway can be granulomatous, fibrous, calcific, inflammatory, or cartilaginous. They can be located supraglottically, in the glottic area (i.e., at the cords), or in the subglottic region (i.e., anywhere in the larynx from the true vocal cords to the cricoid).

Whether supraglottic or subglottic, airway stenoses can make it impossible to pass a regular-diameter ET into the trachea. One particular clinical sign to note is an old tracheostomy scar; if this is present, it is wise to have a couple of smaller-diameter ETs available in case a regular tube cannot be readily passed and to have a surgeon immediately nearby.

REFERENCES

1. Golz A, Goldsher M, Eliachar I, et al: Fatal hemorrhage following a misplaced tracheostomy. J Laryngol Otol 95:529, 1981.
2. Cooper JD: Trachea-innominate artery fistula: Successful management of three consecutive patients. Ann Thorac Surg 4:439, 1977.
3. Heffner JE, Miller KS, Sahn SA: Tracheostomy in the intensive care unit. Part I: Indications, technique, management. Part II: Complications. Chest 90:269, 430, 1986.
4. Carmichael FJ, McGuire GP, Wong DT, et al: Computed tomographic analysis of airway dimensions after carotid endarterectomy. Anesth Analg 83:12, 1996.
5. Stoddart JC: Trauma and the Anaesthetist. London, Balilliere Tindall, 1984.
6. Clark CJ, Reid WH, Telfer BM, Campbell D: Respiratory injury in the burned patient. The role of flexible bronchoscopy. Anaesthesia 38:35, 1983.
7. Eckhauser FE, Billote J, Burke JF, Quinby WC: Tracheostomy complicating massive burn injuries. A plea for conservatism. Am J Surg 127:418, 1974.
8. Goudsouzian N, Szyfelbin SK: Management of upper airway during burns. In Martyn JAJ (ed): Acute Management of the Burned Patient. Philadelphia, WB Saunders, 1990, pp 46–65.
9. Clarke WR, Bonbentura M, Myers W, Kellman R: Smoke inhalation in airway management at a regional burn unit: 1974–1983. II: Airway management. J Burn Care Rehabil 11:121, 1990.

10. Coleman DL: Smoke inhalation. West J Med 135:300, 1981.
11. Peters WJ: Inhalation injury caused by the products of combustion. Can Med Assoc J 125(3):249, 1981.
12. Trunkey DD: Inhalation injury. Surg Clin North Am 58:1133, 1978.
13. Lund T, Goodwin CW, McManus WF, et al: Upper airway sequelae in burn patients requiring endotracheal intubation or tracheostomy. Ann Surg 201:374, 1985.
14. Lukan J, Sandor L, Szabo M: The importance of fiber bronchoscopy in respiratory burns. Acta Chir Plast 32:107, 1990.
15. Denling RH: Fluid replacement in burned patients. Surg Clin North Am 67:15, 1987.
16. Jacobacci S, Towy RM: Anaesthesia for severe burn contractures of the neck. A case report. East Afr Med J 55:543, 1978.
17. Russell R, Judkins KC: The laryngeal mask airway and facial burns. Anaesthesia 45:894, 1990.
18. Othersen HB: The Paediatric Airway. Philadelphia, WB Saunders, 1991, p 102.
19. Weber AL, Grillo HC: Tracheal stenosis: An analysis of 151 cases. Radiol Clin North Am 16:291, 1978.

Chapter 11

Medical Conditions

Affecting the Airway:

A Synopsis*

D. John Doyle and Ramiro Arellano

*Note: This chapter is modified from an earlier review published in Doyle DJ, Arellano R: *Anesthesiology Clinics of North America* 13(3):615–633, 1995.

This chapter summarizes some of the more important medical conditions likely to affect airway management. Our presentation is brief and focused. Numerous rare medical conditions with airway implications are summarized in Table 11–1.

A number of medical conditions may present difficult challenges to the anesthesia practitioner. For instance, infected airway structures may lead to partial airway obstruction, stridor, or even complete airway obstruction. Partial airway obstruction may be mild, as in snoring or nasal congestion, or may be more severe, perhaps requiring the use of airway adjuncts such as a nasopharyngeal airway. Complete airway obstruction is usually managed by prompt intubation, but surgical airways are sometimes needed as a last resort.

TREATMENT OF STRIDOR

Stridor, or noisy inspiration from turbulent gas flow in the upper airway, is often seen in airway obstruction and always commands attention. Wherever possible, attempts should be made to immediately establish the cause of the stridor (e.g., foreign body, vocal cord edema, tracheal compression by tumor).

The first issue of clinical concern in the setting of stridor is whether intubation is immediately necessary. If intubation can be delayed, a number of potential options can be considered, depending on the severity of the situation and other clinical details. These include

- Use of Heliox (70% helium, 30% oxygen)
- Expectant management with full monitoring, oxygen by face mask, and positioning the head of the bed for optimal conditions (e.g., 45 to 90 degrees)
- Use of nebulized racemic epinephrine or cocaine (but not both together) when airway edema may be the cause of the stridor
- Use of dexamethasone (Decadron) 4 to 8 mg intravenously every 8 to 12 hours when airway edema may be the cause of the stridor

Text continued on page 233

Table 11–1   Common and Unusual Medical Conditions with Airway Implications

Medical Condition	Associate Airway Problems	Reference
Achondroplasia	Usually not difficult intubation. Judge endotracheal tube size by weight. Increased prevalence of obstructive sleep apnea.	129, 130, 131
Acromegaly	Macroglossia. Laryngeal stenosis. Increased prevalence of obstructive sleep apnea.	61–65, 132–135
Anderson's syndrome	Severe midfacial hypoplasia. Abnormal shape and structure of mandible. Intubation may be difficult.	129, 136
Apert's syndrome	Variable degrees of cervical spinal fusion possible. Hypoplastic maxilla. Intubation may be difficult.	129, 137–139
Arthrogryposis multiplex	Multiple congenital contractures. May be difficult intubation if mouth opening limited.	129, 140
Beckwith-Wiedemann syndrome	Macroglossia.	129
Behçet's syndrome	Ulceration of mouth. Pharyngeal scarring may make intubation difficult.	129, 141, 142
Carpenter's syndrome	Presence of hypoplastic mandible may make intubation difficult.	129, 137, 138
Cherubism	Oral masses and fibrous dysplasia of mandible and maxilla may make intubation extremely difficult.	129
Chotzen's syndrome	Craniosynostosis may make intubation difficult.	129
Christ-Siemens-Touraine syndrome (anhydrotic ectodermal dysplasia)	Intubation may be difficult because of presence of hypoplastic mandible.	129
Chubby puffer syndrome	Upper airway obstruction may necessitate tracheostomy.	129, 143
Cleft lip and palate	May be associated with subglottic stenosis.	129
Cornelia de Lange's syndrome	May be difficult intubation.	129, 144
Cretinism (congenital hypothyroidism)	Macroglossia may make intubation difficult.	129

Table continued on following page

Table 11-1 Common and Unusual Medical Conditions with Airway Implications *Continued*

Medical Condition	Associate Airway Problems	Reference
Cri du chat syndrome	Micrognathia, laryngomalacia, small larynx, and small epiglottis may make difficult intubation.	129, 145
Crouzon's disease	Tracheomalacia and airway stenosis possible. Hypoplastic maxilla may make intubation difficult.	129, 137, 146
Cystic hygroma	Cysts involving tongue, neck, and mediastinum.	147–152
Down's syndrome	Subglottic stenosis. Large tongue. Atlantoaxial joint instability.	129
Edwards' syndrome	Intubation may be difficult in presence of micrognathia.	129
Ellis–van Creveld syndrome	May have cleft lip, cleft palate, or abnormal maxilla making intubation difficult.	129, 153
Epidermolysis bullosa	Repeated erosions and blisters lead to strictures of pharynx and larynx. Avoid intubation if possible. Lubricate endotracheal tube and laryngoscope blade well.	129, 154, 155
Farber's disease	Sphingomyelin deposition in larynx may make intubation difficult.	129, 156
Fetal alcohol syndrome	Flat maxilla may make intubation difficult.	129, 157–159
Focal dermal hypoplasia	Papillomas may be present in airway.	129
Freeman-Sheldon syndrome	Increased tone and fibrosis of facial muscles prevent relaxation of jaw with neuromuscular blockade making intubation very difficult.	129
Goldenhar's syndrome	Unilateral hypoplasia with mandibular hypoplasia may lead to airway problems and difficult intubation.	129, 160
Gorlin-Goltz syndrome	Mandibular prognathism, multiple jaw cysts, and fibrosarcomas, as well as incomplete segmentation of cervical vertebrae, may make intubation difficult.	129

**Table 11–1   Common and Unusual Medical Conditions with
Airway Implications** *Continued*

Medical Condition	Associate Airway Problems	Reference
Hemophilia	Possible hematoma at intubation or extubation.	129
Hereditary angioneurotic edema	Instrumentation of airway may induce brawny edema.	129, 161–163
Histiocytosis X	Intubation may be difficult if laryngeal fibrosis is present.	129, 164
Hunter's syndrome	Administer large doses of atropine at induction. Infiltration of lymphoid tissue and larynx and copious thick secretions may make intubation difficult.	129, 165–168
Hurler's syndrome	Administer large doses of atropine at induction. Infiltration of lymphoid tissue and larynx and copious thick secretions may make intubation difficult.	129, 165, 166, 169–173
I-cell disease	Limited jaw movement and neck stiffness may make intubation and airway maintenance difficult.	129
Klippel-Feil syndrome	Congenital fusion of cervical vertebrae may make intubation very difficult.	129, 174
Larsen's syndrome	Cleft palate, and poor cartilage in epiglottis, arytenoids, and trachea, may make intubation difficult.	129, 175, 176
Laryngeal papillomatosis	Lesions may obstruct airway.	177
LEOPARD syndrome	Intubation may be difficult.	129
Marfan's syndrome	Intubation may be difficult. Gentle laryngoscopy to avoid cervical spine or temporomandibular joint damage.	129
Meckel's syndrome	Micrognathia and cleft epiglottis may make intubation difficult.	129
Median cleft face syndrome	Cleft lip and palate may make intubation difficult.	129
Möbius' syndrome	Micrognathia may cause intubation difficulties.	129
Morquio's syndrome	Unstable atlantoaxial joint may lead to spinal cord compression. Avoid neck manipulation with intubation.	129, 156, 178

Table continued on following page

Table 11–1 Common and Unusual Medical Conditions with Airway Implications *Continued*

Medical Condition	Associate Airway Problems	Reference
Myositis ossificans	Neck rigidity and limited mouth opening may lead to difficult intubation.	129, 179
Noack's syndrome	Intubation may be difficult.	129, 137
Noonan's syndrome	Micrognathia may lead to intubation difficulties.	129
Opitz-Frias syndrome	Micrognathia, high arched palate, and laryngeal malformations may lead to difficult intubation (prepare small endotracheal tubes).	129, 180
Oral-facial-digital syndrome	Cleft lip and palate, hypoplastic mandible and maxilla, and lobed tongue may lead to airway problems and intubation difficulties.	129
Osteogenesis imperfecta	Must exercise extreme care positioning and intubing. Teeth easily damaged.	129
Patau's syndrome	Micrognathia and cleft lip or palate may make intubation difficult.	129
Pierre Robin syndrome	Cleft palate, micrognathia, and glossoptosis may make intubation very difficult.	129
Pompe's disease	Macroglossia may make intubation difficult.	129, 181
Pyle's disease	Enlarged mandible and craniofacial abnormalities may make intubation difficult.	129
Scleroderma	Scarring of mouth may make intubation difficult.	129
Silver-Russel dwarfism	Micrognathia may make intubation difficult.	129
Sleep apnea syndromes	Mask anesthesia potentially hazardous. May obstruct during induction of anesthesia. Intubation may be difficult (obstructive variety). Monitor closely for apnea postoperatively.	129, 33–41, 182, 183
Smith-Lemli-Opitz syndrome	Micrognathia may lead to intubation problems.	129
Sotos' syndrome	Acromegalic-like skull may cause intubation difficulties.	129

Table 11–1   Common and Unusual Medical Conditions with Airway Implications *Continued*

Medical Condition	Associate Airway Problems	Reference
Stevens-Johnson syndrome	Oral erosions may be worsened by instrumentation and intubation.	129
Thalassemia major		129
Tracheoesophageal fistula	May be associated with subglottic stenosis.	129
Treacher Collins syndrome	Micrognathia and microstomia may lead to intubation difficulties. Increased prevalence of obstructive sleep apnea.	129, 184–185
Trismus-pseudocamptodactyly	Restricted mouth opening may make intubation extremely difficult.	129, 186
Turner's syndrome	Possible micrognathia may make intubation difficult.	129
Urbach-Wiethe disease	Hyaline deposits in pharynx and larynx may make intubation difficult.	129, 164
Wegener's granulomatosis	Macroglossia, laryngeal stenosis, and increased prevalence of obstructive sleep apnea.	177

NONNEOPLASTIC NONINFECTIOUS CONDITIONS WITH AIRWAY IMPLICATIONS

Asthma, Bronchospasm, and Reactive Airway Disease

Dramatic and deadly increases in airway resistance sometimes confront the anesthesia practitioner when an asthmatic patient suffers an episode of bronchospasm.[1-9] Bronchospasm is an exaggerated bronchoconstrictor response to a triggering stimulus and is often seen in susceptible asthmatic patients. Elements in the pathophysiology of asthma (reactive airway disease) include airway inflammation and edema, increased airway secretions, increased contraction of airway smooth muscle, and decreased airway caliber. Exacerbations of asthma are commonly linked to viral illnesses.

Medications used in asthma management include

- β-Agonists
- Theophylline products
- Corticosteroids
- Anticholinergic medications

In addition, a number of anesthetic agents (e.g., halothane, ketamine) have a salutatory effect in asthma.

Inhaled β-adrenergic agonists such as albuterol (salbutamol), terbutaline sulfate, fenoterol hydrobromide, pirbuterol, or salmeterol remain the mainstay of treatment, although their role in the chronic treatment of asthma is in flux, with many clinicians preferring inhaled corticosteroids as first-line therapy, with β-agonists reserved for use as required.

Intravenously administered theophylline products such as aminophylline are waning in clinical popularity since they have a very poor toxic/therapeutic index and do not add significant clinical benefit in patients already receiving β-agonists for an acute exacerbation of asthma. Their main role is in preventing acute attacks in the chronic asthmatic patient, especially at night. In patients with chronic obstructive pulmonary disease, improvements in diaphragmatic function and in mucociliary clearance make theophylline a useful adjunct as well.

Corticosteroids are taking on a new importance in treating patients with asthma as the inflammatory element in asthma is more appreciated. Inhaled corticosteroids are now often used as first-line asthma therapy, whereas intravenous steroids are often used preoperatively in patients with moderately severe asthma or in those previously requiring steroid therapy. However, in contrast to β-agonists, whose clinical effect is almost immediate, intravenous steroids take several hours to work.

Adult Respiratory Distress Syndrome

Adult respiratory distress syndrome (ARDS) is a deadly respiratory condition often found in the intensive care unit, with ventilators straining heroically to push gas into small, stiff lungs.[10–22] The syndrome is similar histologically to respiratory disease of the premature newborn, but rather than resulting from pulmonary immaturity, ARDS is the consequence of many possible clinical insults such as aspiration pneumonitis, massive trauma, or septicemia. ARDS carries with it four major management issues:

- Oxygenation
- Ventilation
- Fluid management
- Intubation

■ Oxygenation

The high degree of pulmonary shunt present in ARDS necessitates that two ventilator parameters (FIO_2 and positive end-expiratory pressure [PEEP]) be adjusted upward jointly to achieve adequate oxygenation (e.g., the arterial oxygen saturation $SaO_2 > 0.9$ or $PaO_2 > 60$ mm Hg). FIO_2 is the fraction of inspired oxygen (e.g., 0.5 for 50% oxygen). PEEP is the positive end-expiratory pressure of minimal lung-distending pressure (e.g., 5 cm H_2O). FIO_2 and PEEP are not adjusted independently but rather jointly, even sometimes by quantitative linking (e.g., PEEP

= 15 F_{IO_2}). Patients who are hypovolemic may tolerate PEEP less well and require less strong linkage to F_{IO_2}.

■ Ventilation

Ventilation may be difficult in ARDS patients because high ventilating pressures are required to achieve normal tidal volumes. The high ventilating pressures required are suspected to be a cause of more lung injury, leading some researchers to advocate the use of "permissive hypercapnia," a ventilating protocol allowing higher P_{CO_2} levels and more acidotic pH levels but with much smaller tidal volumes and airway pressures, and less potential for barotrauma. Special ventilation modes such as inverse ratio ventilation: (I:E ratio < 1), airway pressure release ventilation, and high-frequency jet ventilation are often used with these patients.

■ Fluid Management

ARDS is associated with increases in vascular permeability (leaky capillaries) that mandate special care regarding fluid management. Hypovolemia can be avoided by monitoring urine output and cardiac filling pressures (central venous pressure, pulmonary capillary wedge pressure).

■ Intubation

Patients with ARDS require intubation. High cuff pressures, required when high ventilating pressures are used, may damage tracheal mucosa and cause long-term injury (e.g., tracheal stenosis from scarring). After 10 to 14 days of intubation, consideration is given to a formal tracheostomy. Tracheal suction is also needed to avoid buildup of secretions. Reintubation of patients with ARDS may be necessary because of cuff leaks or because of the buildup of hardened secretions within the lumen of the endotracheal tube (ET).

Guillain-Barré Syndrome

Guillain-Barré syndrome is an acute inflammatory postinfection polyneuropathy involving lymphocytic infiltration and demyelination of spinal and cranial nerves and nerve roots, sometimes with axonal damage.[23] The presence of antibodies directed against neurons and the response to plasmapheresis strongly suggest immune system involvement in Guillain-Barré syndrome.

Clinically, bilateral symmetric weakness occurs, typically ascending from the legs. Loss of diaphragmatic or intercostal muscle power along with possible bulbar involvement in Guillain-Barré syndrome is an indicator of concern about airway management. Prolonged ventilation with or without tracheostomy in an intensive care unit is sometimes necessary, as recovery may take weeks to months.

Diabetes Mellitus

A link between diabetes mellitus and difficult laryngoscopy has been described.[24] About one third of long-term (juvenile-onset) diabetic patients present with laryngoscopic difficulties.[25, 26] This is due at least in part to diabetic "stiff joint syndrome," characterized by short stature, joint rigidity, and tight, waxy skin.[27, 28] The fourth and fifth proximal pharyngeal joints are most commonly involved. Patients with diabetic stiff joint syndrome have difficulty in approximating their palms and cannot bend their fingers backward ("prayer sign"). When the cervical spine is involved, limited atlantooccipital joint motion may make laryngoscopy and intubation quite difficult. Glycosylation of tissue proteins from chronic hyperglycemia resulting in abnormal cross-linking of collagen is believed to be responsible.[29] Joint involvement in diabetic patients is sometimes evaluated using a "palm test," which determines how much of a patient's palm can be made to make contact with a flat surface.[30] Reissell and colleagues studied laryngoscopic conditions in 62 diabetic patients given a fentanyl-thiopental-vecuronium induction for renal transplantation or vitrectomy surgery.[31] Joint stiffness as judged by the palm test was shown to correlate with difficulty in laryngoscopy.[32]

Nichol and Zuck point out that "almost all of the extension of the head on the neck that is helpful to the laryngoscopist takes place at the atlanto-occipital joint."[30] In some patients who present with an "anterior larynx" (which Nichol and Zuck view as a misnomer), head extension is limited by abutment of the occiput against the posterior tubercle of the atlas, with the result that the cervical spine bows forward at laryngoscopy, pushing the larynx anteriorly. The same effect may occur in stiff joint syndrome patients, not because of abutment of the atlas against the occiput, but because of cervical spine joint immobility.

Obstructive Sleep Apnea

Obstructive sleep apnea (OSA) consists of absent nasal and oral airflow during sleep despite continuing respiratory effort. This is generally due to backward tongue movement and pharyngeal wall collapse (glossoptosis) from interference with the normal coordinated contraction of pharyngeal and hypopharyngeal muscles.[33] Enlargement of the tongue, tonsils, or adenoids, or all of these, is often contributory. Obstructive sleep apnea is diagnosed by finding at least 30 episodes of apnea (of duration of at least 10 seconds) in a 7-hour study period. Although OSA is often considered a disease of obese adults,[34–35] it is also common in children with tonsillar adenoidal hypertrophy or craniofacial syndromes.[36–41]

From an anesthetic viewpoint, OSA patients are particularly at risk for airway obstruction during the induction and recovery phases of anesthesia. Management options range from heightened clinical monitoring to the use of artificial airway devices (e.g., nasopharyngeal airway, Guedel airway) to carrying out induction and recovery with the patient in a sitting or semisitting position to minimize pharyngeal wall collapse.

Obesity

Patients 20% over their ideal weight are obese. When they are 100% over this weight they are said to be "morbidly obese."[42] The obese patient has a reduced functional residual capacity with reduced pulmonary oxygen stores, leading to rapid desaturation when apnea occurs.[43–45] The obese patient with a short thick neck, a large tongue, or redundant folds of oropharyngeal tissue may be difficult to intubate and is at increased risk to develop airway obstruction.[46, 47] Positive-pressure ventilation may be more difficult in these patients because of decreased chest wall compliance (restrictive lung defect). The increased work of breathing associated with obesity leads patients to take smaller tidal volumes and breathe at an increased respiratory rate, leading to atelectasis, ventilation-perfusion mismatching, and increased degrees of airway closure. Should a surgical airway become necessary, the situation is made much more difficult as the surgeon attempts to identify the trachea deep in a mound of adipose tissue. Very obese patients are at increased risk of regurgitation and aspiration because of both increased intraabdominal pressure and the high incidence of gastric fluid volumes greater than 25 mL and gastric fluid pH less than 2.5.[48, 49]

Rheumatoid Arthritis

Rheumatoid arthritis is a multisystem autoimmune disease with many anesthetic implications. Patients with rheumatoid arthritis may challenge the anesthesia practitioner at the time of tracheal intubation because of cervical spine instability.[50] In addition, temporomandibular joint[51] or arytenoid joint[50–58] immobility may limit safe access to the airway. The preoperative anesthetic assessment must focus on possible airway difficulties. Patients must be questioned and examined to elicit evidence of neck pain, limitation of cervical spine movement, nerve root impingement, or spinal cord compression. Lateral cervical spine flexion-extension radiographs are potentially helpful in patients with cervical spine symptomatology in order to assess the possibility of cervical spine subluxation. The need for these radiographs in completely asymptomatic patients remains controversial; however, one should keep in mind case reports of neurologic damage following direct laryngoscopy and intubation in asymptomatic patients.[50] Patients with cervical spine instability should generally be intubated and positioned awake before surgery to avoid neurologic injury. The temporomandibular joints must be examined to ensure that mouth opening and anterior subluxation of the mandible will permit direct laryngoscopy. Patients demonstrating stridor or hoarseness require awake direct or indirect laryngoscopy to assess the possibility of arytenoid involvement and determine the size of the glottic opening. Finally, the larynx may be displaced and twisted from its usual location by erosion and generalized collapse of the cervical vertebrae.

To summarize, airway-related concerns in rheumatoid arthritis include concerns about possible cervical spine subluxation, temporomandibular involvement, involvement of the arytenoids, and laryngeal twisting. Other concerns relate to possible systemic involvement with the disease, the possible need for special care in the positioning of the patient, and the fact that the patient may be taking aspirin or other platelet-inhibiting drugs as well as systemic corticosteroids.

Zenker's Diverticulum

Zenker's diverticulum is an esophageal outpouching for which patients sometimes seek surgical repair.[59] Because food and other material may settle in the diverticulum, there is a concern that any pouch material may find itself in the airway with the induction of anesthesia.[60] Some patients can manually empty the pouch themselves; others may benefit from suction catheter placement in the pouch before induction (easier said than done). One key thing to remember, however, is that the application of cricoid pressure (such as is done in a rapid-sequence induction) may actually dislodge any pouch contents into the oropharynx.

Acromegaly

The acromegalic patient suffers from an excess of growth hormone, usually from a pituitary adenoma. If this condition occurs before the closure of the epiphyseal growth plates, giantism may occur. Once the growth plates have fused in adolescence, the patient may take on acromegalic features. From the viewpoint of airway management in the acromegalic patient, three concerns exist: (1) the tongue may be enlarged, resulting in OSA; (2) redundant folds of tissue may be present in the oropharynx; and (3) laryngeal stenosis occurs more frequently than in the general population.[61–65] These factors may make laryngoscopy and intubation somewhat more difficult and increase the likelihood of airway obstruction during anesthetic induction and recovery. Should true giantism be encountered clinically (often when the patient is seen for resection of a pituitary adenoma), the following potential problems should also be considered: (1) an extra-long operating room table may be needed, (2) an extra-large laryngoscope may be needed, (3) ETs may need to be cut longer then usual, and (4) an extra-large face mask may be necessary.

Anaphylaxis

During anaphylactic (or anaphylactoid) reactions, massive release of histamine and other noxious substances from mast cells and basophils produce "leaky capillaries" that result in interstitial fluid buildup (edema).[66–67] When edema of any portion of the airway results, respiratory obstruction can occur. Airway-related clinical manifestations may include dyspnea, stridor, and facial edema. Erythema, urticaria, bronchospasm, and hypotension may also be present. Although many older textbooks advocate establishing a surgical airway, early intubation is now the usual recommendation if the airway appears to be at risk. Another airway-related problem that may occur in anaphylaxis is bronchospasm, sometimes with sufficient severity that air entry is so poor that wheezing is not present and ventilation may be next to impossible. As always, the primary drug treatment in life-threatening anaphylaxis is epinephrine (2 to 4 µg/kg), either intravenously, subcutaneously, or intramuscularly, repeated at 5- to 10-minute intervals based on the patient's clinical response.

NEOPLASTIC CONDITIONS WITH AIRWAY IMPLICATIONS

Airway Polyps

Polyps may be found throughout the airway. Nasal polyps and polyps elsewhere in the airway can lead to partial or complete airway obstruction.[68–69] Vocal cord granulomas and polyps may occur as a result of traumatic intubation, cord irritation from ET movement or lubricant chemicals, and other causes. The problem occurs more frequently in women. Pedunculated granulomas or polyps detected during the investigation of hoarseness are usually removed surgically as they can sometimes lead to airway obstruction. Remember also the potential exacerbation of bronchial asthma in patients with nasal polyps who receive aspirin, ketorolac (Toradol), and other nonsteroidal anti-inflammatory drugs.[8]

Concern about possible nasal polyps or other causes of nasal obstruction requires that the patency of the nasal passages be tested before attempted nasal intubation. This is done by having the patient take deep breaths through each nostril separately. Pledgets soaked with cocaine (or another vasoconstrictor) and inserted into each nostril help shrink the nasal mucosa and reduce the chance of epistaxis with attempted nasal ET insertion. Nasal intubation may become difficult or hazardous when nasal polyps are present, with previous injury to the nose, with a basal skull fracture, or in the presence of a coagulopathy. Fiberoptic nasal endoscopy allows easy study of nasal passages and is faster and less expensive than magnetic resonance imaging. Although routine preoperative nasopharyngeal endoscopy in all patients before intubation has the potential to detect rare but dangerous airway abnormality in asymptomatic patients (and would be educational for anesthesia practitioners), high capital costs and poor reimbursement policies render this procedure impractical.

Carcinoma of the Oral Cavity[70]

Extension of oral carcinoma into the tongue and elsewhere, along with reactive fibrosis, may make laryngoscopy difficult. The mouth and tongue should be examined carefully in such patients to ensure adequate tongue and mandible mobility. Also, there is an increased risk of bleeding, and appropriate precautions should be taken with airway manipulation.

Epiglottic Cysts[71]

Epiglottic cysts may require needle drainage under local anesthesia and other special procedures before intubation is possible. The effect of a cyst in causing airway obstruction may vary with the patient's position as gravity swings the cyst in and out of the glottic opening.

Bronchogenic Cysts[72]

Bronchogenic cysts may be found in a variety of places along the airway, and their clinical presentation varies according to the size and location of the cyst. Histologically, they are thin-walled cysts lined with respiratory epithelium that contains thick mucoid epithelium. Such cysts may be detected incidentally by computed tomography (CT) or magnetic resonance imaging scans in asymptomatic individuals, or in the course of a respiratory workup. These cysts are often situated between the trachea and the esophagus in infants with respiratory distress. Tracheal compression or tracheal deviation may occur.

Bronchogenic Carcinoma[73]

Patients with advanced bronchogenic carcinoma may suffer from intra-luminal or extraluminal mass obstruction of a bronchus or the trachea. The clinical presentation, chest x-ray findings, and a CT scan help determine if one should expect difficulty in passing an ET past the vicinity of a bronchogenic lesion.

Thyroid Goiter[74]

Large thyroid goiters can lead to compression of the trachea and even tracheomalacia. This can worsen in the supine position and with the induction of general anesthesia. Retrosternal extensions of large goiters may act as mediastinal masses (see later).

Laryngeal Papillomatosis[75]

Patients with laryngeal papillomatosis require the frequent application of laser treatment for attempted eradication of the papillomas. Before treatment, the airway may be nearly obstructed from an overgrowth of lesions. During treatment, the inspired oxygen concentration should be kept to the minimum practical amount, with the avoidance of nitrous oxide, to reduce the chance of an airway fire. After treatment, the airway is raw and edematous. Laryngotracheomalacia may also be present, occasionally leading to complete upper airway collapse after extubation.

Mediastinal Masses[76–81]

Airway problems posed by mediastinal masses provide some of the greatest challenges faced by clinical anesthesia practitioners. Anesthesia is needed primarily for diagnostic biopsies and the staging of neoplasms but also occasionally for the relief of acute airway obstruction. The choice of anesthesia is guided by the cause and location of the mass (the extent and effect on adjoining airway or cardiovascular structures). All patients require a meticulous preoperative assessment that includes a careful history and physical examination aimed at delineating symptoms or signs that may indicate compression of major airways, the great vessels, or the heart itself. For emergency relief of airway compromise, one may have to use rigid bronchoscopy as a means of relieving the obstruction and determining the extent of airway compression. Under elective or semielective circumstances, preoperative laboratory investigations should include an electrocardiogram, a chest radiograph, a contrast CT scan of the thorax, and, if indicated by the patient's symptoms or signs, an echocardiogram or pulmonary flow volume loops with the patient sitting and supine (where available). Great clinical judgment must be exercised by the anesthesia practitioner and surgeon in choosing a suitable anesthetic plan. In general, short-acting agents should be used so that the patient returns to a "fully awake" state immediately postoperatively. In instances where the mass is small and does not compress adjoining structures, one may proceed with an intravenous induction and institute positive-pressure ventilation. On the other hand, one must be cognizant that airway or vascular compression may worsen during general anesthesia. Thus a prudent approach may include topical anesthesia of the airway followed by awake fiberoptic intubation of the trachea or inhalational induction and spontaneous ventilation supplemented by manual assistance. Seriously ill patients may require diagnostic biopsy or airway instrumentation with local anesthesia alone, as the risks of general anesthesia may outweigh any possible benefits. In any event, a surgeon experienced with rigid bronchoscopy must be present at induction if the potential for airway compression is substantial. If the airway is "lost" under anesthesia, placing the patient in the lateral decubitus or prone position may relieve the obstruction; however, rapid intubation of the airway with a rigid bronchoscope is usually most effective.

Significant obstruction of the superior vena cava (SVC) by tumor (SVC syndrome) is indicated by cyanosis, engorged veins, or edema of the upper body, or all of these. Patients with SVC syndrome are especially prone to airway obstruction, hypotension, and massive hemorrhage. Ideally, patients should be kept in a semiupright position to reduce airway edema; diagnostic tissue should be obtained under local anesthesia; packed red blood cells should be available in the operating room; large-bore intravenous access should be obtained in the lower extremities; and an arterial catheter should be inserted preoperatively.

■ Practical Points

1. Evaluation of the patient should center around the following clinical questions:
   - Is there superior vena cava (SVC) obstruction?
   - Is there tracheal compression?

- Is the pulmonary artery involved?
- Is the heart involved?

2. These questions must be investigated with the following tools:
   - Clinical presentation (signs, symptoms, and clinical findings; *most important*)
   - Chest radiograph
   - CT scan of chest
   - Flow-volume loops (ideally, both sitting and supine)

3. Signs and symptoms indicating *airway compromise* often include stridor, orthopnea, dyspnea, cyanosis, cough, decreased breath sounds, and wheezes. Signs and symptoms indicating critical *cardiovascular compression* may include fatigue, neck or facial edema, faintness, jugular venous distention, headache, papilledema, dyspnea, pulsus paradoxus, orthopnea, postural changes in blood pressure, and pallor.

4. With an anterior mediastinal mass, the mass compresses the mediastinal structures to varied degrees. Compression is maximal with the patient lying supine and would be expected to be less with the patient lying prone or on the side. If the patient seems to be getting into trouble when positioned supine, consider placing the patient on the side, or even prone.

5. With SVC obstruction, the face may become edematous and venous engorgement is present. The edema is a concern from the viewpoint of airway management, and special concern must be given to these patients when they are extubated. The venous engorgement is potentially a problem when nasal intubation is being considered (popular for fiberoptic intubation); the engorgement of nasopharyngeal veins may lead to troublesome epistaxis. Also, if there is SVC obstruction, do not place an intravenous line in the upper extremities; the principal source of venous return is the inferior vena cava, so the main intravenous line should be placed in a lower extremity.

6. The patient's history (especially symptoms when supine) often tells most of the story. That, together with a CT scan of the thorax and a chest radiograph, provides the most important information. Echocardiography evaluates myocardial contractility and assesses tumor encasement of the heart and great vessels. Differences between sitting and supine flow volume loops can help differentiate intrathoracic or extrathoracic obstruction. (However, most pulmonary function laboratories are not set up to do flow-volume loops with the patient in the supine position.) Fiberoptic bronchoscopy also evaluates dynamic airway obstruction. Finally, never forget that patients who are asymptomatic while awake may become obstructed after the administration of anesthetic.

7. In emergency situations when there is no time for a more complete assessment, increased emphasis must be placed on the

clinical findings, especially signs and symptoms in the supine position. Options to consider in this case are (1) awake fiberoptic bronchoscopy for intubation, checking for dynamic airway collapse, and (2) the maintenance of spontaneous breathing throughout (muscle relaxants may lead to airway loss).

8. When appropriate, preoperative radiation or chemotherapy should be considered to shrink sensitive tumors and alleviate symptoms.

SOME INFECTIOUS CONDITIONS WITH AIRWAY IMPLICATIONS

Tonsillitis and Other Tonsillar Disorders[82]

Tonsillectomy may be required in adults and children either because tonsillar hypertrophy is causing partial airway obstruction or because of the nuisance of repeated tonsillar infections. Less commonly, tonsillar malignancy may require radical craniofacial surgery, and occult hypertrophic tonsillar masses in completely asymptomatic individuals may rarely lead to fatal airway obstruction with the routine induction of general anesthesia.

Airway considerations for general anesthesia for tonsillectomy include determining that the intubation will likely be easy and extubating the patient at the end of the procedure only when the patient is wide awake with a good cough reflex.

Bleeding following tonsillectomy may necessitate a return to the operating room. A number of important considerations apply in this setting. The stomach contains blood, so the patient is at risk of aspiration, and a rapid sequence induction may be needed. The act of laryngoscopy may lead to torrential tonsillar bleeding. The patient may also be hypovolemic if the bleeding has been extensive. Finally, the possibility of coagulopathy should also be entertained with unexpected bleeding.

Epiglottitis[83–110]

Epiglottitis is the most dreaded of airway infections, especially in children. Victims are usually children aged 2 to 6 years, often infected with *Haemophilus influenzae*. These children may appear to be systemically ill ("toxic"), perhaps with a fever, or perhaps sitting up in a "tripod" position and drooling from difficulty with swallowing. Examining the child's airway may exacerbate the problem (by increasing airway edema), so tongue depressors and laryngoscopy are not options in the initial management.* Anything that might make the child cry (for example, needles) should be avoided. Consequently (and for other

---

*However, that has not stopped photographs of the epiglottis from being taken. With epiglottitis, the epiglottis looks like a bright red cherry. The airway is narrowed to an orifice only 2 to 3 mm in diameter.

reasons), the usual approach to management involves a careful inhalational induction with the child sitting in the anesthetist's lap and intubation of the child while he or she is breathing spontaneously under deep halothane anesthesia. If at laryngoscopy the orifice through the epiglottis cannot be identified, one trick is to have someone compress the child's chest, thus generating a small bubble in the epiglottis that the anesthetist can aim for. In the past, patients were managed by emergency tracheostomy; however, contemporary management of children includes short-term nasal intubation and intravenous antibiotic therapy.

Epiglottitis can occur in adults, too (George Washington is said to have died of it), but the situation is less dreadful here because the adult airway is larger. Most operators use awake fiberoptic laryngoscopy to secure the airway when necessary in this situation. There is considerable disagreement concerning airway management of the adult; however, there seems to be a growing consensus that the majority of adults are adequately treated in an intensive care unit with inhaled mist, antibiotics, and corticosteroids and that tracheal intubation is necessary only if symptoms of respiratory distress develop.

Airway in Human Immunodeficiency Virus–Infected Patients

With increasing frequency, clinicians are becoming aware of airway-related problems in human immunodeficiency virus–infected individuals. For example, Kaposi's sarcoma in acquired immunodeficiency syndrome patients has been reported to result in airway obstruction.[111] Similarly, opportunistic infections can also result in airway obstruction.[112, 113] A review by Judson and Sahn provides additional information.[114]

Ludwig's Angina[115–120]

Ludwig's angina is a multispace infection of the floor of the mouth. The infection starts with infected mandibular molars and spreads to sublingual, submental, buccal, and submandibular spaces. The tongue becomes elevated and displaced posteriorly, which may lead to loss of the airway, especially when the patient is placed in the supine position. An additional concern is the potential for abscess rupture into the hypopharynx (with possible lung soiling) either spontaneously or with attempts at laryngoscopy and intubation. Airway management options depend on the clinical severity, surgical preferences, and other factors (e.g., CT findings), but elective tracheostomy before incision and drainage remains the classic treatment modality (although many experts advocate fiberoptic intubation if at all possible).

Retropharyngeal Abscess[121]

Retropharyngeal abscess formation may occur from bacterial infection of the retropharyngeal space secondary to tonsillar or dental infections. Untreated, the posterior pharyngeal wall may advance anteriorly into the oropharynx, resulting in dyspnea and airway obstruction. Other clinical findings may include difficulty in swallowing, trismus, and a fluctuant posterior pharyngeal mass. An abscess cavity may be evident on lateral neck radiographs with anterior displacement of the esophagus and upper pharynx. Airway management may be complicated by trismus or airway obstruction. Because abscess rupture can lead to soiling of the trachea, contact with the posterior pharyngeal wall during laryngoscopy and intubation should be minimized. Incision and drainage is the mainstay of treatment. Tracheostomy is often required.

PRINCIPLES OF LASER AIRWAY SURGERY[122-128]

The word *laser* is an acronym for *light amplification by stimulated emission of radiation.* Light radiation emitted from conventional light sources (e.g., the incandescent lamp) is composed of many wavelengths that diverge with increasing distance from the source. In contrast, laser radiation is monochromatic (one color), characterized by the emission of photons that have the same energy, frequency, and wavelength traveling in exactly the same direction.

The energy from laser light is converted to thermal energy when the beam strikes human tissues. In airway surgery, lasers are used to vaporize pathologic lesions of the upper airway, vocal chords, trachea, and bronchi (Table 11–2). Compared with other ablative techniques, lasers offer the advantages of sterility, precision, and hemostasis while minimizing postoperative pain and edema.

Anesthesia practitioners must be aware of the risks of thermal injury or fire that may occur in laser airway surgery: (1) an airway fire caused by ignition of an endotracheal tube in the presence of nitrous oxide or oxygen-enriched air, (2) the ignition of drapes or other material in the operation room, and (3) thermal injury to the patient or operating room staff caused by inappropriate use of the laser.

Operating Room Hazards

Whenever lasers are used, safety precautions must be instituted to prevent the ignition of flammable substances in the operating room or unintentional injury to the patient or operating room personnel (Table 11–3).

Anesthetic Considerations for Laser Airway Surgery

Airway laser surgery may be performed with or without an ET in situ. If a rubber or plastic ET is used, special precautions must be used to prevent an ET fire. The incidence of airway fires is estimated at 0.4% to 0.6%, and a death following an airway fire has been reported. Several methods of endotracheal tube protection have been advocated to reduce the incidence of this complication (Table 11–4). In addition, the cuff of the ET should be filled with saline dyed with methylene blue. Saline will reduce the likelihood of ET ignition in the event the laser beam strikes the cuff, and leakage of the dye will alert the surgeon to termi-

Table 11–2 Lasers Used in Airway Surgery

Type of Laser	Use in Airway Surgery	Characteristics
Carbon dioxide laser	Wide variety of otolaryngologic procedures	Infrared radiation (invisible); therefore used with visible helium-neon (red) laser for aiming
		Energy absorbed by first 200 μm of all tissues
		CO_2 laser radiation cannot be transmitted through fiberoptic bundles
		May damage cornea No risk to retina
Neodymium-yttrium-aluminum-garnet laser (Nd-YAG)	Coagulation and deep thermal destruction of obstructing bronchial lesions	Infrared radiation (invisible)
		Absorption enhanced by blue and black pigments
		Nd-YAG radiation may be transmitted through fiberoptic bundles
		High energy levels may perforate bronchial structures or large blood vessels

Table 11–3 Safety Precautions for Laser Surgery

Level of Application	Safety Precaution
Laser	Set on "off" or "standby" modes unless firing.
	Use in "pulsed" mode rather than "continuous" mode whenever possible (limits energy output).
	Avoid aiming at reflective surfaces (matte finished or black instruments are often used in laser surgery).
Patients	Tape patient's eyes shut and cover with moistened eye pads.
	Minimize use of surgical drapes since paper and cloth drapes are flammable and may cause severe burns or inhalational smoke injury if ignited.
	Place moistened cloth drapes near surgical field to reduce combustibility.
Operating room personnel	Wear protective eyeglasses with side guards (contact lenses are *not* protective): Nd-YAG laser (green with maximal absorption at 1.064 μm); argon laser (orange); CO_2 laser (clear).
Operating room	Place sign on door leading to operating room warning of laser use.
	Place appropriate protective eyeglasses outside operating room for personnel entering while procedure is underway.
	Nd-YAG and argon lasers may penetrate glass (cover any windows in operating room).

Table 11–4 Strategies That Reduce the Incidence of Endotracheal Tube Fires

Method	Advantages	Disadvantages
Plastic or rubber endotracheal tubes Wrap shaft of combustible* endotracheal tube with metallic foil tape	Inexpensive technique	Endotracheal tubes may be ignited by heating of gases or material in the endotracheal tube.
		Incendiary characteristics of different brands of metallic tapes vary.
		Flammability of every batch of tape must be evaluated before use since changes in manufacture of metallic foil tapes may occur without prior notice to physicians.
		Metallic foil tapes are not made for medical applications, and none have been sanctioned by FDA.
		Metallic foil tape does not protect internal surface of ETs or distal end beyond cuff.
Wrap shaft of combustible* endotracheal tube with Merocel Laser-Guard (Mystic, Conn) ET protective coating	Consists of rectangular sheet of silver foil covered by Merocel sponge layer that is applied to external surface of combustible ETs	Does not protect entire length of ET shaft.
		Does not protect internal surface of ETs or distal end beyond cuff.
	Easier to apply than metallic foil tape	
Specialty endotracheal tubes Xomed Laser-Shield I Endotracheal Tubes (Xomed, Jacksonville, Fla)	Composed of nonreflective silicone-containing metallic materials	May be perforated by CO_2 laser operated at high energy settings.
	Effective when used with CO_2 laser in pulsed mode	In enriched O_2 environment ignition may result in blowtorch fire and disintegration of tube.
		Expensive and approved for single use only.

Table continued on following page

Table 11–4   Strategies That Reduce the Incidence of Endotracheal Tube Fires *Continued*

Method	Advantages	Disadvantages
Biona Fome-Cuf Laser Endotracheal Tubes (Biona, Gary, Ind)	Flexible aluminum shaft covered with silicone Effective when used with CO_2 laser in pulsed mode	Fome-Cuf made from polyurethane foam covered with silicone. If pilot tube or cuff is perforated it may be impossible to deflate Fome-Cuf. Polyurethane may ignite if Fome-Cuf is not filled with saline and is struck by laser beam. Silicone covering may ignite under extreme circumstances. Expensive; single use only.
Mallinckrodt Laser-Flex Endotracheal Tubes (Mallinckrodt, Glen Falls, NY)	Flexible stainless steel shaft with two PVC cuffs at distal end For use with CO_2 and KTP lasers	PVC cuffs are combustible. Expensive; single use only.
Norton Laser Endotracheal Tubes (A. V. Mueller, Chicago, Ill)	Cuffless, flexible stainless steel shaft May be autoclaved and reused	Thick-walled and stiff; inconvenient to position in airway. May leak anesthetic gases unless separate combustible cuff is attached to distal end.
Alternatives to endotracheal tubes Venturi jet lung ventilation	Oxygen from 50 psig (pounds per square inch gauge) source is directed down rigid bronchoscope or operating laryngoscope through small catheter No risk of airway fire from combustion of foreign material Provides unobstructed view for surgeon	Oxygen concentration delivered to patient is unknown since pure oxygen from catheter mixes with air that is entrained through bronchoscope. Impossible to measure end-tidal CO_2 concentration reliably. Requires total intravenous anaesthesia to anesthetize patient. Risk of barotrauma. No protection against pulmonary aspiration of stomach contents or debris from laser procedure.

**Table 11–4 Strategies That Reduce the Incidence of
Endotracheal Tube Fires** *Continued*

Method	Advantages	Disadvantages
Intermittent apneic technique	Lung ventilation with mask or endotracheal tube followed by period of apnea in which artificial airway is removed and laser therapy is performed. Sao_2 determines frequency of ventilation No risk of airway fire from combustion of foreign material Provides unobstructed view for surgeon	Cannot measure end-tidal CO_2 during period of apnea. Requires total intravenous anesthesia to anesthetize patient. No protection against pulmonary aspiration of stomach contents or debris from laser procedure.

*Included rubber and plastic ETs.
ET, endotracheal tube; FDA, Food and Drug Administration; PVC, polyvinyl chloride.

nate operation of the laser. Nitrous oxide should be avoided during airway laser surgery since it supports combustion as readily as oxygen. Oxygen blended with air or helium should be administered at the lowest fraction of inspired oxygen that will support satisfactory arterial oxygen hemoglobin saturation. Although high concentrations of the halogenated volatile agents (halothane, enflurane, and isoflurane) are flammable, the clinical concentrations normally employed will not affect combustion.

Management of an Airway Fire

All personnel associated with laser endoscopic surgery should be well versed with procedures to rapidly extinguish fires localized to the site

Table 11–5 Laser Airway Fire Protocol

Cease ventilation and turn off all anesthetic gases, *including oxygen.*

Extinguish flames with saline solution.*

Remove endotracheal tube after deflating cuff.* Be certain entire endotracheal tube has been removed.

Ventilate patient's lungs by mask after all burning material has been removed and extinguished.

Examine airway for burns and foreign bodies such as fragments of endotracheal tube or packing material.

*These steps should be taken simultaneously by the anesthetist and the surgeon.
Modified from Benumof JL: Anesthesia for special elective therapeutic procedures. In Anesthesia for Thoracic Surgery, 2nd ed. Philadelphia, WB Saunders, 1995, p 520.

of airway surgery or elsewhere in the operating room. In the event of an airway fire, immediate, appropriate actions taken by the anesthetist may prevent what would otherwise result in serious injury (Table 11–5).

REFERENCES

1. Abou-Shala N, MacIntyre N: Emergent management of acute asthma. Med Clin North Am 80:677, 1996.
2. Alberts WM, do Pico GA: Reactive airways dysfunction syndrome. Chest 109:1618, 1996.
3. Beveridge RC, Grunfeld AF, Hodder RV, Verbeek PR: Guidelines for the emergency management of asthma in adults. CAEP/CTS Asthma Advisory Committee. Canadian Association of Emergency Physicians and the Canadian Thoracic Society. Can Med Assoc J 155:25, 1996.
4. Craig TJ: Drugs to be used with caution in patients with asthma. Am Fam Physician 54:947, 957, 1996.
5. Kamada AK, Szefler SJ: The role of theophylline in the treatment of asthma. Ann Allergy Asthma Immunol 77:1, 1996.
6. Wasserfallen JB, Baraniuk JN: Clinical use of inhaled corticosteroids in asthma. J Allergy Clin Immunol 97:177, 1996.
7. Weinberger M, Hendeles L: Theophylline in asthma. N Engl J Med 334:1380, 1996.
8. Haddow GR, Riley E, Isaacs R, McSharry R: Ketorolac, nasal polyposis, and bronchial asthma: A cause for concern. Anesth Analg 76:420, 1993.
9. Kardon EM: Acute asthma. Emerg Med Clin North Am 14:93, 1996.
10. Bigatello LM, Zapol WM: New approaches to acute lung injury. Br J Anaesth 77:99, 1996.
11. Cole FJ Jr, Shouse BA: Alternative modalities of ventilation in acute respiratory failure. Surg Ann 27:55, 1995.
12. Fulkerson WJ, MacIntyre N, Stamler J, Crapo JD: Pathogenesis and treatment of the adult respiratory distress syndrome. Arch Intern Med 156:29, 1996.
13. Hudson LD: New therapies for ARDS. Chest 108(2 suppl):79S, 1995.
14. Kollef MH, Schuster DP: The acute respiratory distress syndrome. N Engl J Med 332:27, 1995.
15. Lessard MR: New concepts in mechanical ventilation for ARDS. Can J Anaesth 43(5, part 2):R42, 1996.
16. Macnaughton PD, Evans TW: Management of adult respiratory distress syndrome. Lancet 339:469, 1992.
17. Marinelli WA, Ingbar DH: Diagnosis and management of acute lung injury. Clin Chest Med 15:517, 1994.
18. Repine JE: Scientific perspectives on adult respiratory distress syndrome. Lancet 339:466, 1992.
19. Schuster DP, Kollef MH: Acute respiratory distress syndrome. Dis Mon 42:270, 1996.
20. Sessler CN, Bloomfield GL, Fowler AA 3rd: Current concepts of sepsis and acute lung injury. Clin Chest Med 17:213, 1996.
21. Steltzer H, Krafft P, Fridrich P, Hammerle AF: Severity and outcome of ARDS: The present place of extracorporeal lung assist (ECLA). Int J Artif Organs 18:607, 1995.
22. Fields AI: Newer modes of mechanical ventilation for patients with adult respiratory distress syndrome. Crit Care Med 21(9 suppl):S367, 1993.
23. Fulghan JR, Wijdicks EF: Guillain-Barré syndrome. Crit Care Clin 13:1, 1997.
24. Salzarulo HH, Taylor LA: Diabetic "still joint syndrome" as a cause of difficult endotracheal intubation. Anesthesiology 64:366, 1986.
25. Eleborg L, Norberg AA: Are diabetic patients difficult to intubate? Acta Anaesthesiol Scand 32:508, 1988.
26. Hogan K, Rusy D, Springman SR: Difficult laryngoscopy and diabetes mellitus. Anesth Analg 67:1162, 1988.
27. Grfic A, Rosenbloom AL, Weber FT, et al: Joint contracture in childhood diabetes. N Engl J Med 292:372, 1975.

28. Seibold JR: Digital sclerosis in children with insulin-dependent diabetes mellitus. Arthritis Rheum 25:1357, 1982.
29. Buckingham B, Uitto J, Sandborg C, et al: Scleroderma-like syndrome and the non-enzymatic glycosylation of collagen in children with poorly controlled insulin dependent diabetes (IDDM). Pediatr Res 5:A626, 1981.
30. Nichol H, Zuck D: Difficult laryngoscopy—The "anterior" larynx and the atlanto-occipital gap. Br J Anaesth 55:120, 1983.
31. Reissell E, Orko R, Maunuksela EL, Lindgren L: Predictability of difficult laryngoscopy in patients with long-term diabetes mellitus. Anaesthesia 45:1024, 1990.
32. Chapple M, Jung RT, Francis J, et al: Joint contractures and diabetic retinopathy. Postgrad Med J 59: 291, 1983.
33. Cadieux RJ, Kales A, Santen RJ, et al: Endoscopic findings in sleep apnea associated with acromegaly. J Clin Endocrinol Metab 55:18, 1982.
34. Horner RL, Mohiaddin RH, Lowell DG, et al: Sites and sizes of fat deposits around the pharynx in obese patients with obstructive sleep apnoea and weight matched controls. Eur Respir J 2:613, 1989.
35. Suratt PM, McTier RF, Findley LJ, et al: Changes in breathing and the pharynx after weight loss in obstructive sleep apnea. Chest 92:631, 1987.
36. Davies SF, Lber C: Obstructive sleep apnea associated with adult-acquired micrognathia from rheumatoid arthritis. Am Rev Respir Dis 127:245, 1983.
37. Dodds C, Ryall DM: Tonsils: Obesity and obstructive sleep apnoea. Br J Hosp Med 47:62, 1992.
38. Goldstein SJ, Wu RH, Thorpy MJ, et al: Reversibility of deficient sleep entrained growth hormone secretion in a boy with achondroplasia and obstructive sleep apnea. Acta Endocrinol 116:95, 1987.
39. Johnston C, Taussig LM, Koopmann C, et al: Obstructive sleep apnea in Treacher-Collins syndrome. Cleft Palate J 18:39, 1981.
40. Schmidt-Nowara WW: Continuous positive airway pressure for long-term treatment of sleep apnea. Am J Dis Child 138:82, 1984.
41. Shapiro J, Strome M, Crocker AC: Airway obstruction and sleep apnea in Hurler and Hunter syndromes. Ann Otol Rhinol Laryngol 94:458, 1985.
42. Bray GA, Gray DS: Obesity. Part 1: Pathogenesis. West J Med 149:429, 1988.
43. Buckley FP, Robinson NB, Simonowitz DA, Dellinger EP: Anaesthesia in the morbidly obese. A comparison of anaesthetic and analgesic regimens for upper abdominal surgery. Anaesthesia 38:840, 1983.
44. Farebrother MJB: Respiratory function and cardiorespiratory response to exercise in obesity. Br J Dis Chest 73:211, 1979.
45. Luce JM: Respiratory complications of obesity. Chest 78:626, 1980.
46. Lee JJ, Larson RM, Buckley JJ, Roberts AB: Airway maintenance in the morbidly obese. Anesthesiol Rev 7:33, 1980.
47. Norton ML, Brown ACD: Evaluating the patient with a difficult airway for anesthesia. Otolaryngol Clin North Am 23:771, 1990.
48. Baughn RW, Bauer S, Wise L: Volume and pH of gastric juice in obese patients. Anesthesiology 43:686, 1975.
49. Kallar SK, Everett LL: Potential risks and preventive measures for pulmonary aspiration: New concepts in preoperative fasting. Anesth Analg 77:171, 1993.
50. Schneller S: Medical considerations and perioperative care for rheumatoid surgery. Hand Clin 5:115, 1989.
51. Redlund-Johnell I: Upper airway obstruction in patients with rheumatoid arthritis and temporomandibular joint destruction. Scand J Rheumatol 17:273, 1988.
52. Brazeau-Lamontagne L, Charlin B, Levesque RY, Lussier A: Cricoarytenoiditis: CT assessment in rheumatoid arthritis. Radiology 158:463, 1986.
53. Funk D, Raymon F: Rheumatoid arthritis of the cricoarytenoid joints: An airway hazard. Anesth Analg 54:742, 1975.
54. Geterud A, Bake B, Berthelsen B, Bjelle A, Ejnell H: Laryngeal involvement in rheumatoid arthritis. Acta Otolaryngol 111:990, 1991.
55. Geterud A, Ejnell H, Mansson I, et al: Severe airway obstruction caused by laryngeal rheumatoid arthritis. J Rheumatol 13:948, 1986.

56. Leicht MJ, Harrington TM, Davis DE: Cricoarytenoid arthritis: A cause of laryngeal obstruction. Ann Emerg Med 16:885, 1987.
57. McGeehan DF, Crinnion JN, Strachan DR: Life-threatening stridor presenting in a patient with rheumatoid involvement of the larynx. Arch Emerg Med 6:274, 1989.
58. Vassallo CL: Rheumatoid arthritis of the cricoarytenoid joints: Cause of upper airway obstruction. Arch Intern Med 117:273, 1966.
59. McCredie JA (ed): Basic Surgery. New York, Macmillan, 1977.
60. Meyer GW, Castell DO: Evaluation and management of diseases of the esophagus. Am J Otolaryngol 2:336, 1981.
61. Goldhill DR, Dalgleish JG, Lake RH: Respiratory problems and acromegaly. An acromegalic with hypersomnia, acute upper airway obstruction and pulmonary oedema. Anaesthesia 37:1200, 1982.
62. Hassan SZ, Matz GJ, Lawrence AM, Collins PA: Laryngeal stenosis in acromegaly: A possible cause of airway difficulties associated with anesthesia. Anesth Analg 55:57, 1976.
63. Mezon BJ, West P, MaClean JP, Kryger MH: Sleep apnea in acromegaly. Am J Med 69:615, 1980.
64. Singelyn FJ, Scholtes, JL: Airway obstruction in acromegaly: A method of prevention. Anaesth Intensive Care 16:491, 1988.
65. Ziemer DC, Dunlap DB: Relief of sleep apnea in acromegaly by bromocriptine. Am J Med Sci 295:49, 1988.
66. Gaba DM, Fish KJ, Howard SK: Crisis Management in Anesthesiology. New York, Churchill Livingstone, 1994.
67. Levy JH: Anaphylactic Reactions in Anaesthesia and Intensive Care, 2nd ed. Boston, Butterworth, 1986.
68. Lund VJ: Diagnosis and treatment of nasal polyps. BMJ 311:1411, 1995.
69. Bernstein JM, Gorfien J, Noble B: Role of allergy in nasal polyposis: A review. Otolaryngol Head Neck Surg 113:724, 1995.
70. Hindle I, Downer MC, Speight PM: The epidemiology of oral cancer. Br J Oral Maxillofac Surg 34:471, 1996.
71. Wijayaweera ND, Ganepala SR: Epiglottic cyst aspiration before induction of anaesthesia. Ceylon Med J 38:137, 1993.
72. Aktogu S, Yuncu G, Halilcolar H, et al: Bronchogenic cysts: Clinicopathological presentation and treatment. Eur Respir J 9:2017, 1996.
73. Dartevelle P, Macchiarini P: Carinal resection for bronchogenic cancer. Semin Thorac Cardiovasc Surg 8:414, 1996.
74. Licker M, Schweizer A, Nicolet G, et al: Anesthesia of a patient with an obstructing tracheal mass: A new way to manage the airway. Acta Anaesthesiol Scand 41:84, 1997.
75. Gardner GM, Benninger MS: Adult onset laryngeal papillomatosis. Ear Nose Throat J 75:404, 1996.
76. Amaha K, Okutsu Y, Nakamuru Y: Major airway obstruction by mediastinal tumour. A case report. Br J Anaesth 45:1082, 1973.
77. Bray RJ, Fernandes FJ: Mediastinal tumour causing airway obstruction in anaesthetized children. Anaesthesia 37:571, 1982.
78. Mackie AM, Watson CB: Anaesthesia and mediastinal masses. Anaesthesia 39:899, 1984.
79. Piro AJ, Weiss DR, Hellman S: Mediastinal Hodgkin's disease: A possible danger for intubation anesthesia. Int J Radiat Oncol Biol Phys 1:415, 1976.
80. Neuman GG, Weingarten AE, Abramowitz RM, et al: The anesthetic management of the patient with an anterior mediastinal mass. Anesthesiology 60:144, 1984.
81. Prakash UBS, Abel MD, Hubmay RD: Mediastinal mass and tracheal obstruction during general anesthesia. Mayo Clin Proc 63:1004, 1988.
82. Dodds C, Ryall DM: Tonsils, obesity and obstructive sleep apnoea. Br J Hosp Med 47:62, 1992.
83. Benjamin B, O'Reilly B: Acute epiglottitis in infants and children. Ann Otol Rhinol Laryngol 85:565, 1976.

84. Trollfors B, Nylen O, Strangert K: Acute epiglottitis in children and adults in Sweden 1981–3. Arch Dis Child 65:491, 1990.
85. Vernon DD, Sarnaik AP: Acute epiglottitis in children: A conservative approach to diagnosis and management. Arch Intern Med 14:23, 1986.
86. Claesson B, Trollfors B, Ekström-Jodal B, et al: Incidence and prognosis of acute epiglottitis in children in a Swedish region. Pediatr Infect Dis J 3:534, 1984.
87. Adair JC, Ring WH: Management of epiglottitis in children. Anesth Analg 54:622, 1975.
88. Arndal H, Andreassen UK: Acute epiglottis in children and adults. Nasotracheal intubation, tracheostomy or careful observation? Current status in Scandinavia. J Laryngol Otol 102:1012, 1988.
89. Baines DB, Wark H, Overton JH: Acute epiglottis in children. Anaesth Intensive Care 13:25, 1985.
90. Battaglia JD, Lockhart CH: Management of acute epiglottitis by nasotracheal intubation. Am J Dis Child 129:334, 1975.
91. Blanc VF, Weber ML, Leduc C, et al: Acute epiglottitis in children: Management of 27 consecutive cases with nasotracheal intubation, with special emphasis on anaesthetic considerations. Can J Anaesth 24:1, 1977.
92. Breivik H, Klaastad O: Acute epiglottitis in children. Review of 27 patients. Br J Anaesth 50:505, 1978.
93. Butt W, Shann F, Walker C, et al: Acute epiglottitis: A different approach to management. Crit Care Med 16:43, 1988.
94. DiTirro FR, Silver MH, Hengerer AS: Acute epiglottitis: Evolution of management in the community hospital. Int J Pediatr Otorhinolaryngol 7:145, 1984.
95. Gonzalez C, Reilly JS, Kenna MA, Thompson AE: Duration of intubation in children with acute epiglottitis. Otolaryngol Head Neck Surg 95:477, 1986.
96. Greenberg LW, Schisgall R: Acute epiglottitis in a community hospital. Am Fam Physician 19:123, 1979.
97. Sendi K, Crysdale WS: Acute epiglottitis: Decade of change—A 10-year experience with 242 children. J Otolaryngol 16:196, 1987.
98. Andreassen UK, Husum B, Tos M, Leth N: Acute epiglottitis in adults. A management protocol based on a 17-year material. Acta Anaesthesiol Scand 28:155, 1984.
99. Carenfelt C: Etiology of acute infectious epiglottitis in adults: Septic vs local infection. Scand J Infect Dis 21:53, 1989.
100. Crosby E, Reid D: Acute epiglottitis in the adult: Is intubation mandatory? Can J Anaesth 38:914, 1991.
101. Deeb ZE, Yenson AC, DeFries HO: Acute epiglottitis in the adult. Laryngoscope 95:289, 1985.
102. Fontanarosa PB, Polsky SS, Goldman GE: Adult epiglottitis. J Emerg Med 7:223, 1989.
103. Khilanani U, Khatib R: Acute epiglottitis in adults. Am J Med Sci 287:65, 1984.
104. MayoSmith MF, Hirsch PJ, Wodzinski SF, Schiffman FJ: Acute epiglottitis in adults. An eight-year experience in the state of Rhode Island. N Engl J Med 314:1133, 1986.
105. McNelis FL: Medical and legal management of adult acute epiglottitis. Laryngoscope 95:125, 1985.
106. Rivron RP, Murray JA: Adult epiglottitis: Is there a consensus on diagnosis and treatment? Clin Otolaryngol 16:338, 1991.
107. Stair TO, Hirsch BE: Adult supraglottitis. Am J Emerg Med 3:512, 1985.
108. Stanley RE, Liang TS: Acute epiglottitis in adults (the Singapore experience). J Laryngol Otol 102:1017, 1988.
109. Tveteras K, Kristensen S: Acute epiglottitis in adults: Bacteriology and therapeutic principles. Clin Otolaryngol 12:337, 1987.
110. Wurtele P: Nasotracheal intubation—A modality in the management of acute epiglottitis in adults. J Otolaryngol 13:118, 1984.
111. Greenberg JE, Fischl MA, Berger JR: Upper airway obstruction secondary to acquired immunodeficiency syndrome–related Kaposi's sarcoma. Chest 88:638, 1985.

112. Berlinger NT, Freeman TJ: Acute airway obstruction due to necrotizing tracheo-bronchial aspergillosis in immunocompromised patients: A new clinical entity. Ann Otol Rhinol Laryngol 98:718, 1989.

113. Imoto EM, Stein RM, Shellito JE, Curtis JL: Central airway obstruction due to cytomegalovirus-induced necrotizing tracheitis in a patient with AIDS. Am Rev Respir Dis 142:884, 1990.

114. Judson MA, Sahn SA: Endobronchial lesions in HIV-infected individuals. Chest 105:1314, 1992.

115. Patterson HC, Kelly JH, Strome M: Ludwig's angina: An update. Laryngoscope 92:370, 1982.

116. Fritsch DE, Klein DG: Ludwig's angina. Heart Lung 21:39, 1992.

117. Sethi DS, Stanley RE: Deep neck abscesses—Changing trends. J Laryngol Otol 108:138, 1994.

118. De Heyn G, Mullier JP, De Smet JM: Etiology and therapy of Ludwig's angina. Acta Otorhinolaryngol Belg 33:235, 1979.

119. Holland CS: The management of Ludwig's angina. Br J Oral Surg 13:153, 1975.

120. Schwartz HC, Bauer RA, Davis NJ, Guralnick WC: Ludwig's angina: Use of fiberoptic laryngoscopy to avoid tracheostomy. J Oral Surg 2:608, 1974.

121. Gidley PW, Ghorayeb BY, Stiernberg CM: Contemporary management of deep neck space infections. Otolaryngol Head Neck Surg 116:16, 1997.

122. Burgess GE, LeJeune FE Jr: Endotracheal tube irrigation during laser surgery of the larynx. Arch Otolaryngol 105:561, 1979.

123. Cozine K, Stone JG, Shulman S, et al: Ventilatory complications of carbon dioxide laryngeal surgery. J Clin Anesth 3:20, 1991.

124. Le Jeune FE Jr, Guice C, Letard F, et al: Heat sink protection against lasering endotracheal tube cuffs. Ann Otol Rhinol Laryngol 91:606. 1982.

125. Sosis M, Dillion FX: Saline filled cuffs help prevent laser-induced tracheal tube cuff ignition. Anesth Analg 72:197, 1991.

126. Pashayan AG, Gravenstein JS: Helium retards endotracheal tube fires from carbon dioxide lasers. Anesthesiology 62:274, 1985.

127. Leonard PF: The lower limits of flammability of halothane enflurane and isoflurane. Anesth Analg 54: 238, 1975.

128. Ossoff RH: Laser safety in otolaryngology–head and neck surgery: Anesthetic and educational considerations for laser laryngeal surgery. Laryngoscope 99(8 part 2, suppl 48):1, 1989.

129. Steward DJ: Manual of Pediatric Anesthesia, 3rd ed. New York, Churchill Livingstone, 1990.

130. Mayhew JF, Katz J, Miner M, et al: Anaesthesia for the achondroplastic dwarf. Can J Anaesth 33:216, 1986.

131. Stokes DC, Phillips JA, Leonard CO, et al: Respiratory complications of achondroplasia. J Pediatr 102:534, 1983.

132. Southwick JP, Katz J: Unusual airway difficulty in the acromegalic patient—Indications for tracheostomy. Anesthesiology 51:72, 1979.

133. Kitahata LM: Airway difficulties associated with anaesthesia in acromegaly. Three case reports. Br J Anaesth 43:1187, 1971.

134. Burn JM: Airway difficulties associated with anaesthesia in acromegaly. Br J Anaesth 44:413, 1972.

135. Trotman-Dickenson B, Weetman AP, Hughes JM: Upper airflow obstruction and pulmonary function in acromegaly: Relationship to disease activity. Q J Med 79:527, 1991.

136. Gorlin RJ, Pindborg JJ, Cohen MM Jr (eds): Syndromes of the Head and Neck, 2nd ed. New York, McGraw-Hill, 1976.

137. Andersson H, Gomes SP: Craniosynostosis: Review of the literature and indications for surgery. Acta Paediatr Scand 57:47, 1968.

138. Davies DW, Munro IR: The anesthetic management and intraoperative care of patients undergoing major facial osteotomies. Plast Reconstr Surg 55:50, 1975.

139. Kreiborg S, Barr M Jr, Cohen MM Jr: Cervical spine in the Apert syndrome. Am J Med Genet 43:704, 1992.

140. Friedlander HL, Westin GW, Wood WL: Arthrogryposis multiplex congenita: A review of 45 cases. J Bone Joint Surg Am 50:89, 1968.
141. Chamberlain MA: Behçet's syndrome in 32 patients in Yorkshire. Ann Rheum Dis 36:491, 1977.
142. Turner ME: Anaesthetic difficulties associated with Behçet's Syndrome. Br J Anaesth 44:100, 1972.
143. Stool SE, Eavey RD, Stein NL, Sharrar WG: The chubby puffer syndrome: Upper airway obstruction and obesity, with intermittent somnolence and cardiorespiratory embarrassment. Clin Pediatr 16:43, 1977.
144. Smith DW: The compendium on shortness of stature. J Pediatr 70:463, 1967.
145. Rudolf Am, Hoffman J, Axelrod S (eds): Pediatrics, 18th ed. East Norwalk, Conn, Appleton-Century-Crofts, 1987.
146. Sagehashi N: An infant with Crouzon's syndrome with a cartilaginous trachea and a human tail. J Craniomaxillofac Surg 20:21, 1992.
147. Seashore JH, Gardiner LJ, Ariyan S: Management of giant cystic hygromas in infants. Am J Surg 149:459, 1985.
148. Evans P: Intubation problem in a case of cystic hygroma complicated by a laryngotracheal haemangioma. Anaesthesia 36:696, 1981.
149. Ricciardelli EJ, Richardson MA: Cervicofacial cystic hygroma. Patterns of recurrence and management of the difficult case. Arch Otolaryngol Head Neck Surg 117:546, 1991.
150. Myer CM, Bratcher GO: Laryngeal cystic hygroma. Head Neck Surg 6:706, 1983.
151. Hamoir M, Remacle M, Youssif A, et al: Surgical management of parapharyngeal cystic hygroma causing sudden airway obstruction. Head Neck Surg 10:406, 1988.
152. Emery PJ, Bailey CM, Evans JN: Cystic hygroma of the head and neck. A review of 37 cases. J Laryngol Otol 98:613, 1984.
153. Ellis RWB, Van Creveld S: A syndrome characterized by ectodermal dysplasia, polydactyly, chondrodysplasia and congenital morbus cordis: Report of 3 cases. Arch Dis Child 15:65, 1940.
154. Reddy ARR, Wong DHW: Epidermolysis bullosa: A review of anesthetic problems and case reports. Can J Anaesth 19:536, 1972.
155. James I, Wark H: Airway management during anesthesia in patients with epidermolysis bullosa dystrophica. Anesthesiology 56:323, 1982.
156. Gilbertson AA, Boulton TB: Anaesthesia in difficult situations: Influence of disease on pre-op preparation and choice of anesthetic. Anaesthesia 22:607, 1967.
157. Clarren SK, Smith DW: The fetal alcohol syndrome. N Engl J Med 298:1063, 1978.
158. Finucane BT: Difficult intubation associated with the fetal alcohol syndrome. Can J Anaesth 27:574, 1980.
159. Usowicz AG, Golabi M, Curry C: Upper airway obstruction in infants with fetal alcohol syndrome. Am J Dis Child 140:1039, 1986.
160. Aoe T, Kohchi T, Mizuguchi T: Respiratory inductance plethysmography and pulse oximetry in the assessment of upper airway patency in a child with Goldenhar's syndrome. Can J Anaesth 37:369, 1990.
161. McKusick VA: Mendelian Inheritance in Man, 5th ed. Baltimore, Johns Hopkins University Press, 1983.
162. Hopkinson RB, AJ Sutcliffe: Hereditary angioneurotic oedema. Anaesthesia 34:183, 1979.
163. Gibbs PS, LoSasso AM, Moorthy SS, Hutton CE: The anesthetic and perioperative management of a patient with a documented hereditary angioneurotic edema. Anesth Analg 56:571, 1977.
164. Lieberman PH, Dargeon HWK, Begg CF: A reappraisal of eosinophilic granuloma of bone. Hand-Schuller-Christian syndrome and Letterer-Siwe syndrome. Medicine 48:375, 1969.
165. Kempthorne PM, Brown TC: Anaesthesia and the mucopolysaccharidoses: A survey of techniques and problems. Anaesth Intensive Care 11:203, 1983.
166. Herrick IA, Rhine EJ: The mucopolysaccharidoses and anaesthesia: A report of clinical experience. Can J Anaesth 35:67, 1988.
167. Brama I, Gay I, Feinmesser R, Springer C: Upper airway obstruction in Hunter syndrome. Int J Pediatr Otorhinolaryngol 11:229, 1986.

168. Saki CT, Ruiz R, Gaito R Jr, et al: Hunter's syndrome: A study in airway obstruction. Laryngoscope 97:280, 1987.

169. Sjogren P, Pedersen T: Anaesthetic problems in Hurler-Scheie syndrome. Report of two cases. Acta Anaesthesiol Scand 30:484, 1986.

170. Baines D, Keneally J: Anaesthetic implications of the mucopolysaccharidoses: A fifteen-year experience in a children's hospital. Anaesth Intensive Care 11:198, 1983.

171. Adachi K, Chole RA: Management of tracheal lesions in Hurler syndrome. Arch Otolaryngol Head Neck Surg 116:1205, 1990.

172. Myer CM: Airway obstruction in Hurler's syndrome—Radiographic features. Int J Pediatr Otorhinolaryngol 22:91, 1991.

173. Peters ME, Arya S, Langer LO, et al: Narrow trachea in mucopolysaccharidoses. Pediatr Radiol 15:225, 1985.

174. Daum RE, Jones DJ: Fibreoptic intubation in Klippel-Feil syndrome. Anaesthesia 43:18, 1988.

175. Grundfast KM, Mumtaz A, Kanter R, Pollack M: Tracheomalacia in an infant with multiplex congenita (Larsen's) syndrome. Ann Otol Rhinol Laryngol 90:303, 1981.

176. Rock MJ, Green CG, Pauli RM, Peters ME: Tracheomalacia and bronchomalacia associated with Larsen syndrome. Pediatr Pulmonol 5:55, 1988.

177. Katz J, Benumof J, Kadis L: Anesthesia and Uncommon Diseases, 3rd ed. Philadelphia, WB Saunders, 1990.

178. Birkinshaw KJ: Anesthesia in a patient with an unstable neck: Morquio's syndrome. Anaesthesia 30:46, 1975.

179. McKusick VA: Heritable Disorders of Connective Tissue, 8th ed. Baltimore, The Johns Hopkins University Press, 1988.

180. Bolsin SN, Gillbe C: Opitz-Frias syndrome: A case with potentially hazardous anaesthetic implications. Anaesthesia 40:1189, 1985.

181. Cox JM: Anesthesia and glycogen-storage disease. Anesthesiology 29:1221, 1968.

182. Chung F, Crago RR: Sleep apnea syndrome and anaesthesia. Can J Anaesth 29:439, 1982.

183. Phillipson EA: Control of breathing during sleep. Am Rev Resp Dis 118:909, 1978.

184. Shprintzen RJ, Croft C, Berkman MD, Rakoff SJ: Pharyngeal hypoplasia in Treacher Collins syndrome. Arch Otolaryngol 105:127, 1979.

185. Rasch DK, Browder F, Barr M, Greer D: Anaesthesia for Treacher Collins and Pierre Robin syndromes: A report of three cases. Can J Anaesth 33:364, 1986.

186. Vaghadia H, Blackstock: Anesthetic implications of the trismus pseudocamptodactyly (Dutch-Kentucky or Hecht Beals) syndrome. Can J Anaesth 35:80, 1988.

Chapter 12

The Difficult Pediatric Airway

Melissa Wheeler

Two landmark reviews of critical anesthesia incidents, collected from settled lawsuits (American Society of Anesthesiologists [ASA] Closed Claims Project: Pediatric Data[1]) and voluntary reports to a central monitoring body (the Australian Incident Monitoring Study[2]), underscore the importance that a skilled and knowledgeable approach to pediatric airway management has to the delivery of safe pediatric anesthesia. Pediatric claims represented approximately 10% of all claims reviewed for both the ASA Closed Claims Project (238 pediatric claims, 2262 adult claims) and the Australian Incident Monitoring Study (207 pediatric claims, 1793 adult claims). Findings for pediatric claims were also different than for adult claims in both studies. The salient findings of the ASA Closed Claims Project were as follows: (1) There was a greater percentage of respiratory events in the pediatric population (43% versus 30%; $P = .01$). Also, in contrast to adults, these children were healthy and not obese. (2) There was a greater mortality rate in the pediatric population (50% versus 35%; $P = .01$). (3) There was more frequent brain damage in the pediatric population (30% versus 11%; $P = .01$). (4) Care was more frequently judged to be substandard in the pediatric population (54% versus 44%; $P = .01$). (5) Complications were more frequently thought to be preventable with better monitoring in the pediatric population (45% versus 30%; $P = .01$). (6) A higher percentage of patient injuries was attributed to inadequate ventilation in the pediatric population (20% versus 9%; $P = .01$). The salient findings of the Australian Incident Monitoring Study were that in the pediatric population, incidents were more likely to be related to respiratory system and airway management and that the availability of skilled assistance and specific protocols was felt to be more likely to minimize the impact of incidents.[2]

The ASA Difficult Airway Algorithm[3] is one such protocol that may be used as a framework for managing the child with a difficult airway; however, there are special considerations for the pediatric patient. The specific approaches and techniques that are suitable for children are outlined in this chapter.

RECOGNITION AND EVALUATION OF THE DIFFICULT PEDIATRIC AIRWAY

History

There are conditions that are more frequently or are exclusively found in the pediatric population. Conditions that are unique to or more common in children and are associated with difficult airways fall into two broad categories: congenital syndromes and hereditary diseases (Table 12–1) and acquired abnormalities (Table 12–2). Although airway management is potentially adversely affected when any of these conditions are present, some generalizations can be made.

A primary feature of many syndromes associated with the difficult airway is micrognathia. Micrognathia results in a decreased potential displacement space for laryngoscopy and therefore increases the likelihood that the glottis will be difficult to visualize by rigid laryngoscopy. These patients often have a history of obstructive apnea, snoring, or previous difficult airway management. Patients with syndromes associated with obstructing masses, micrognathia, or limited mouth opening may have both challenging mask airways and difficult intubations. Awake techniques or those that preserve spontaneous ventilation should be considered. Patients with syndromes that are associated with maxillary or midface hypoplasia tend to have challenging mask airways but may not necessarily be difficult to intubate by rigid laryngoscopy. An exception to this generalization is patients with Treacher Collins syndrome, in whom the combination of micrognathia and pharyngeal hypoplasia often makes both mask ventilation and rigid laryngoscopy difficult. Patients with potential cervical instability or immobility require intubation techniques that can be accomplished without neck manipulation.

Patients with airway trauma or an abnormality at risk for bleeding are usually not good candidates for fiberoptic airway management because blood may interfere with visualization. Patients with Hurler's or Hunter's syndrome have distortion of facial features and macroglossia secondary to the progressive accumulation of abnormally metabolized mucopolysaccharides. Their airways become increasingly compromised as they age, and both mask ventilation and rigid laryngoscopy are extremely difficult. Techniques to secure the airway that preserve spontaneous ventilation are recommended.

Old anesthesia records are an invaluable source of information for the patient with a difficult airway. It is important to carefully document for future caretakers the technique, the ability to ventilate by mask (if tested), and difficulties encountered.

The Medic Alert National Registry for difficult airway and intubation should be used by all practitioners who encounter a patient with a difficult airway.[4]

The following historical findings should also alert the practitioner to the possibility of airway management difficulty:

- Snoring
- "Noisy breathing"
- Difficulty feeding secondary to coughing or cyanosis
- Difficulty breathing with an upper respiratory infection
- Recurrent croup
- History of previous problems with airway management

Physical Examination (Table 12–3)

No studies that evaluate physical predictors of difficult intubation have been completed in children. Physical examination to predict the potentially difficult airway must be guided by extrapolation from adult studies and knowledge of normal anatomy and physiology and of the causes of the syndrome-related difficult pediatric airway.

Most examination criteria are subjective; experience and consistent application of examination criteria improve the ability to predict the potentially difficult airway. Difficulty with cooperation may make some portions of the physical examination impossible or useless. The validity of the Mallampati score in children has never been confirmed. Berry suggests that an acceptable submandibular distance as measured from the middle of the inside of the mentum to the hyoid bone is 1.5 cm (approximately one finger breadth) in infants and changes proportionally with age to the adult distance of 3 cm (two fingerbreadths).[7] However, this is subjective and unconfirmed.

Following is a review of normal infant and child airway anatomy and physiology and implications for airway management (Fig. 12–1).[5, 6]

■ Upper Airway

- In infants, a large occiput compared with the body size results in automatic anatomic sniffing position without elevation of the occiput.
- Infants and toddlers have a short neck compared with adults; therefore, posterior laryngeal pressure is more frequently required in this age range.
- Infants have small nares and nasal passages (approximately the diameter of the cricoid). They are obligate nasal breathers until 5 to 6 months of age (see the later discussion of the epiglottis). Avoid elective nasotracheal intubation in this age group.
- Infants have a large tongue relative to oropharyngeal size. This

Table 12-1 Selected Congenital Syndromes and Hereditary Diseases Associated with the Difficult Airway: Grouped by Features That May Cause Difficult Airway Management

Micrognathia and/or Mandibular Hypoplasia	Macroglossia	Cervical Instability or Limited Cervical Mobility	TMJ Syndrome or Limited Mouth Opening	Midface or Maxillary Hypoplasia	Obstructing Mass	Enlarged Mandible or Distortion of Facial Features
Carpenter's syndrome	Beckwith-Wiedemann syndrome	Arnold-Chiari malformation	Arthrogryposis	Anderson's syndrome	Cherubism (tumors)	Acromegaly
Christ-Siemens-Touraine syndrome	*Down's syndrome (trisomy 21)	*Down's syndrome (trisomy 21)	Behçet's syndrome	Apert's syndrome	Encephalocele	Gaucher's disease
Cornelia de Lange's syndrome	*Farber's disease	*Hurler's syndrome (type I mucopolysaccharidosis)	Cockayne-Touraine syndrome (dystrophic epidermolysis bullosa)	Crouzon's syndrome	*Farber's disease (laryngeal tumors)	Hunter's syndrome (type II mucopolysaccharidosis)
Cri du chat syndrome	*Hurler's syndrome (type I mucopolysaccharidosis)	*Juvenile rheumatoid arthritis (Still's disease)	CREST syndrome	*Hallermann-Streiff syndrome (oculomandibulofacial syndrome)	Kasabach-Merritt syndrome (hemangioma)	*Hurler's syndrome (type I mucopolysaccharidosis)
DiGeorge's syndrome	Pompe's disease (type II glycogen storage disease)	Klippel-Feil syndrome	Epidermolysis bullosa	Oral-facial-digital syndrome	Neurofibromatosis (fibroma)	*Maroteaux-Lamy syndrome (type VI mucopolysaccharidosis)
Edwards' syndrome (trisomy 18)		*Larsen's syndrome	*Freeman-Sheldon syndrome (whistling face syndrome)	Pfeiffer's syndrome	Stevens-Johnson syndrome (bullae)	*Morquio's syndrome (type IV mucopolysaccharidosis)
*Freeman-Sheldon syndrome (whistling face syndrome)		Marfan's syndrome	*Juvenile rheumatoid arthritis (Still's disease)	Rieger's syndrome	Sturge-Weber syndrome (hemangioma)	Pyle's disease

Goldenhar's syndrome	*Maroteaux-Lamy syndrome (type VI mucopolysaccharidosis)	Myositis ossificans	*Treacher Collins syndrome	Saethre-Chotzen-Sanfilippo syndrome (type III mucopolysaccharidosis)
*Hallermann-Streiff syndrome (oculo-mandibulofacial syndrome)	*Morquio's syndrome (type IV mucopolysaccharidosis)	Scleroderma		Sotos' syndrome
Hemifacial microsomia	*Osteochondro-dystrophies (dwarfism)			
King-Denborough syndrome				
*Larsen's syndrome				
Miller's syndrome				
Möbius' syndrome				
Nager's syndrome				
Noonan's syndrome				
*Osteochondro-dystrophies (dwarfism)				
Pierre Robin syndrome				
*Treacher Collins syndrome				
Turner's syndrome				

*Listing at more than one site.
TMJ, temporomandibular joint.

**Table 12–2 Acquired Abnormalities Associated with
the Potentially Difficult Airway**

Laryngotracheobronchitis (infectious croup)
Epiglottitis
Trauma (facial and cervical)
Obstructive sleep apnea
Foreign body aspiration or ingestion
Laryngeal papillomatosis
Retropharyngeal or peritonsillar abscess
Anterior mediastinal tumor
Obesity

may make visualization of the larynx more difficult. There is
also less room for endotracheal tube (ET) placement and manipulation.

- Tonsils are small in the newborn but grow to maximal size at 4
  to 7 years of age. "Kissing tonsils" may completely obscure the
  view of the larynx and make mask ventilation difficult.
- The infant epiglottis is large, stiff, and omega shaped and sits at
  a 45-degree angle to the anterior pharyngeal wall (extending
  over the larynx). Use of a straight blade to pick up the relatively
  large and obliquely angled infant epiglottis facilitates vocal cord
  visualization.
- The tip of the epiglottis lies at C1 (adult at C3); therefore, the
  epiglottis can touch the soft palate, separate the esophageal inlet
  from the laryngeal inlet, and allow simultaneous breathing and
  swallowing. This also interferes with oral breathing; thus, infants are obligate nasal breathers. At 5 to 6 months of age, the
  epiglottis descends; the "skill" of breathing and swallowing at
  the same time is lost, and the infant is no longer an obligate nasal breather.
- In infants and young children, there is a higher vagal tone and
  prominent innervation of the epiglottis; therefore, there is an in-

Table 12–3 Physical Examination of the Airway

Neck length and range of motion

Mouth opening and temporomandibular joint mobility

Presence of loose teeth or absence of teeth (especially in children 5–10 years
of age)

Submandibular space

Micrognathia

Mallampati classification or macroglossia

Signs of respiratory distress (retractions, tachypnea, nasal flaring, cyanosis)

ADULT

INFANT

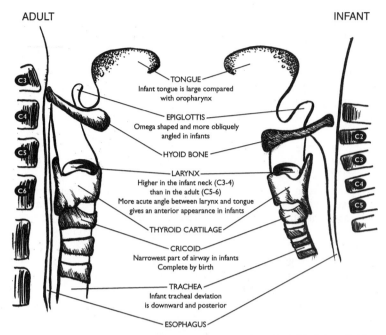

Figure 12–1 Adult versus pediatric airway. (Adapted from Coté CJ, Todres ID: The pediatric airway. *In* Coté CJ, Ryan JF, Todres ID, Goudsouzian NG [eds]: A Practice of Anesthesia for Infants and Children, 2nd ed. Philadelphia, WB Saunders, 1993, p 55.)

creased risk of bradycardia when the epiglottis is picked up during intubation.

- The larynx lies in a more cephalic position: C3–4 at birth, C4–5 by 2 years of age, C5–6 by adulthood. A cephalic or superior position in infants creates a more acute angle between the glottic opening and the base of the tongue, leading to the appearance at laryngoscopy of an "anterior" larynx; therefore, a straight laryngoscopic blade allows better visualization in infants.
- The vocal cords are angled until 2 years of age (the anterior attachment is more caudal).
- The larynx is funnel shaped versus cylindric until 6 to 8 years of age.
- The cricoid cartilage (versus the glottic opening in adults and older children) is the narrowest part of the airway until approximately 6 to 8 years of age; therefore, an ET that passes easily through the glottis may be too large to pass beyond the cricoid cartilage.
- The cricoid cartilage is complete by birth, so cricoid pressure for

rapid sequence induction and intubation can be used even in the newborn.

■ Lower Airways and Chest

- The trachea in infants is short, narrow, and angled posteriorly in the chest; therefore, there is an increased risk of accidental endo-bronchial intubation or extubation with changes in head position.

- Viscosity of mucus in the newborn is increased compared to that in adults and older children; with the requisite small ET size, this can lead to frequent and rapid ET obstruction.

- The ribs in neonates are horizontal with decreased anterior-posterior and cephalic movement and therefore increased diaphragmatic breathing. Increased intraabdominal pressure has a relatively greater deleterious effect on the airway in neonates because of a dependence on diaphragmatic breathing.

- The chest wall is more compliant; therefore, there is a prominent intercostal tug, with any degree of airway obstruction resulting in a "flail chest" appearance.

- Infants have a higher percentage of type II fibers (fast twitch, low oxidative) in their respiratory musculature. This approaches adult levels by 2 years of age. This greater proportion of immature musculature leads to an increased risk of fatigue.

- There are 25 million alveoli at birth. This reaches 360 million by 8 years of age.

- The alveoli are less stable at birth, especially in preterm infants (aided by surfactant treatment).

Diagnostic Evaluation

Diagnostic evaluation implies that a difficult airway is anticipated, either by history or by physical examination. There are three general approaches: endoscopic evaluation, radiographic evaluation, and consultation with other physicians.

- Endoscopic evaluation (flexible fiberoptic endoscopy) can be useful in infants and in older cooperative children for evaluation before intubation when glottic abnormality is suspected or when glottic visualization is anticipated to be difficult (see the later discussion of fiberoptic airway management).

- Radiographic evaluation is particularly useful for suspected foreign body aspiration or ingestion. Magnetic resonance imaging and computed tomography may be helpful to evaluate mass lesions.

- Consultation with other physicians may be useful. An otolaryngologist may be consulted for a second opinion about the airway and for surgical backup (for tracheotomy if required). A pulmonologist may be helpful to assist with pulmonary function testing.

TECHNIQUES FOR DIFFICULT VENTILATION

Oropharyngeal and Nasopharyngeal Airways

Both oropharyngeal and nasopharyngeal airways can improve mask ventilation by providing space for gas exchange between the tongue and the posterior pharynx. Choosing the appropriate size is necessary, or airway obstruction may be worsened rather than improved (Fig. 12–2).

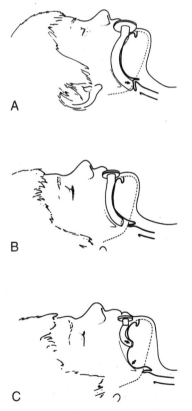

Figure 12–2 Choosing the appropriate oral airway. *A*, Too large. *B*, Appropriate size. *C*, Too small. (Adapted from Coté CJ, Todres ID: The pediatric airway. *In* Coté CJ, Ryan JF, Todres ID, Goudsouzian NG [eds]: A Practice of Anesthesia for Infants and Children, 2nd ed. Philadelphia, WB Saunders, 1993, p 68.)

Two- and Three-Handed Mask Ventilation

In two- and three-handed mask ventilation, one person uses both hands to maintain an adequate mask fit and a second person compresses the ventilation bag (two-handed technique). Occasionally, the second person must assist with the mask fit (three-handed technique) (Fig. 12–3).

Laryngeal Mask Airway (Table 12–4)

Laryngeal mask airway (LMA) use has been described as a tool in the ASA Difficult Airway Algorithm.[8, 9] Its use has been described in the awake patient (LMA insertion in awake infants with Pierre Robin syndrome[10]) and in the anesthetized patient with a known or suspected difficult airway. For the anesthetized patient, it can be used in either the nonemergency (can ventilate, cannot intubate) or the emergency (cannot ventilate, cannot intubate) pathway of the ASA Difficult Airway Algorithm. It can be used as the definitive airway in some circumstances or as a conduit for intubation (see later).[11]

■ Insertion Techniques

The traditional LMA insertion technique described for adults is also recommended in children (see Chapter 8). The rotational or reverse technique for children has been advocated as being simpler and more successful than the traditional placement technique (Fig. 12–4). The LMA is placed in the mouth with the cuff facing the hard palate (opposite of the traditional technique). It is then advanced and rotated into position simultaneously. A partial inflation technique has also been

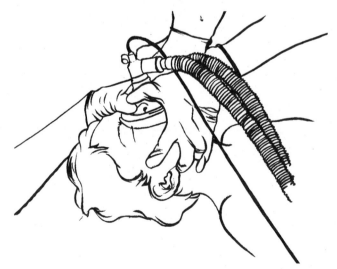

Figure 12–3 Three-handed mask ventilation technique.

Table 12–4   Laryngeal Mask Airway: Recommendations for Choice of Laryngeal Mask Airway, Endotracheal Tube, and Fiberoptic Bronchoscope Sizes

LMA Size	Patient Size (kg)	Cuff Volume (mL)	Largest ET (ID, mm)	Largest FB Inside ET (mm)
1	<5	2–4	3.5	2.7
1.5	5–10	4–7	4.0	3.0
2	10–20	7–10	4.5	3.5
2.5	20–30	10–14	5.0	4.0
3	30–70	15–20	6.0 cuffed	5.0
4	>70	25–30	6.0 cuffed	5.0
5	>90	35–40	7.0 cuffed	6.5

LMA, laryngeal mask airway; ET, endotracheal tube; FB, fiberoptic bronchoscope.

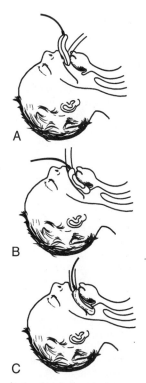

Figure 12–4   Reverse or rotational technique for laryngeal mask airway insertion. *A,* Oral axis. *B,* Tracheal axis. *C,* Pharyngeal axis.

advocated as more successful than the traditional technique. The LMA is left partially inflated to smooth the edges of the mask and then is inserted as usual.[12]

■ Potential Problems

The most common cause of failure is using an LMA that is too small. With the traditional insertion technique, the LMA often hangs up in the posterior pharynx, making proper positioning impossible. The epiglottis frequently overlies the laryngeal inlet, even when the LMA is effective for ventilation.[13] Attempting to place the LMA when the level of anesthesia is too light may make advancement impossible or result in laryngospasm. Removal of the LMA may also be problematic. Experts have advocated both awake and deep-anesthesia removal. Deep removal avoids excessive airway reactivity and potential laryngospasm but may increase the risk of aspiration. Awake removal ensures a return of protective reflexes but with the attendant problems of airway reactivity. Lubrication of the cuff with 2% lidocaine jelly or the addition of intravenous (IV) narcotic to the anesthetic may reduce coughing on emergence.[12]

■ Use in Infants

A review of the use of a no. 1 LMA in 50 infants cautions that the LMA may migrate over time even after apparent correct initial placement (delayed airway obstruction occurred in 12 infants after apparently successful placement). Vigilance is required to prevent the loss of the airway.[14]

The LMA has been used successfully for neonatal resuscitation. Some suggest that this is an easier skill to acquire than bag-mask ventilation.[15]

Cricothyrotomy, Percutaneous Needle Cricothyrotomy, and Transtracheal Jet Ventilation[16, 17]

In children, percutaneous needle cricothyrotomy is recommended over surgical cricothyrotomy because there is less risk of injury to vital structures such as the carotid arteries or jugular veins. In addition, most practitioners can more rapidly perform the percutaneous procedure.

Percutaneous needle cricothyrotomy can be performed using commonly available medical materials. However, because of the high resistance created by the relatively small-bore needle, ventilation is limited. Oxygenation can be maintained for a limited period of time while a definitive course of action is pursued. Be aware that if upper airway obstruction is present (for example, after multiple unsuccessful attempts at rigid laryngoscopy), there will be a limited pathway for the egress of air and oxygen, and barotrauma may result from insufflation of oxygen or attempts at ventilation.[6] In addition, there is a risk of kinking the catheter. Special catheters designed for needle cricothyrotomy are stiffer than angiocatheters and may decrease the incidence of this problem.

Alternatively, several commercially available percutaneous dilatational cricothyrotomy kits are designed for use in pediatric patients. These may create an airway that allows reasonable ventilation as well as oxygenation (3.0-mm internal diameter [ID] minimal size required).

■ Technique (Fig. 12–5)[6]

- The head is extended with a shoulder roll and the trachea stabilized with the right hand.
- The cricothyroid membrane is located with the forefinger of the left hand.
- A 12- or 14-gauge IV catheter is inserted through the membrane.

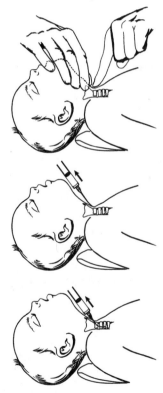

Figure 12–5 Percutaneous needle cricothyrotomy. (Adapted from Coté CJ, Todres ID: The pediatric airway. *In* Coté CJ, Ryan JF, Todres ID, Goudsouzian NG [eds]: A Practice of Anesthesia for Infants and Children, 2nd ed. Philadelphia, WB Saunders, 1993, p 55.)

- Air is aspirated, the catheter is advanced, and the needle is discarded.
- Air is again aspirated to confirm correct placement.
- A 15-mm connector from a 3.0-mm ET is attached to the IV catheter, or a 15-mm connector from an 8.0-mm ET can be inserted into a 3-mL syringe.
- Oxygenation is accomplished by attaching a circuit with a standard 22-mm connector.
- Alternatively, a jet ventilation system with a Luer-Lok connector can be attached directly to the IV catheter.

■ Risks and Possible Problems

Risks and possible problems associated with percutaneous needle cricothyrotomy and transtracheal jet ventilation include

- Barotrauma
- Pneumothorax
- Subcutaneous emphysema
- Mediastinal emphysema
- Esophageal puncture
- Bleeding and hematoma
- Vascular injury
- Hemoptysis
- Hypercarbia
- Kinking of the catheter

Combitube

The Combitube airway management equipment is available for adult-sized patients only.

TECHNIQUES FOR DIFFICULT INTUBATION

Rigid Laryngoscopy

■ Indications

If a second look is attempted after an unexpected failed intubation, something about the approach should be changed to improve visualization. Suggestions are reviewed later. In certain circumstances, rigid laryngoscopy may be chosen as a first-look technique when mask ventilation is easy and the difficulty of rigid intubation is uncertain. Awake rigid intubation is a traditional approach to the problematic infant airway.

■ Tips and Techniques

Head Position[18]

Because the larynx in infants and children to 2 years of age is relatively more cephalic (i.e., located higher in the neck than in adults) and because the head size in infants is larger, the ideal position is head extension without elevation of the head or shoulders (Fig. 12–6). At 6 years of age the position of laryngeal structures more closely mirrors that of adults; slight elevation of the occiput (5 to 10 cm) improves laryngeal visualization (Fig. 12–7).

External Posterior Laryngeal Pressure

External posterior laryngeal pressure is particularly helpful for infants and also for children with syndromes causing abnormal cervical vertebrae (resulting in immobile or shortened necks).[7, 18] Note that this is pressure applied to the larynx, not the cricoid, and the maneuver should be performed during the intubation attempt to maximize visualization.

Flexible Stylets

Flexible stylets or a gum elastic bougie can be used in the blind placement of the ET under the epiglottis.

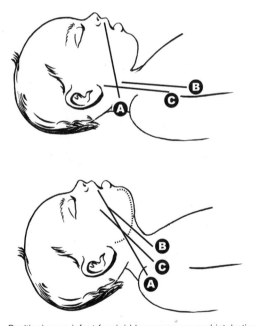

Figure 12–6 Positioning an infant for rigid laryngoscopy and intubation. Note that the increased occiput size creates an "automatic anatomic" elevation of the head, in contrast to the case in older children and adults (see Fig. 12–7). *A,* Oral axis; *B,* tracheal axis; *C,* pharyngeal axis.

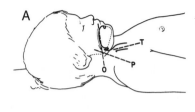

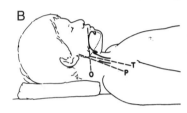

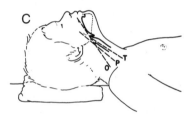

Figure 12–7 Positioning a child for rigid laryngoscopy and intubation. *A,* The oral (O), tracheal (T), and pharyngeal (P) axes lie in three different planes when the head is in neutral position. *B,* Elevation of the occiput aligns the tracheal (T) and pharyngeal (P) axes. *C,* Extension of the head aligns all three axes. (Adapted from Coté CJ, Todres ID: The pediatric airway. *In* Coté CJ, Ryan JF, Todres ID, Goudsouzian NG [eds]: A Practice of Anesthesia for Infants and Children, 2nd ed. Philadelphia, WB Saunders, 1993, p 55.)

Oxyscope

The Oxyscope is a Miller no. 1 laryngoscope blade with an insufflation channel along its length so that it may be attached to an oxygen source. It is used for laryngoscopy in spontaneously breathing infants in whom prolonged laryngoscopy attempts are anticipated; it maintains oxygen saturation and makes airway instrumentation safer.[19]

Tongue Suture

A tongue suture may be more effective in improving obstructed laryngeal visualization than simply pulling the tongue forward manually and may interfere less with laryngoscopy than the use of forceps.

Dental Mirror

Patil and colleagues used a short-handled dental mirror (no. 3, Stortz Instrument Company, Manchester, Mont.) to assist in the indirect visualization of the larynx of a 10-week-old infant.[20] Laryngoscopy was impossible with a Miller no. 1 blade. Therefore, the patient was returned to spontaneous ventilation and a MacIntosh no. 1 blade was used to expose the pharynx and the mirror used to visualize the larynx. A styletted ET was then passed into the glottis under indirect vision.

Retromolar, Paraglossal, or Lateral Approach Using a Straight Blade[21, 22]

This technique may allow glottic visualization when the classic rigid intubation technique fails, particularly when the difficulty is due to a large glottis or small mandible, or both. A no. 1 Miller blade is introduced into the extreme right side of the mouth. It is advanced in the space between the tongue and the lateral pharyngeal wall; the tongue is swept completely to the left and is essentially bypassed. The blade is advanced while staying to the right, overlying the molars, until the epiglottis or the glottis is visualized. If the epiglottis is seen, it is elevated with the blade tip to expose the glottis. At this point it may be possible to bring the proximal end of the blade toward the midline to increase room for ET placement and manipulation. If the glottis is not visualized, the head can be rotated to the left and the blade can be kept lateral to improve visualization. An assistant is helpful to help pull back the right corner of the mouth to increase the space for ET placement. The ET should be styletted with a hockey stick configuration to assist in placement, particularly if the view of the glottis is only partial.

Several mechanisms are responsible for the improved view of the glottis. The technique allows a reduced need for soft tissue displacement and compression because the lateral placement of the blade bypasses the tongue and because a straight blade requires less tissue compression and displacement than a curved blade does. There is a lowered proximal end of the line of sight because the incisors and maxillary structures are bypassed by lateral blade placement and by shifting the head to the left. Also, the use of a straight blade avoids the possible intrusion of the curved blade into the line of sight.

Anterior Commissure Scope and Rigid Ventilating Bronchoscope[23]

Two pieces of equipment used by otolaryngologists that can assist in visualizing the larynx and providing a method of ventilation are the anterior commissure scope and rigid ventilating bronchoscope. The technique to place the anterior commissure scope and the advantages for visualization are similar to those described for the straight blade used with the retromolar approach.

■ Advantages

- Most familiar piece of airway equipment
- Most universally available piece of airway equipment
- Allows the possibility of direct visualization

■ Disadvantages

- Some anatomic features are completely unfavorable for success, despite the application of appropriate tips and techniques.
- Repeated unsuccessful attempts can lead to airway trauma and edema. Infants and children already have limited airway spaces and are susceptible to a rapid progression to the can't ventilate, can't intubate scenario.

Direct Fiberoptic Laryngoscopy[24, 25]

■ Indications

All indications for fiberoptic airway management in adult patients may also be applied to pediatric patients.

■ Equipment

Fiberscopes

The availability of an ultrathin fiberoptic endoscope with a directable tip allows the use of a fiberoptic approach to airway management even in neonates requiring endotracheal tubes as small as 2.5 mm ID.[26]

Ancillary Equipment

Commercially available are the Frei endoscopy mask[27] and the Patil-Syracuse endoscopy masks. The Patil-Syracuse masks are available in a child size but are too large for most children younger than 4 years. "Homemade" endoscopy masks similar to the commercially available endoscopic mask designed by Frei can also be made using a disposable face mask, corrugated tubing, and a silicon diaphragm.[27, 28] Alternatively, an endoscopy mask with swivel adapter can be constructed by two methods.[29] In the first method, a commercially available swivel adapter can be attached directly to a disposable clear anesthesia mask. The fiberscope can be introduced through the adapter and into either the nasal or the oral cavity. In the second method, a swivel adapter designed for placement on an ET can be adapted by using a 15- to 22-mm adapter between the swivel adapter and the face mask.

No intubating airways are available for use in pediatric patients; however, Guedel airways can be modified for this use.[29] A strip is cut from the convex surface of the airway to create a channel for the placement of the fiberscope. This may be used to maintain a midline approach to the glottis; however, it is ineffective as a bite block. Goskowicz and colleagues[30] modified a standard nipple for bottle feeding to act as an oropharyngeal conduit to assist with awake fiberoptic intubation in a 7-month-old infant with cervical instability. An 8-mm hole was cut obliquely at the tip and a mark made at the rim to facilitate the orientation of the hole inferiorly. Topical anesthetic (2% lidocaine) was applied directly to the glottis via a working channel.

■ Techniques for Direct Fiberoptic Intubation

Equipment preparation for fiberoptic intubation should include checking the fiberscope, light source, and related supplies as well as preparing the rigid laryngoscopy equipment, masks, the circuit, appropriate drugs, ETs, and stylets. The practitioner should choose a fiberoptic scope that passes easily through the appropriately sized ET for the patient but also fits with relatively little play between the ET and the scope. A fiberoptic scope that is too small for the ET increases the likelihood that the ET will not easily pass into the glottis (because the tube tip hangs up on laryngeal structures) or that the insertion cord of the fiberoptic scope may be flipped out of position, resulting in esophageal intubation.

The position of the patient's head should usually be neutral or extended to obtain the best angle for visualization of the larynx; however, occasionally a more classic sniffing position can improve visualization or ET passage, or both. An antisialagogue should be administered either intramuscularly or intravenously before proceeding with the fiberoptic intubation. The airway should be suctioned before proceeding and during endoscopy if necessary. If there is no working channel (as for some small scopes), suction catheters prepared with tape over the thumb control port and hooked up to a suction source allow one-hand operation if necessary.

A method for delivering supplemental oxygen should also be available. The method used depends on the airway management technique. For spontaneously breathing patients, oxygen can be delivered blow-by from the circuit, by nasal cannula, by the working channel, or by an endoscopy mask. For patients who are paralyzed, an endoscopy mask or a laryngeal mask airway may be used in conjunction with the fiberscope to provide oxygen and allow ventilation.

An assistant is necessary to aid in the safe monitoring of the patient and to provide a jaw thrust. A jaw thrust is necessary to elevate the tongue off the posterior pharynx and facilitate visualization of the vocal cords (Fig. 12–8). Occasionally, the tongue must be pulled forward with gauze, clamps, or a tongue suture to allow visualization.

One should keep in mind several anatomic differences between adults and children that affect the fiberoptic technique. The airway distances are much shorter in neonates, infants, and young children than in adults; structures come into view very quickly; the operator should advance the scope only when recognizable landmarks are seen. The fiberscope is advanced by using the fingers of the right hand while directing the fiberscope tip with the thumb of the left hand. When needed, the body of the fiberscope may be rotated to change the orientation of the tip. If the view through the fiberscope is a pink mass, the operator should pull back the fiberscope, and recognizable structures usually come into view. The most common mistake is to advance the fiberscope too deep, thus entering the esophagus, particularly if the operator is accustomed to adult airways.

Because neonates and infants have a larynx and vocal cords that are more acutely angled and because they are small in relation to the size

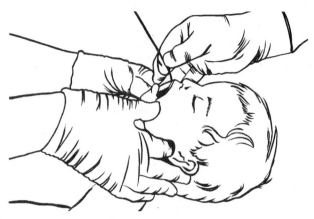

Figure 12–8 Technique for maintaining the fiberoptic scope in the midline position during oral direct fiberoptic intubation in infants or children and method for assisting with mouth opening and jaw thrust.

of the fiberscope, it is critical that the larynx be approached from the midline position, not from the sides of the mouth. If the approach is not midline, the insertion cord may not pass easily through the glottis.

Because the cricoid cartilage is the narrowest portion of the airway in children, as opposed to the glottic opening in adults, uncuffed ETs are usually used. This presents a problem unique to children: an inability to effectively ventilate or protect the airway after ET placement because the inserted ET is too small! The following options may be considered:

- A ventilating ET changer can be used to switch to an ET a half-size larger. The fiberscope can then be used to confirm correct placement of the new ET.
- The fiberscope can be loaded with the new ET and the tip directed to the larynx. An assistant can then withdraw the old tube as the fiberscope is directed through the glottis. The new ET is then advanced into the trachea and the fiberscope removed as usual.
- A small, cuffed ET can be used for the first attempt.

If the ET will not thread over the scope into the glottis, the operator should pull the tube back and rotate it 90 degrees counterclockwise and advance. If still unsuccessful, the operator should rotate the ET an additional 180 degrees. If there is still great difficulty, the operator must *stop*! The ET may be too big! The following steps may be taken:

- Place a guide wire down the working channel and use this to place a smaller ET or to replace the fiberscope after loading it with a smaller ET.
- Abut the ET against the glottis and pass a guide wire or ET

changer into the glottis through this ET. Remove the large ET, and then change to a smaller ET by passing it over the guide.

- Regroup and start over.

Oral Versus Nasal Approach

Disadvantages of the oral compared with the nasal approach are that it is difficult to stay in the midline in patients who are too small to have an oral guide, and sedated patients may bite the scope. One method to maintain a midline position during an oral approach is to rest the right hand on the patient's face and hold the insertion cord of the fiberscope in the midline position.

Advantages of the oral over the nasal approach are that the potential problems of shearing adenoid tissue and of creating a nasal bleed are avoided and that it may be less stimulating and better tolerated than the nasal approach. If a nasal approach is chosen in a young child, phenylephrine (Neo-Synephrine) or oxymetazoline (Afrin) drops may be used to vasoconstrict the nasal passages. This may ease placement and decrease the possibility of bleeding.

■ Advantages

Advantages of direct fiberoptic laryngoscopy are that the technique does not require extensive head manipulation and the flexible instrument conforms to a variety of abnormal airways; therefore, the technique is very versatile. Also, it is well tolerated by the spontaneously breathing patient.

■ Disadvantages

Disadvantages of direct fiberoptic laryngoscopy are that it has limited use in the presence of blood or copious secretions, it requires experience and practice in normal airways first, and the equipment is fragile and expensive.

■ Learning Direct Fiberoptic Intubation Techniques

At our hospital we compared the time to intubation and complications in 20 normal infants intubated conventionally using a rigid Miller no. 1 laryngoscope and in 20 normal infants intubated by using an Olympus LF-P fiberscope. The time to intubation was 13.6 ± 0.9 seconds in the conventional group and 22.8 ± 1.7 seconds in the fiberoptic group. There was no difference in complications. We conclude that routine use of the fiberscope for intubation in normal infants is a safe and reasonable method to gain skills with this technique.[26]

Another study evaluated the Olympus LF-P for use in oral intubation in 40 anesthetized, spontaneously breathing children aged 6 months to 7 years. The intubations were accomplished via a "homemade" ventilating mask, using a split Guedel airway or a no. 7 Great Ormand Street tracheotomy as an intubating guide.[31] The authors found a 12% failure rate and 25% complication rate. Two patients had laryngospasms and required conventional laryngoscopy; in seven patients the fiberscope flipped out of the trachea (three required conventional laryngoscopy); four patients had oxygen desaturations (two less than 94%, two less than 90%); and in one patient the initial ET size was wrong. The authors felt that although the LF-P gave a good field of vision it was very "whippy." It easily curled up in the back of the pharynx, and although the vocal cords could be visualized, maneuvering the fiberscope through the vocal cords and into the trachea was more difficult to achieve than with the larger and more rigid LF-1. A plausible explanation for the difficulty with the maneuvering of the scope and ET passage is the age of patients studied. For older children who required an ET size greater than 4.5 mm ID, the LF-1 fiberscope would have been a better choice. Also, the operators had virtually no experience with the LF-P. A better approach to gaining skills is to practice on paralyzed infants first (as per our study) and then proceed to intubations in the spontaneously breathing patient.

Other Fiberoptic Techniques

■ Two-Stage Fiberoptic Intubation Technique[32]

The two-stage fiberoptic intubation technique is a method used in infants and small children when the fiberscopes available are too large to pass through the appropriate-size endotracheal tube. It requires a fiberscope with a working channel and a standard cardiac catheter and guide wire with the proximal connector removed.

- The cardiac catheter guide wire is passed through the working channel of the fiberscope to within 1 inch of its tip, and the fiberscope is then introduced into the mouth and positioned at the top of the vocal cords.

- The guide wire is advanced under direct observation through the glottis into the trachea. The fiberscope is removed, leaving the guide wire in place.

- The patient is ventilated by mask while an assistant passes the cardiac catheter over the guide wire (used to stiffen the guide wire to facilitate passing the endotracheal tube). The ET is threaded over the catheter–guide wire combination, which is then removed, leaving the ET in place.

This technique has been utilized for the intubation of two infants with the Pierre Robin syndrome.[33, 34] However, these authors found that threading of the cardiac catheter over the guide wire was unnecessary.

A modification of this technique when the fiberscope has no working channel has also been described.[35] The authors used an 8 Fr red rubber catheter attached by waterproof tape to the insertion cord of the fiberscope. The larynx was visualized with the fiberscope, and a guide wire was threaded through the rubber catheter into the trachea. With the guide wire in position, the fiberscope was withdrawn and an ET was passed over the guide wire into the trachea.

■ Three-Stage Fiberoptic Intubation Technique[36]

The three-stage fiberoptic intubation technique can be used when the available fiberscope both is too large and lacks a working channel.

- The fiberscope is loaded with an ET and then used to visualize the larynx. The ET (which is larger than the larynx of the infant) is advanced over the fiberscope and positioned on top of the vocal cords.
- The fiberscope is then removed, and a tube changer or catheter is advanced into the trachea through the ET.
- The larger tube is then removed, and the appropriate-size ET is threaded over the tube changer or catheter into the trachea.

This technique was used successfully in a 6-month-old infant whose operation had been previously canceled because of failure to intubate.

■ Intubation Under Fiberoptic Observation[37, 38]

Intubation under fiberoptic observation is another alternative for intubation when the fiberscope is too large to pass through the appropriate-size ET. The fiberscope is introduced through one naris to visually aid the placement of the ET that is passed through the other naris and manipulated into the glottis.

Alternatively, if the observed ET is not easily passed into the glottis, a small catheter may be more easily manipulated into the glottis to be used as a stylet to pass the ET into the trachea. Spontaneous ventilation is preserved and O_2 administered via the ET tube during the intubation.

A disadvantage of this technique is that a minimum of two people, and ideally a third person, is needed to perform the manipulations. This technique was used successfully in two neonates, one with congenital fusion of the jaws and a second with Dandy-Walker syndrome associated with Klippel-Feil syndrome, micrognathia, hypoplasia of the soft palate, and anteversion of the uvula.[37, 38]

Blind Nasotracheal Intubation

Blind nasotracheal intubation requires adequate sedation, topical anesthesia and vasoconstriction, or general anesthesia with preservation of spontaneous ventilation. The head is positioned as for rigid laryngoscopy. The ET is directed into the glottis by listening for maximal breath sounds, by observing fogging of the ET, or by capnograph tracing. The ET, the patient's head, and the larynx are manipulated (the last with external maneuvers) as needed for successful placement. Forming the ET into an exaggerated curve and preserving the shape by placing the ET in ice has been suggested by some.[39] Berry describes placing a stylet with a 30-degree angle at the distal end into the ET after it is in the nasopharynx. The proximal end of the ET and stylet are maneuvered posteriorly, thus displacing the distal end of the ET anteriorly and into the glottis.[7] Elective blind nasotracheal intubation of a prone neonate with Pierre Robin syndrome has also been described. The technique was used twice for the same infant, after unsuccessful attempts at rigid laryngoscopy by otolaryngologists and anesthesiologists.[40]

Tactile or Digital Intubation

Tactile or digital intubation may be performed either orally or nasally. The nasal technique is a variation of the blind nasotracheal technique. An ET is placed nasally into the pharynx. The practitioner inserts the second and third fingers into the patient's mouth and behind the tongue until the epiglottis is palpated. The ET is then directed into the glottis, between the practitioner's two fingers. The nasal technique has been used successfully in an infant with Treacher Collins syndrome.[41] The oral technique is similar to the nasal technique, except the ET is introduced through the mouth after identification of the epiglottis.

Retrograde Guide Wire

A retrograde guide wire has been advocated for situations in which there is no pediatric fiberoptic scope or when blood or secretions limit the use of fiberoptic techniques. The following technique may be used in infants.[42] See Chapter 6 for a description of a technique that may be used in older children. The technique requires sedation or general anesthesia. Topical anesthetic is applied to the nasopharynx and oropharynx, and local anesthetic to the neck over the cricothyroid membrane. The neck is hyperextended with a shoulder roll. A 16-gauge red rubber catheter with a 2–0 silk suture attached is passed through the nose, and the free suture end retrieved through the mouth. A cricothyrotomy is performed with a 20-gauge angiocatheter attached to a saline-filled syringe. The tip is directed superiorly toward the glottis. Correct placement is confirmed by aspiration of air. The intravenous catheter is left in place and a 0.021-cm flexible-tip guide wire is passed superiorly and retrieved from the mouth. The wire and suture are tied together and the wire is pulled through the nasopharynx. The wire is passed through the Murphy eye of a lubricated ET and advanced into the trachea. The guide wire is removed.

Lightwand[43]

The Lightwand uses a high-intensity light that transmits through the skin as a red glow when advanced into the trachea. Smaller sizes are now available for ETs as small as 2.5 mm (Fiberoptic Medical Products, Allentown, Pa.).

■ Technique

After the Lightwand and ET are lubricated, the Lightwand tip is placed so that it remains just inside the ET tip, and then the ET is shaped into a 90- to 120-degree angle. Room lights are dimmed. The ET-wand combination is placed into the mouth and advanced in the midline, behind the tongue to the glottis. A slight jaw thrust may be helpful. A red glow should be visible through the skin at the midline; the ET-wand is advanced until the glow is below the level of the cricoid cartilage (or at the sternal notch). The wand is withdrawn and the ET left in place.

■ Pitfalls

- Esophageal intubation, usually indicated by complete or transient loss of the glowing tip as it is advanced in the midline. The operator should withdraw and try again, maintaining the tip firmly against the anterior neck.
- ET-wand combination hangs up in the midline. This usually means the epiglottis is in the way; the operator should pull back and advance the wand slightly posteriorly.

■ Indications

- In general, when there is no intrinsic laryngeal or airway abnormality, but visualization is difficult
- Facial trauma
- Micrognathia
- Small mouth or limited temporomandibular joint movement
- Cervical spine disease (instability or fusion)

■ Advantages

- Usually rapid (in skilled hands)
- Less costly than the fiberscope
- Can be used in bloody airways
- Can be used orally or nasally

■ Problems

Problems with this technique can be grouped into three categories:

1. Equipment shortcomings (these vary by manufacturer)
   - Light source too bright or too dim
   - Stylet too flexible or too stiff
   - Fragile or expensive, or both
   - May need external light source
2. Contraindications
   - Mass lesions or tumors
   - Vocal cord paresis or paralysis
   - Retropharyngeal or tonsillar abscess
3. Disadvantages compared with other techniques
   - Inability to directly visualize the glottis-larynx

- Inability to visually confirm ET placement
- Necessity to dim room lights in most cases
- Requires experience

Bullard Laryngoscope (Fig. 12–9)

A pediatric model of the Bullard laryngoscope is available.

■ Technique[44]

The Bullard laryngoscope uses indirect visualization of the glottis. The ET is loaded onto the intubating stylet of the scope. The scope is held in the left hand and parallel to the patient as the blade is inserted into the mouth. The blade is then advanced while the handle is moved perpendicular to the patient.

Once the blade tip is behind the epiglottis, the glottis can be visualized and the ET passed off the stylet and into the trachea.

■ Advantages

- Can be inserted into a relatively limited mouth opening
- Requires little temporomandibular joint or cervical spine movement
- Can be used in awake patients with topical anesthesia

■ Disadvantages

- Must use oral approach
- Requires extensive practice in normal airways first

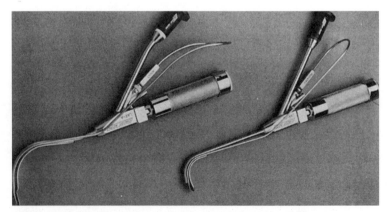

Figure 12–9 The adult *(left)* and pediatric *(right)* Bullard scopes. (Courtesy of Circon Corporation.)

Laryngeal Mask Airway as a Conduit for Intubation

■ Techniques

- Fiberoptic scope–assisted;[10] LMA insertion was performed in two awake infants with Pierre Robin syndrome; a fiberoptic scope was used in the second case to place an ET through the LMA (see Table 12–4)
- Blind intubation[45]
- Retrograde wire–assisted[46]
- Antegrade passage of an airway exchange catheter (ventilating stylet)

Combined Techniques

■ Retrograde Wire and Fiberoptic Scope[47]

A case series reports the use of a retrograde wire and fiberoptic scope in 20 children aged 1 day to 17 years. Equipment required is a ventilating endoscopic mask, a guide wire of suitable length, a fiberscope with a working channel, and grabbing forceps. Tips for success with the technique are to preserve spontaneous ventilation, use transtracheal lidocaine as necessary, and remove the guide wire in the caudal direction. This technique may improve success over that with retrograde intubation alone, because the fiberscope allows visualization and is a stiffer guide for the ET tube. Also, this technique may improve success over that with the fiberscope alone because the glottis is more readily found, even in the presence of secretions.

■ Rigid Laryngoscope and Fiberoptic Scope[48]

The rigid laryngoscope blade can be used to facilitate exposure so that a fiberscope can be used to visualize the larynx.

■ Fiberoptic Scope Used in a Retrograde Manner

A fiberoptic scope was used in a retrograde manner in a 4-year-old child with Nager's syndrome who presented for tracheocutaneous fistula closure after decannulation of a tracheostomy placed as an infant for severe airway obstruction due to micrognathia. After failed attempts at rigid and direct fiberoptic ET placement, a fiberoptic scope was placed in a retrograde fashion, using direct vision, through the fistula, past the vocal cords, into the nasopharynx, and out the naris. It was then used as a stylet for ET placement.[49] The clinical scenario is unusual, but the technique was successful for this child.

DIFFICULTY WITH PATIENT COOPERATION OR CONSENT[24]

Psychologic Preparation

Both the child and the family must be involved in planning and preparation. For the child, a thoughtful and age-appropriate explanation of the procedures and of the need for cooperation can greatly improve success when the awake-sedated approach is planned.

Sedation and Anesthesia

■ Benzodiazepine-Narcotic Combinations

Benzodiazepine-narcotic combinations are effective for adolescents and mature preteens. Most practitioners are familiar with providing sedation with these medications, and details of their use are discussed elsewhere. For younger and less cooperative patients, the addition of small doses of droperidol adds a neuroleptic dimension and may improve success with this technique. This drug also decreases the incidence of nausea and vomiting, which can occur in the extremely anxious child. However, one should keep in mind that this medication, unlike a benzodiazepine or narcotic, has no reversal agent. Unfortunately, benzodiazepine-narcotic sedation (even with the addition of droperidol) may only serve to disinhibit an already frightened young child. "Enough" sedation to ensure compliance of a 2-year-old child with fiberoptic endoscopy may be "too much" to preserve adequate spontaneous ventilation. There are, however, safe and effective alternatives to the benzodiazepine-narcotic combinations.

■ Ketamine

Ketamine is a potent hypnotic as well as analgesic agent that produces a dissociative anesthesia. It may be used for infants, young children, or mentally delayed older children or adolescents.

Advantages

- It usually preserves adequate spontaneous ventilation while providing adequate anesthesia to prevent reaction to airway manipulation.
- There are many routes for administration. If an IV line is difficult or impossible to obtain, a small intramuscular, intranasal, oral, or rectal dose can be used. An IV line can then be secured, and further sedation, if necessary, may be given intravenously.
- It may be used alone or in conjunction with midazolam.

Potential Disadvantages (and Reasons Why It's Still OK to Use Ketamine!)

- Although there is a high incidence of psychomimetic emergence reactions in adults, these reactions are less common in children, particularly if the drug is combined with midazolam.
- It can produce increased upper airway secretions that might interfere with fiberoptic airway management. However, a preoperative antisialagogue in conjunction with pre-endoscopy suctioning of the airway alleviates this problem.
- There are anecdotal reports of "hyperreactive" airway reflexes when ketamine is used. However, adequate doses combined with good suctioning and skilled airway management are the best defense against airway reactivity. Ketamine is a commonly described anesthetic agent for management of children with dif-

ficult airways (including fiberoptic endoscopy), and no problems with increased airway reactivity have been noted.

■ Propofol

An infusion of propofol is titrated to provide a more profound degree of sedation (essentially general anesthesia) and to maintain spontaneous ventilation.

Advantages

- Quick awakening after the infusion is discontinued, unlike with titrated doses of ketamine
- Useful for those patients for whom conscious sedation is not an option
- Useful when utilizing the combined technique of laryngeal mask airway with fiberoptic endoscopy

Disadvantages

- Risk of apnea
- Pain on injection (use a larger vein or mix lidocaine with the propofol)

Inhalation Induction

Inhalation induction is an alternative technique for those patients in whom sedation is not an option. However, the disadvantages of this technique must be carefully considered before this approach is undertaken. These disadvantages include the risks of apnea, laryngospasm, and loss of the airway.

■ Technique

Halothane should be used; it is least irritating to the airway. The relative merits of using N_2O should be considered; it speeds and smoothes induction but diminishes the fraction of inspired oxygen (FIO_2). Induction should be smooth, careful, and gradual. Controlled ventilation may be gradually assumed to ensure that the child's airway can be managed by mask. If mask ventilation is easily performed, a muscle relaxant can be given and intubation begun. This obviates the risk of laryngospasm or of sudden patient movement. However, the time allowable for each intubation attempt will be decreased because of the patient's apnea.

If the use of a muscle relaxant is unadvisable and maintaining spontaneous ventilation increases the safety for the patient, an adequate depth of anesthesia must be ensured before airway manipulation.

Lidocaine can be sprayed on the vocal cords to prevent or minimize the incidence and severity of laryngospasm before the advancement of the ET into the trachea.

Topical Anesthesia

For tracheal intubation performed with the patient under sedation and general anesthesia with spontaneous ventilation, topical anesthesia of the airway is absolutely necessary. It improves the patient's acceptance, prevents laryngospasm, and increases the success rate by decreasing airway reflexes. In general, all techniques that are used in adults may be used in children, with a few caveats. Children are smaller; therefore, the volumes and amounts of local anesthetic that can be used must be limited (Table 12–5).

Cetacaine spray, Americaine ointment, and Hurricaine ointment, gel, and spray may cause methemoglobinemia because of their ingredient benzocaine. It is best to avoid them in infants and young children. Translaryngeal injection is technically difficult in infants younger than 6 months and should therefore be avoided in this age group. Nebulized lidocaine is useful in young children. Many children have used nebulizers in the treatment of asthma or bronchospastic disease and therefore readily accept the lidocaine nebulizer. Suggested volumes and total lidocaine doses based on weight are given in Table 12–6.

INTRODUCING NEW TECHNIQUES INTO THE PRACTICE

Reading

It is essential to learn about a new technique by reviewing pertinent literature about the methods of use, reasonable applications and limitations, and the associated equipment.

Table 12–5   Topical Anesthetics: Maximal Recommended Dosages

Formulation	Active Anesthetic Agent	Maximal Anesthetic Dosage (mg/kg)	Maximal Formulation Dosage (mL/kg)
Lidocaine 2% gel	2% lidocaine	4	0.2
Lidocaine 4% solution	4% lidocaine	4	0.1
Lidocaine 2% solution	2% lidocaine	4	0.2
Cetacaine spray*	2% tetracaine 14% benzocaine	0.25 (tetracaine) 2.5 (benzocaine)	No more than 1-sec spray
3:1 mixture of 4% lidocaine and 1% phenyl-ephrine	3% lidocaine	4	0.13

*Not advisable for children <40 kg because of the inability to deliver a nontoxic dose.

Table 12–6 Lidocaine Nebulizer: Suggested Doses

Patient Weight (kg)	4% Lidocaine (mL)	0.9% NaCl
10–14.9	0.5	0.5
15–19.9	1.0	1.0
20–24.9	1.5	0.5
25–29.9	2.0	—
30–34.9	2.5	—
35–39.9	3.0	—
40–44.9	3.5	—
45 and up	4.0	—

Workshops

A variety of workshops devoted to airway management and special airway techniques are held each year. These give the opportunity to learn about the techniques, get hands-on experience, and have questions answered by colleagues with more experience with these methods.

Practice in Normal Patients

Virtually all techniques should be practiced in normal airways before application in the patient with a difficult airway. Several papers have confirmed the safety of practicing special airway techniques in normal children.[26, 50, 51]

PEDIATRIC AIRWAY—SPECIAL CIRCUMSTANCES

Epiglottitis

■ Pathophysiology

Epiglottitis is an acute infectious process of the supraglottic structures causing inflammation and edema that can rapidly progress to complete airway obstruction. It is usually a bacterial infection, historically caused by *Haemophilus influenzae*, type b (Hib), that occurs in children, aged 2 to 6 years. More recently, more cases are being seen in older children and adults secondary to *Staphylococcus aureus* infection, primarily because of the impact of the Hib vaccine. The first Hib vaccine was introduced in 1985. Immunization guidelines now recommend the use of the Hib vaccine for infants and children up to 5 years of age. This policy has resulted in a dramatically decreased incidence of infectious epiglottitis in children.[52, 53]

■ Presentation and Diagnosis

Children present without a viral prodrome and complain of worsening sore throat. Within 4 to 8 hours of initial symptoms, most appear lethargic and toxic and usually have a fever greater than 38°C. This acute presentation is usually in contrast to that of croup. Dysphagia, dysphonia, and drooling occur as the disease progresses. Children often assume the "tripod" position to relieve airway obstruction: sitting upright with the neck extended and leaning forward on their arms. Diagnosis is primarily clinical. Radiographs should be obtained only in confusing cases when a child is stable. An expert in pediatric airway management should accompany the child to the study. Confirmation of the diagnosis is made by direct vision after preparation for definitive airway management, ideally in the operating room with an anesthesiologist and an otolaryngologist in attendance (see the later section on management).[54]

■ Treatment and Airway Management

The following protocol is adapted from the Acute Supraglottitis Protocol (Children's Memorial Hospital, Chicago).

- When a patient with suspected acute supraglottitis arrives in the emergency room,
    - *If the patient is moribund,* positive-pressure ventilation is administered by mask and 100% oxygen, and a pulse oximeter is placed on the patient immediately to monitor oxygen saturation.
    - *If the airway is adequate,* a pulse oximeter should also be applied. The child should be made comfortable and not disturbed, since this may make airway obstruction worse. The patient may be most comfortable *sitting* on a parent's lap. Attempts to examine the larynx, start an IV line, measure blood gases, and administer oxygen by face mask can all precipitate acute airway obstruction.
- The resident on call in the emergency room
    - Calls the otolaryngology resident and attending physician
    - Calls the anesthesiology resident, who will then call his or her attending physician
    - Calls the pediatric intensive care resident and the attending physician, who will ensure pediatric intensive care unit bed and nursing availability for the period of evaluation and the patient's stay
- From the time a patient has been identified as suspected of having supraglottitis, the patient cannot be left without personnel trained in airway management in attendance.
- If the patient is stable and the airway expert is at the bedside, lateral neck films can be taken in the emergency room. The patient should not go to the radiology department.
- If the patient's condition doesn't require immediate intervention (intubation), the anesthesia resident sets up the operating room. Appropriate equipment includes a wide selection of ETs with stylets, as well as a selection of blades, oral and nasal airways,

suction, at least two laryngoscope handles, and syringes of atropine and succinylcholine.

- Once all the required personnel are present and ready, the patient is transported to the operating room for direct laryngoscopy under general anesthesia.

- In the operating room, monitoring with a chest stethoscope, blood pressure cuff, pulse oximeter, capnograph, and electrocardiograph is begun. Relative merits of inserting an IV cannula are considered.

- Inhalation induction with halothane-oxygen or halothane with O_2-N_2O follows, with the patient assuming the position that allows the most effective air exchange.

- An IV cannula is inserted before laryngoscopy is attempted if this was not done earlier. As the patient is anesthetized, upper airway obstruction may occur. Gentle application of positive pressure usually corrects this.

- After an adequate level of anesthesia is attained, direct rigid laryngoscopy is performed. If the patient has supraglottitis, an oral tube (often one-half size smaller than the size usually used) is inserted. This may subsequently be exchanged for a nasal tube, often using nondepolarizing muscle relaxation.

- After the tube is secured, anesthesia is discontinued, and the patient is transferred to the pediatric intensive care unit. The anesthesia team does not leave the patient until the managing service is present to assume care of the patient.

This protocol for the management of patients with epiglottitis is similar to others described in the literature and can be adapted for use in a nontertiary medical center.[55]

Croup (Laryngotracheobronchitis)[54]

■ Pathophysiology, Presentation, and Diagnosis

Croup is a common viral illness in children aged 3 months to 3 years. It usually occurs in the early fall or winter and may be confused with epiglottitis or a laryngeal foreign body; however, the onset is usually gradual in contrast to that in the other diagnoses. Croup is also associated with a low-grade fever, barky or croupy cough, and stridor.

■ Treatment and Airway Management

In contrast to patients with epiglottitis, these patients rarely require intubation. Treatment usually consists of cool mist therapy, supplemental oxygen, racemic epinephrine nebulizers, and dexamethasone (0.5 to 1 mg/kg). In the rare case when airway obstruction is severe and symptomatic therapy fails, airway management is rarely problematic, but a smaller ET should be selected because subglottic edema is universally present.

Foreign Body Ingestion or Aspiration[56]

■ Location

The locations, listed from most to least common, are esophageal > right bronchial > left bronchial > tracheal > laryngeal > pharyngeal.

Laryngeal and pharyngeal locations are most dangerous because they may easily dislodge and cause complete airway obstruction.

■ Presentation

History

- *Initial event.* This is usually coughing, choking, or gagging. Partial airway obstruction may also occur. This may be missed or minimized by parents.

- *Asymptomatic interval.* This stage, when the airway reflexes have fatigued, is of variable duration and is responsible for most cases of delayed diagnosis.

- *Complications.* At this stage, children may present with airway obstruction, erosion, or infection.

Symptoms

These vary by the location of the foreign body.

- Patients with esophageal-pharyngeal foreign bodies present with dynophagia and dysphagia or failure to thrive in infants.

- Patiens with tracheal-bronchial foreign bodies present with coughing, wheezing, or stridor. This may be misdiagnosed as asthma.

- Laryngeal foreign bodies may be immediately fatal. Children with partial obstruction may present with croup, hoarseness, cough, stridor, and dyspnea or occasionally with odynophagia.

■ Evaluation and Management

Chest radiographs often confirm or increase the suspicion of the presence of a foreign body. These should be reviewed for evidence of air trapping or a mediastinal shift; N_2O should then be avoided in these cases. Most foreign bodies are *not* an acute emergency and should wait until an appropriate nothing-by-mouth time has elapsed (6 hours for solids, 2 hours for clear liquids).

There are four situations that *are* an acute emergency:

- Actual or potential airway obstruction.

- Dried beans or peas in the airway. These will absorb moisture, increase in size, and thus create greater obstruction and become more difficult to retrieve.

- Disc batteries in the esophagus. Mucosal damage occurs in 1 hour and can progress to perforation within 8 to 12 hours.
- Esophageal perforation.

■ Anesthetic and Airway Management

A review of the results of a survey study summarizes management techniques for children (838 of 1342 questionnaires sent to members of the Society of Pediatric Anesthesiologists were returned).[57] Most respondents secure an IV line before induction. In general, an IV induction is used for an esophageal foreign body, and inhalation induction without cricoid pressure for a tracheobronchial foreign body, regardless of the type of object (pin versus coin) or location, *except* 14.5% choose awake-sedated fiberoptic endoscopy for a foreign body in the supraglottic location. Inhalation induction is more frequently chosen by the more experienced clinicians.

An alternative approach using an LMA is described in a case report of a 2-year-old child with a screw in the left main bronchus.[58] The authors used an inhalation induction followed by a relaxant, then placement of a size 2 LMA. This allowed the use of a no. 6 fiberoptic bronchoscope to retrieve the foreign body. The child maintained 100% saturation and an ETCO$_2$ of 35 to 45 mm Hg throughout. It is important to remember that the LMA does not protect against aspiration.

Caustic Ingestion[59]

■ Pathology and Presentation

Esophageal, pharyngeal, and laryngeal injury can occur from the ingestion of bases (lye in drain cleaners, ammonia in household cleaners, low-phosphate detergents, hair straighteners), acids, or bleach. Bases produce the most severe injury. Small amounts ingested can lead rapidly to severe edema and upper airway obstruction, necessitating immediate endotracheal intubation. Children who present with a history of caustic ingestion should be carefully monitored for the development of airway obstruction, and intubation should be considered at the first signs of distress.

■ Airway Management

Most children with caustic ingestion present to the operating room for laryngoscopy and esophagoscopy. Management should proceed assuming a full stomach and the possibility of marked edema of airway structures. The decision between rapid sequence induction versus gentle inhalation induction should be based on the child's present degree of respiratory distress and the perceived risk of aspiration. Often an ET should be left in place until there is resolution of edema or, because of the severity of injury, a tracheostomy is required.

Laryngeal Papillomatosis[60]

■ Pathophysiology

Laryngeal papillomatosis is infection of the airway by the human papillomavirus, resulting in wartlike epithelial growths involving the true and false vocal cords, larynx, and subglottis with rare spread to the trachea and bronchi; it is probably transmitted from mother to infant at birth and presents commonly after 2 years of age; presentation in infancy is associated with a poor prognosis.

Children have voice changes (muffled or hoarse, or both) and dyspnea that worsen as the lesions enlarge. Complete airway obstruction can occur.

■ Treatment, Airway Management, and Anesthetic Techniques

Treatment primarily relies on laser ablation of the lesions. Lesions are almost always recurrent; therefore, children present repeatedly for laser ablation under general anesthesia.

Usually, the induction technique should preserve spontaneous ventilation, or airway obstruction can occur. Inhalation induction is often the most effective method to achieve this goal. However, in older children or when obstruction is already severe, an inhalation technique may be ineffective or impossible. IV propofol can be used to supplement the inhalation agent or replace the inhalation technique, but the risk of apnea is higher. If total obstruction occurs, positive pressure may or may not be effective. Proceeding directly to laryngoscopy and passing a ventilating bronchoscope may be the only effective method to reestablish the airway. Once an adequate depth of anesthesia is ensured, there are several possible approaches to maintaining anesthesia and providing oxygenation and ventilation during the procedure: jet ventilation, apneic technique, passage of a red rubber ET wrapped in a protective metal tape (usually copper) or of an articulated metal endotracheal tube, or an insufflation technique.

The apneic technique is an option when the patient has lesions that are obscured by the ET and it is difficult both to maintain an adequate degree of anesthesia and to preserve spontaneous ventilation. The patient is ventilated with 100% oxygen and anesthetic gas until maximal oxygen saturations are achieved and the end-tidal CO_2 is in the upper 20s. Laser ablation of lesions that are inside the laryngeal inlet can proceed for up to 2 minutes or until the first sign of desaturation occurs. The trachea is reintubated, and the process is repeated as needed.

The insufflation technique requires the preservation of spontaneous ventilation and careful placement of the insufflation catheter to maintain anesthesia and oxygenation without inflating the stomach. The tip of the catheter should lie just above the laryngeal inlet. These techniques can be used for other laryngeal lesions and surgeries.[61, 62]

Laryngomalacia[63]

■ Pathology and Presentation

Laryngomalacia is the most common congenital anomaly of the larynx. Laryngomalacia results from abnormally flaccid supraglottic laryngeal cartilages that fold in paradoxically with inspiration. The cause of this flaccidity remains unclear. Relative immaturity of airway structures or central respiratory control centers may play a role, yet the incidence of this disorder is not increased in premature infants. Infants present with high-pitched inspiratory stridor that classically worsens with crying. Most outgrow the disorder by 12 to 24 months of age.

■ Treatment and Airway Management

Infants may present for diagnostic laryngoscopy and bronchoscopy or rarely with acute airway obstruction. Positive pressure applied to the airway is usually effective in temporarily correcting obstruction. Treatment in severe cases may consist of laser supraglottoplasty (partial laser excision of redundant tissue), suturing the epiglottis to the base of the tongue, or rarely tracheotomy.

Anterior Mediastinal Mass

■ Pathology and Presentation

Most lesions are lymphomas (both Hodgkin's and non-Hodgkin's), teratomas, or neuroblastomas. Symptoms on clinical presentation reflect a mass effect of the lesion on nearby structures: the tracheobronchial tree, superior vena cava, heart, and great vessels.

■ Airway Management

Preoperative Evaluation

Preoperative evaluation should include a review of symptoms, physical examination, computed tomography, pulmonary function testing, and determination of the optimal position to minimize symptoms. The focus has been on finding predictors that can be used to determine which patients will experience severe and sudden cardiovascular and respiratory collapse under general anesthesia. This is a well-described phenomenon, which is notoriously refractory to efforts at resuscitation. Pulmonary function tests, specifically the peak expiratory flow rate (PEFR), have been advocated by some authorities to determine which patients may be at risk for arrest under general anesthesia.[64] These authors recommend that when PEFR is less than 50% of predicted, general anesthesia should be avoided. Although they did not specifically evaluate whether impaired PEFR would be predictive of respiratory collapse during general anesthesia, because all with such low PEFRs were excluded and operated on under local anesthesia, all children with PEFR greater than 50% tolerated general anesthesia.

Airway Management Strategies[65]

When there is a suspicion of marked cardiovascular or respiratory compromise, general anesthesia should be avoided. If general anesthesia is necessary, consideration should be given to the use of a femoral-femoral bypass. Conservatively, spontaneous ventilation should be preserved and muscle relaxants avoided, although they may be safe to use in the asymptomatic patient with good pulmonary function test results.

Techniques

Techniques to manage respiratory collapse include resuming spontaneous ventilation; stenting the trachea with a rigid bronchoscope or by placing an ET past any obstruction and into the bronchus; placing traction on the airway with a rigid scope or by changing the patient to a lateral or prone position; and femoral-femoral bypass.

Pediatric Trauma and Emergency Airway Management

Often emergency airway management in children is performed by paramedical personnel or by nonanesthesiologist physicians. Outcome reviews in the emergency medicine literature underscore the problems associated with this management.[66–68] Airway complications are common during emergency ET intubation and are more frequent and more severe if intubation is attempted in the field. In one study, complications were less severe for intubations performed at a children's hospital than at a community hospital, but the complication rates were the same. Drugs used for emergency airway management were often inappropriately omitted (particularly drugs for increased intracranial pressure). In addition, errors in technique contributed significantly to morbidity. However, despite management errors, patients who present apneic but with a pulse have an excellent survival rate (96.9%). These authors recommend increased emphasis on rapid sequence induction techniques in Pediatric Advanced Life Support courses to decrease mistakes and associated morbidity.

■ Suggested Steps in Emergency Pediatric Airway Management

- Quickly assess the airway and breathing status of the patient.
- Oxygenate and, if needed, establish adequate ventilation by mask. It is rare that endotracheal intubation needs to be performed before restoring adequate oxygenation and ventilation.
- Drugs are useful for assisting intubation in the pediatric patient who has an adequate cardiac output, although they are not used in a patient without vital signs (see the later list of drug dosages).
- Assistance should be directed to help with the intubation. This includes
  - One person to apply cricoid pressure and hand the ET to the operator
  - One person to apply in-line stabilization (without traction) for patients with suspected cervical spine instability
  - One person to inject and flush medications
  - One person to watch the monitors
- After intubation,

- Confirm the ET position
- Note the length marker of the ET at the gum line
- Recheck the ET position after taping
- Medications
  - Atropine—10 μg/kg intravenously before intubation
  - Sedative-hypnotic-analgesic, depending on cardiovascular or central nervous system status

    Ketamine—1 to 2 mg/kg

    Thiopental—1 to 5 mg/kg

    Midazolam—0.05 to 0.1 mg/kg

    Lidocaine—1 to 1.5 mg/kg

    Fentanyl—1 to 2 μg/kg

  - Muscle relaxant

    Succinylcholine—2 mg/kg

    Rocuronium—1.5 mg/kg

    Pancuronium—0.1–0.2 mg/kg (for maintenance of paralysis only)

Extubation of the Child with a Difficult Airway

Unless a child who has difficult airway management requires a tracheostomy for long-term management, the child will require extubation! Preparation for extubation begins shortly after the airway is secured. Equipment used to secure the airway should be rechecked, quickly returned to functional status, and then left in the operating room until successful extubation.

Patients who had prolonged attempts at intubation or who will have procedures that may lead to airway edema may benefit from a dose of dexamethasone (0.5 to 1 mg/kg). If significant airway edema is suspected either because of airway management or the type of surgery, one should consider leaving the patient intubated postoperatively until this resolves. The patient must be fully awake and have full return of strength and adequate ventilatory effort before extubation is attempted. Consideration should be given to extubation over a ventilating stylet. This can be used for oxygenation and ventilation and as a guide to reinsert the ET if the patient's ventilatory efforts are inadequate. A case report describes the successful use of this technique in a child with difficult airway.[69]

In circumstances in which the patient will remain intubated for a prolonged period of time after surgery, it is advisable to have the patient return to the operating room for extubation. Both an otolaryngologist who is prepared to perform rigid bronchoscopy or tracheotomy, or both, and an anesthesiologist who is familiar with the techniques used for the airway management should be in attendance.

CONCLUSION

A challenge of pediatric anesthesia is the great variety in the patients' age, size, and maturity. The skill this challenge requires is most evident when faced with a child who has a potential airway problem. A thoughtful and well-prepared approach that takes into consideration the child's age, size, and maturity as well as the specific airway problem will result in the best possible outcome.

REFERENCES

1. Morray JP, Geiduschek JM, Caplan RA, et al: A comparison of pediatric and adult anesthesia closed malpractice claims. Anesthesiology 78:461, 1993.
2. Van der Walt JH, Sweeney DB, Runciman WB, Webb RK: The Australian Incident Monitoring Study. Paediatric incidents in anaesthesia: An analysis of 2000 incident reports. Anaesth Intensive Care 21:655, 1993.
3. Practice guidelines for management of the difficult airway. A report by the American Society of Anesthesiologists Task Force on Management of the Difficult Airway. Anesthesiology 78:597, 1993.
4. Mark LJ, Beattie C, Ferrell CL, et al: The difficult airway mechanisms for effective dissemination of critical information. J Clin Anesth 4:247, 1992.
5. Eckenhoff JE: Some anatomic considerations of the infant larynx influencing endotracheal anesthesia. Anesthesiology 12:401, 1951.
6. Coté CJ, Todres ID: The pediatric airway. *In* Coté CJ, Ryan JF, Todres ID, Goudsouzian NG (eds): A Practice of Anesthesia for Infants and Children, 2nd ed. Philadelphia, WB Saunders, 1993, p 55.
7. Berry FA: Anesthesia for the child with a difficult airway. *In* Berry FA (ed): Anesthetic Management of Difficult and Routine Pediatric Patients, 2nd ed. New York, Churchill Livingstone, 1990, p 167.
8. Benumof JL: Laryngeal mask airway and the ASA Difficult Airway Algorithm. Anesthesiology 84:686, 1996.
9. Brain AI: The laryngeal mask airway—A possible new solution to airway problems in the emergency situation. Arch Emerg Med 1:229, 1984.
10. Markakis DA, Sayson SC, Schreiner MS: Insertion of the laryngeal mask airway in awake infants with the Robin sequence. Anesth Analg 75:822, 1992.
11. Heard CM, Caldicott LD, Fletcher JE, Selsby DS: Fiberoptic-guided endotracheal intubation via the laryngeal mask airway in pediatric patients: A report of a series of cases. Anesth Analg 82:1287, 1996.
12. O'Neill B, Templeton JJ, Caramico L, Schreiner MS: The laryngeal mask airway in pediatric patients: Factors affecting ease of use during insertion and emergence. Anesth Analg 78:659, 1994.
13. Dubreuil M, Laffon M, Plaud B, et al: Complications and fiberoptic assessment of size 1 laryngeal mask airway. Anesth Analg 76:527, 1993.
14. Mizushima A, Wardall GJ, Simpson DL: The laryngeal mask airway in infants. Anaesthesia 47:849, 1992.
15. Paterson SJ, Byrne PJ, Molesky MG, et al: Neonatal resuscitation using the laryngeal mask airway. Anesthesiology 80:1248, 1994.
16. Benumof JL, Scheller MS: The importance of transtracheal jet ventilation in the management of the difficult airway. Anesthesiology 71:769, 1989.
17. Silverman BK: APLS: The Pediatric Emergency Medicine Course, 2nd ed. Elk Grove Village, Ill, American Academy of Pediatrics/American College of Emergency Physicians, 1993.
18. Westhorpe RN: The position of the larynx in children and its relationship to the ease of intubation. Anaesth Intensive Care 15:384, 1987.
19. Ledbetter JL, Rasch DK, Pollard TG, et al: Reducing the risks of laryngoscopy in anaesthetised infants. Anaesthesia 43:151, 1988.
20. Patil VU, Sopchak AM, Thomas PS: Use of a dental mirror as an aid to tracheal intubation in an infant. Anesthesiology 78:619, 1993.

21. Henderson JJ: The use of paraglossal straight blade laryngoscopy in difficult tracheal intubation. Anaesthesia 52:552, 1997.
22. Bonfils P: Difficult intubation in Pierre-Robin children, a new method: The retromolar route. Anaesthesist 32:363, 1983.
23. Loudermilk EP, Hartmannsgruber M, Stoltzfus DP, Langevin PB: A prospective study of the safety of tracheal extubation using a pediatric airway exchange catheter for patients with a known difficult airway. Chest 111:1660, 1997.
24. Wheeler M, Ovassapian A: Pediatric fiberoptic intubation. In Ovassapian A (ed): Fiberoptic Endoscopy and the Difficult Airway, 2nd ed. Philadelphia, Lippincott-Raven, 1996, p 105.
25. Ovassapian A, Wheeler M: Fiberoptic endoscopy-aided techniques. In Benumof JL (ed): Airway Management Principles and Practice. St Louis, Mosby–Year Book, 1996, p 282.
26. Roth AG, Wheeler M, Stevenson GW, Hall SC: Comparison of a rigid laryngoscope with the ultrathin fibreoptic laryngoscope for tracheal intubation in infants. Can J Anaesth 41:1069, 1994.
27. Frei FJ, àWengen DF, Rutishauser M, Ummenhofer W: The airway endoscopy mask: Useful device for fibreoptic evaluation and intubation of the paediatric airway. Pediatr Anaesth 5:319, 1995.
28. Frei FJ, Ummenhofer W: A special mask for teaching fiber-optic intubation in pediatric patients. Anesth Analg 76:458, 1993.
29. Wilton NC: Aids for fiberoptically guided intubation in children [letter]. Anesthesiology 75:549, 1991.
30. Goskowicz R, Colt HG, Voulelis LD: Fiberoptic tracheal intubation using a nipple guide. Anesthesiology 85:1210, 1996.
31. Wrigley SR, Black AE, Sidhu VS: A fibreoptic laryngoscope for paediatric anaesthesia: A study to evaluate the use of the 2.2 mm Olympus (LF-P) intubating fibrescope. Anaesthesia 50:709, 1995.
32. Stiles CM: A flexible fiberoptic bronchoscope for endotracheal intubation of infants. Anesth Analg 53:1017, 1974.
33. Howardy-Hansen P, Berthelsen P: Fibreoptic bronchoscopic nasotracheal intubation of a neonate with Pierre Robin syndrome. Anaesthesia 43:121, 1988.
34. Scheller JG, Schulman SR: Fiber-optic bronchoscopic guidance for intubating a neonate with Pierre-Robin syndrome. J Clin Anesth 3:45, 1991.
35. Ford RW: Adaptation of the fiberoptic laryngoscope for tracheal intubation with small diameter tubes. Can Anaesth Soc J 28:479, 1981.
36. Berthelsen P, Prytz S, Jacobsen E: Two-stage fiberoptic nasotracheal intubation in infants: A new approach to difficult pediatric intubation. Anesthesiology 63:457, 1985.
37. Alfery DD, Ward CF, Harwood IR, Mannino FL: Airway management for a neonate with congenital fusion of the jaws. Anesthesiology 51:340, 1979.
38. Gouverneur JM, Veyckemans F, Licker M, et al: Using a ureteral catheter as a guide in difficult neonatal fiberoptic intubation. Anesthesiology 66:436, 1987.
39. Brett CM, Zwass MS, France NK: Eyes, ears, nose, throat, and dental surgery. In Gregory GA (ed): Pediatric Anesthesia, 3rd ed. New York, Churchill Livingstone, 1994, p 652.
40. Populaire C, Lundi JN, Pinaud M, Souron R: Elective tracheal intubation in the prone position for a neonate with Pierre Robin syndrome. Anesthesiology 62:214, 1985.
41. Sklar GS, King BD: Endotracheal intubation and Treacher-Collins syndrome. Anesthesiology 44:247, 1976.
42. Borland LM, Swan DM, Leff S: Difficult pediatric endotracheal intubation: A new approach to the retrograde technique. Anesthesiology 55:577, 1981.
43. Fisher QA, Tunkel DE: Lightwand intubation of infants and children. J Clin Anesth 9:275, 1997.
44. Cooper SD, Benumof JL, Ozaki GT: Evaluation of the Bullard laryngoscope using the new intubating stylet: Comparison with conventional laryngoscopy. Anesth Analg 79:965, 1994.
45. Rabb MF, Minkowitz HS, Hagberg CA: Blind intubation through the laryngeal

mask airway for management of the difficult airway in infants. Anesthesiology 84:1510, 1996.

46. Harvey SC, Fishman RL, Edwards SM: Retrograde intubation through a laryngeal mask airway. Anesthesiology 85:1503, 1996.

47. Audenaert SM, Montgomery CL, Stone B, et al: Retrograde-assisted fiberoptic tracheal intubation in children with difficult airways. Anesth Analg 73:660, 1991.

48. Haas JE, Tsueda K: Direct laryngoscopy with the aid of a fiberoptic bronchoscope for tracheal intubation. Anesth Analg 82:438, 1996.

49. Przybylo HJ, Stevenson GW, Vicari FA, et al: Retrograde fibreoptic intubation in a child with Nager's syndrome. Can J Anaesth 43:697, 1996.

50. Erb T, Marsch SU, Hampl KF, Frei FJ: Teaching the use of fiberoptic intubation for children older than two years of age. Anesth Analg 85:1037, 1997.

51. Lopez-Gil M, Brimacombe J, Cebrian J, Arranz J: Laryngeal mask airway in pediatric practice: A prospective study of skill acquisition by anesthesia residents. Anesthesiology 84:807, 1996.

52. Rhine EJ, Roberts D: Acute epiglottitis—revisited. Paediatr Anaesth 5:345, 1995.

53. Gonzalez Valdepena H, Wald ER, Rose E, et al: Epiglottitis and *Haemophilus influenzae* immunization: The Pittsburgh experience—A five-year review. Pediatrics 96:424, 1995.

54. Cressman WR, Myer CM: Diagnosis and management of croup and epiglottitis. Pediatr Clin North Am 41:265, 1994.

55. Parsons DS, Smith RB, Mair EA, Dlabal LJ: Unique case presentations of acute epiglottic swelling and a protocol for acute airway compromise. Laryngoscope 106:1287, 1996.

56. Holinger LD: Foreign bodies of the airway and esophagus. *In* Holinger LD, Lusk RP, Green CG (eds): Pediatric Laryngology and Bronchoesophagology. Philadelphia, Lippincott-Raven, 1997, p 233.

57. Kain ZN, O'Connor TZ, Berde CB: Management of tracheobronchial and esophageal foreign bodies in children: A survey study. J Clin Anesth 6:28, 1994.

58. Tatsumi K, Furuya H, Nagahata T, et al: Removal of a bronchial foreign body in a child using the laryngeal mask. Masui 42:441, 1993.

59. Holinger LD: Caustic ingestion, esophageal injury and stricture. *In* Holinger LD, Lusk RP, Green CG (eds): Pediatric Laryngology and Bronchoesophagology. Philadelphia, Lippincott-Raven, 1997, p 295.

60. Andrews SE: Laser ablation of recurrent laryngeal papillomas in children. AORN J 61:532, 1995.

61. Weisberger EC, Emhardt JD: Apneic anesthesia with intermittent ventilation for microsurgery of the upper airway. Laryngoscope 106:1099, 1996.

62. Weisberger EC, Miner JD: Apneic anesthesia for improved endoscopic removal of laryngeal papillomata. Laryngoscope 98:693, 1988.

63. Holinger LD: Congenital laryngeal anomalies. *In* Holinger LD, Lusk RP, Green CG (eds): Pediatric Laryngology and Bronchoesophagology. Philadelphia, Lippincott-Raven, 1997, p 137.

64. Shamberger RC, Holzman RS, Griscom NT, et al: Prospective evaluation by computed tomography and pulmonary function tests of children with mediastinal masses. Surgery 118:468, 1995.

65. Pullerits J, Holzman R: Anaesthesia for patients with mediastinal masses. Can J Anaesth 36:681, 1989.

66. Nakayama DK, Gardner MJ, Rowe MI: Emergency endotracheal intubation in pediatric trauma. Ann Surg 211:218, 1990.

67. Nakayama DK, Waggoner T, Venkataraman ST, et al: The use of drugs in emergency airway management in pediatric trauma. Ann Surg 216:205, 1992.

68. Schoenfeld PS, Baker MD: Management of cardiopulmonary and trauma resuscitation in the pediatric emergency department. Pediatrics 91:726, 1993.

69. Chipley PS, Castresana M, Bridges MT, Catchings TT: Prolonged use of an endotracheal tube changer in a pediatric patient with a potentially compromised airway. Chest 105:961, 1994.

Chapter 13

The Difficult Obstetric

Airway

Anita Giezentanner and Carin A. Hagberg

The care of the obstetric patient is always a challenge for the anesthesia practitioner because of the very nature of caring for two patients simultaneously. The difficult obstetric airway is a particular challenge as a result of the many anatomic and physiologic changes that occur in women during pregnancy. Decisions and management strategies may negatively impact the fetus yet be necessary for the safety of the mother. The dictum "mother's safety first," although undeniably correct, is nevertheless unpalatable when one is faced with actual implementation of difficult decisions. The two outstanding differences in the care of the obstetric patient include (1) consideration of the needs of the fetus and (2) dramatically reduced maternal oxygen reserves in the presence of greater metabolic requirements. It is hoped that with careful evaluation and preparation, most of the difficult airway situations may be handled in such a way as to provide a desirable outcome for both patients.

SIGNIFICANCE OF OBSTETRIC AIRWAY MANAGEMENT

Statistics and Overall Maternal Mortality

Airway management has always been the primary responsibility of the anesthesia practitioner. Mismanagement or mishaps involving the airway have traditionally accounted for up to 30% of general anesthetic procedure–related deaths.[1] Morbidity figures for airway complications also are sobering and must cause a deep and abiding respect for the potential for serious complications. The absolute necessity for preparation and a decisive plan of action in the case of an inability to achieve endotracheal intubation is never more evident than in the obstetric population. The incidence of difficult obstetric intubation has been quoted as approximately eight times higher than in the general population, with a frequency of approximately 1 in 300.[2] Although this figure alone is frightening, the physiologic changes that accompany the obstetric airway make the consequences more severe than in the general population. Morbidity with difficult intubation is 13 times higher in obstetric patients than in the general population.[2] Further, the incidence of an airway mishap in emergency procedures and in the morbidly obese patient is recognized to be dramatically higher than during routine care.[3] In the practice of obstetric anesthesia, the frequency of both emergency situations and morbidly obese patients is higher. Obstetric patients are usually healthy young women, and their care is for the most part without incident. However, a false sense of security may develop and is refuted by the continuing unpredictability of these patients. An obstetric anesthesia practitioner should never let his or her guard down in anticipating difficulties with the management of the obstetric patient.

Anesthetic-Related Morbidity and Mortality

Current figures on maternal mortality in the United States quote an incidence of 9.1 per 100,000 deliveries.[4] Anesthesia-related deaths accounted for approximately 4% to 7% depending on the study, with airway mishaps representing at least one third of the deaths. Maternal death associated with general anesthesia is usually of a respiratory nature.[1] Fatal complications arise from difficulty with intubation, esophageal intubation, aspiration, and inadequate ventilation. Significant developments during the past few decades have greatly reduced anesthesia-related deaths. First, recognition of the high incidence of pulmonary aspiration in these patients and a cautious approach with the use of sedation and inhalational anesthetics in the obstetric patient caused a dramatic reduction in complications. In the following years, increased awareness and knowledge of maternal physiology prompted increased caution and monitoring along with careful titration of local anesthetics. Finally, technologic monitoring advances such as pulse oximetry and end-tidal CO_2 monitoring in the past decade have dramatically reduced maternal mortality. Unfortunately, a 7% maternal anesthesia-related mortality remains.

Regional Anesthesia Versus General Anesthesia

Regional anesthesia, especially with abiding respect for the inherent potential toxicities of local anesthetics, appears to be associated with lower morbidity and mortality in the obstetric population. A 1972 study in England and Wales revealed a maternal mortality four times higher in the general anesthesia group than in those who received regional anesthesia.[5] This confidential inquiry series further revealed that of 155 maternal deaths attributable to anesthesia, complications with general anesthesia were responsible for 148 deaths, whereas regional anesthesia was implicated in only 7 deaths. This difference is directly related to careful fluid management, monitoring, and incremental dosing of local anesthetics.

DIFFERENCES IN OBSTETRIC AIRWAYS

Recognition and Evaluation

The recognition and evaluation of the obstetric airway is very similar to the evaluation of any other patient's airway and must never be omitted (see Chapter 2 for a detailed discussion). A simple three-step method of airway evaluation may be performed that includes an assessment of (1) the mouth opening and the visibility of posterior pharyngeal structures (supine versus sitting), (2) the mandibular length, and (3) the neck mobility. False indicators of the Mallampati score, such as evaluating the patient in the supine position and encouraging phonation or arching of the tongue, should be avoided. In the obstetric patient, it is also prudent to attempt to estimate the severity of the local edema and friability of mucosal tissues. Also, evaluation of the airway may need to be repeated, since changes may occur throughout pregnancy as well as during the course of labor.[6] The key to any approach is to realize that any and all external assessments are at best estimates or educated guesses as to what will actually be visualized on direct laryngoscopy of the sedated and paralyzed patient. Difficult or impossible intubations will occur, and the only safe way to manage them is to be well prepared. Vigilance is the key, along with backup plans and the availability of any necessary equipment in case of difficulty.

Maternal Anatomic Differences

Standard evaluation of the airway is essentially the same in all patients; however, there are anatomic differences in the obstetric patient that make intubation more likely to be difficult. These include, but are not limited to, weight gain, breast enlargement, mucosal engorgement, and an increased risk of pulmonary aspiration. Preexisting conditions that appear in the nonobstetric population such as a small mandible, protruding incisors, limited mouth opening or neck extension, short neck, high-arched palate, large breasts, and misapplied cricoid pressure, as well as inadequate anesthesia or muscle relaxation, may also complicate airway management in the obstetric population (Table 13–1). Several systemic diseases such as rheumatoid arthritis, diabetes mellitus, dwarfism, systemic sclerosis, sarcoidosis, ankylosing spondylitis, and tumors of the neck and throat may hinder mouth opening or neck extension in the obstetric patient. Additional causes of limited neck extension may include previous injury or surgery on the face, mandible, or neck. Also, asthma may worsen in pregnancy and indirectly complicate airway management. Finally, increased abdominal contents raise the diaphragm and alter the normal anatomic alignment of the upper airway.

Maternal Physiologic Differences

The physiologic changes of pregnancy are numerous and play a multitude of roles in contributing to the increased morbidity and mortality of the obstetric patient in the presence of difficult airway management (Table 13–2).[7] Although anatomic changes enhance the likelihood of difficulty, it is the physiologic changes that make the consequences so much more severe. The arterial oxygen tension increases and the carbon

Table 13–1   Anatomic Factors that May Complicate the Ability to Intubate the Obstetric Patient

Breast enlargement
Coagulopathy
Edema
High arched palate
Inadequate muscle relaxation
Limited mouth opening
Limited neck extension
Protruding incisors
Short neck
Small mandible
Risk of aspiration
Weight gain

Table 13-2   Physiologic Factors that May Affect the Obstetric Airway

Decreased functional residual capacity
    Cephalad displacement of diaphragm
    Supine position for labor
Increased oxygen consumption (20–30%)
    Increased fetal metabolic requirements
    Increased work of breathing
Increased risk of aspiration
Increased shunt fraction
Increased total body water
Labor
Preexisting chemically induced weakness
Pregnancy-induced hypertension

dioxide level declines because of a first-trimester increase in alveolar ventilation, peaking at 70% by term. The obstetric patient has a 20% to 30% higher oxygen consumption at term. This increase is due to increased maternal work of breathing and fetal metabolic requirements. The onset of labor along with painful contractions may raise the oxygen consumption as much as 80% over control values. The obstetric patient has not only an increased oxygen consumption but also a decreased oxygen reserve or supply. In the obstetric patient, the functional residual capacity is decreased by the cephalad displacement of the diaphragm even in the upright position. The functional residual capacity is further compromised in the supine position, the standard position for a patient in labor. There may be airway closure at tidal volume in the supine position, which increases the shunt fraction and furthers the potential for hypoxemia. Obstetric patients who have a preexisting neuromuscular disease and receive narcotics for pain relief during labor, or magnesium sulfate for preterm labor or pregnancy-induced hypertension (PIH), may become weak and be more prone to inadequate minute ventilation. The clinical effect of these physiologic changes is *rapid desaturation during apnea.* Thus obstetric patients benefit from supplemental oxygen therapy, and early oxygenation and ventilation is necessary when difficulty with laryngoscopy or intubation, or both, occurs.

Several additional factors play a role in the physiologic changes that complicate airway management in the obstetric patient. One factor is the increased potential for aspiration. All obstetric patients are at increased risk of pulmonary aspiration and should receive aspiration chemoprophylaxis before any manipulation of the airway. Also, precautions against aspiration should be taken if the ability to protect the airway is compromised in any fashion. Although opinions vary as to whether gastric aspiration precautions are necessary in early pregnancy, most obstetric anesthetists practice routine prophylaxis and airway protection after approximately 20 weeks of gestation until 48 hours into the puerperium.[8] Nonetheless, all obstetric patients in labor or requiring emergency surgery should be considered to have a full stomach, irrespective of the duration of fasting. The increased potential for aspiration is initially the result of hormonal changes that occur early in pregnancy. Elevated levels of progesterone cause gastric emptying to be delayed and lower esophageal sphincter pressure to be decreased, and placental gastrin causes gastric acid production to increase. These changes occur early and are clinically significant by 10 to 12 weeks of gestation. By 20 weeks of gestation, the gravid uterus exerts physical pressure on the stomach causing its upward displacement and rotation, which alters the angle of the gastroesophageal junction and increases intragastric pressure. Intragastric pressure is further increased in the presence of polyhydramnios, a multiple gestation, morbid obesity, the lithotomy position, or applied fundal pressure. Overall, there are numerous factors including decreased gastric motility and food absorption, lowered esophageal sphincter tone, and increased gastric volume and acid production that place the obstetric patient at significantly increased risk of pulmonary aspiration of gastric contents. Not only is the obstetric patient more likely to experience aspiration, but the associated mortality is seven times higher than in the nonpregnant patient population.[1] This poorer outcome from aspiration in the obstetric population may be related to increased permeability and interstitial water in the lung and to decreased colloid osmotic pressure and lymphatic clearance.[9]

The fact that total body water is increased in the obstetric patient is also important with respect to the airway. An increase in total body water leads to mucosal engorgement of the entire respiratory tree including the larynx, nasopharynx, and vocal cords. This engorgement may be worsened by conditions that accompany pregnancy such as concurrent respiratory tract infection, PIH, or a prolonged or strenuous labor.[6, 10, 11] The patient receiving oxytocin may be even more prone to fluid overload due to its antidiuretic side effect. Obviously, these changes may pose problems in the instrumentation of the mouth or nasopharynx for intubation. It is prudent to be alert for these changes and prepare for them by having smaller-sized endotracheal tubes and vasoconstriction agents readily available on the obstetric unit.

The weight gain that accompanies pregnancy is frequently 20 kg or more. This may cause problems not only with endotracheal intubation but also with the maintenance of satisfactory mask ventilation during general anesthesia. Excessive weight gain is associated with an increased incidence of both postdate deliveries and cesarean section; thus the need for either regional or general anesthesia often arises. The breast enlargement that accompanies pregnancy is more pronounced in the presence of excessive weight gain. Intubation of the obstetric patient with enlarged breasts is facilitated by the use of a short-handled laryngoscope and breast retraction during laryngoscopy. Proper positioning of the patient facilitates intubation attempts and increases the likelihood of success. Regional anesthesia may also be more difficult to perform, and extra-long needles (spinal or epidural) should be available. Ultrasonography may help locate the intervertebral spaces in the obese obstetric patient.

Morbid Obesity

Morbid obesity is a condition that affects a significant percentage of obstetric patients.[12] Anesthetic management of the morbidly obese patient is extremely challenging, including obtaining intravenous access, positioning for adequate fat and uterine displacement, and administration of regional or general anesthesia (Table 13–3). Chest compliance is often poor, and intubation or mask ventilation may prove to be difficult. Furthermore, morbidly obese patients have a higher incidence of other complicating medical conditions such as diabetes mellitus, chronic hypertension, and PIH. These patients are also more likely to require cesarean section and to have prolonged surgical times with more bleeding and attendant complications. In one study of obstetric patients who weighed more than 300 pounds, cesarean section was required three times as often as in controls.[12] Even more alarming was the finding that the incidence of emergent cesarean section was almost 50% as compared with 9% in the control group. It is well established that complications with emergency airway management are higher in all types of cases in morbidly obese patients, particularly in the obstetric population. In this same study, regional anesthesia was successful in almost equal percentages, although it took longer to perform and the epidural had to be repeated more often in the morbidly obese group because of migration of the catheter as a result of excess adipose tissue. This study speaks strongly for adequate proactive preparation of these patients in anticipation of problems. Good communication and cooperation between the obstetric and anesthetic team is never more important than when dealing with these patients.

Morbid obesity has been implicated as a contributing factor in up to 80% of anesthesia-related maternal deaths. It is in these patients that some of the airway "gadgets" and alternative laryngoscopes should be considered and alternative methods of securing the airway become important. The ability to use these devices may be lifesaving for both the mother and the fetus.

Table 13–3 Complications of Morbid Obesity in Parturients

Difficulty in basic medical management
    Intravenous access
    Positioning
    Regional or general anesthesia
Associated medical conditions
    Diabetes mellitus
    Chronic hypertension
    Pregnancy-induced hypertension
Higher cesarean section rate
    Elective
    Emergent
Longer duration of surgery
Increased amount of surgical bleeding
Increased maternal mortality

MANAGEMENT OPTIONS AND PLANS

Recognized Difficult Intubation

■ Early Recognition and Planning

Difficult airway management can occur in a variety of circumstances and patients. The key to proper management of any airway is anticipation of difficulty, adequate preparation (patient and equipment), and a detailed plan of action should problems arise. Management of the obstetric patient must also take into account the condition of the fetus and the urgency of the operative procedure. A difficult airway may be either recognized or unrecognized before intubation, and airway management varies accordingly (Fig. 13–1).

Most difficult intubations may be predicted with adequate preoperative screening and evaluation of the airway. All patients on an obstetric unit should have a full anesthetic evaluation including assessment of their airway. Their evaluation should include a record of prior surgeries and anesthesia, as well as their current weight and the amount of weight gained during their pregnancy. Patients who have had a previous cesarean section should be evaluated for the precipitating factors that led to cesarean section, since it may provide insight into the likelihood of another operative delivery. The interview allows the initial establishment of rapport between the anesthesia practitioner and the patient. This communication will be invaluable in terms of patient cooperation should emergency or invasive procedures, such as awake intubation, become necessary. An emergency situation is not the time to be meeting a patient or discussing potential airway complications with the obstetrician for the first time. An aggressive policy of patient evaluation allows the anticipation of potential difficulties, the preparation of equipment, and the notification of appropriate personnel.

The safest method of induction may be selected if general anesthesia is necessary, although it may be avoided with the use of a carefully administered regional anesthetic. Management decisions are best worked out with a team approach between the patient, obstetrician, and anesthesia practitioner.

■ Regional Anesthesia

Aspiration chemoprophylaxis with a nonparticulate antacid and gastric motility enhancer or H_2 blocker, or both, minimizes the potential for any aspiration. Regional anesthesia is a controversial solution in the presence of a recognized potentially difficult airway. Admittedly, undertaking regional anesthesia is not and must never be considered a failsafe "out" for dealing with an airway that appears difficult to manage. The possibility for seizures or a high block resulting in respiratory arrest is always present. There is no excuse for not having a plan of action for any of these mishaps. Preparatory disclaimers aside, we believe that regional anesthesia, undertaken in experienced and careful hands, is a very acceptable technique in these situations. Indeed, many patients with recognizable difficult airways have had elective cesarean

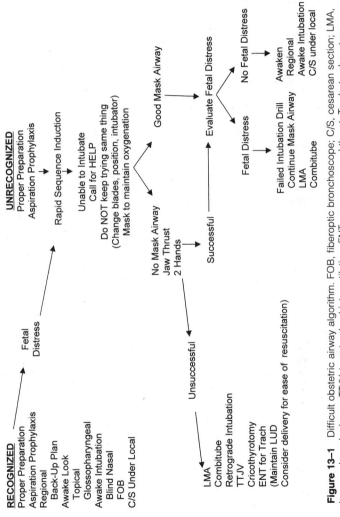

Figure 13–1 Difficult obstetric airway algorithm. FOB, fiberoptic bronchoscope; C/S, cesarean section; LMA, laryngeal mask airway; TTJV, transtracheal jet ventilation; ENT, ears, nose, and throat; Trach, tracheostomy; LUD, left uterine displacement. (Adapted from Practice Guidelines for Management of the Difficult Airway. A report by the ASA task force on management of the difficult airway. Anesthesiology 78:597–602, 1993.)

sections performed successfully under regional anesthesia. This option may be preferable to letting these patients labor, which may result in fetal distress requiring an emergency cesarean section.

The type of regional anesthesia for cesarean section is also controversial. There are valid arguments for and against both epidural and spinal anesthesia in any type of case. The advantage of epidural anesthesia is that it allows slow titration of the level of anesthetic, thus avoiding major hemodynamic shifts or respiratory compromise. A disadvantage of epidural anesthesia, however, is that it has a higher incidence of inadvertent intravascular injection and injection of local anesthetic into a place other than the intended space (subarachnoid space), compared with spinal anesthesia. In fact, a high block or "total spinal" requiring emergency intubation is more frequently a complication of an epidural anesthetic than a planned subarachnoid block that ended with a higher dermatomal level than anticipated. Undoubtedly, the safest way to proceed depends on the experience of the anesthesia practitioner. Nonetheless, it is best not to try something new on a patient with potential airway difficulties. In some patients, regional anesthesia may not be feasible because of the anesthesia practitioner's or patient's preference, anatomic limitations of the spine, or a poor coagulation status.

Safety of the mother is the primary concern for the anesthesia practitioner. This is the standard dictum, and it cannot be disputed. Even in the case of fetal distress, a mother who presents with a potentially difficult airway is not a candidate for a rapid sequence or "crash" induction. Maternal hypoxemia is not going to help either the mother or the fetus and may prove fatal to both. The true controversy arises in the wide spectrum of potential difficult airways. It is obvious in some patients, such as those with anatomic limitations or a history of difficult failed intubation, that they would be impossible to intubate under standard conditions. In these patients, therapeutic options, as mentioned previously, must be used as quickly as possible in order to achieve control of the airway. The majority of patients, however, fall somewhere in between having the ideal or the impossible airway. Each case should be treated separately by the anesthesia practitioner based on his or her experience and judgment. The difficult airway combined with fetal distress is the nightmare of every anesthesia practitioner. A plan of action should be detailed beforehand and followed once the situation occurs.

■ Awake Intubation

Patients who present with a recognized potentially difficult airway are best managed with a conservative approach and awake intubation. If there is a question about the amount of difficulty, an "awake look" may be undertaken, remembering that in the awake patient, all muscle tone is still intact and the full effect of the relaxed oropharyngeal tissue cannot be appreciated unless the patient is paralyzed. An awake look may be undertaken with topical spray applied to the oropharynx or a glossopharyngeal nerve block, or both, in order to facilitate tolerance of the laryngoscope in the oropharynx. The glossopharyngeal nerve provides sensory innervation to the posterior third of the tongue, vallecula, anterior surface of the epiglottis, posterior and lateral walls of the pharynx, and tonsillar pillars. Blocking this nerve, especially if this is combined with topicalization of the oral cavity, may allow the patient to tolerate attempts at awake visualization of the oropharynx.[13–15] Further topicalization of the vocal cords should be performed before intubation if this technique allows such visualization.

Awake intubation is the gold standard for conservative management of a recognized difficult airway. This is usually accomplished by the use of a flexible fiberoptic bronchoscope. In the obstetric patient, the oral route is preferred because of mucosal engorgement of the nose and the tendency of the nasal membranes to bleed. The insertion of anything by way of the nose, including a nasal airway, a nasogastric tube, or a nasotracheal tube, may result in epistaxis. Awake intubation, by the oral route, is fully described in Chapter 4. It requires adequate topicalization and may be performed with the aid of an oral intubating airway, a laryngeal mask airway (LMA),[16] a lightwand, or a rigid fiberoptic laryngoscope (Bullard, Upsher, or Wu). Whether to medicate the obstetric patient for fear of placental transfer and fetal sedation is controversial. This is a valid concern since benzodiazepines and narcotics readily cross the placenta. However, the effects are usually short-lived and should not be problematic if the neonatal care team is aware of the circumstances. Although it is undeniably best to avoid or minimize the medications offered to the obstetric patient, the comfort of the mother and her ability to cooperate with the procedure are the primary considerations.

■ Cesarean Under Local Anesthesia

A last resort for a required operative procedure in an obstetric patient with a recognizable difficult airway is for the obstetrician to perform the operation using local anesthesia. This is certainly possible but may not be the most pleasant option for either the obstetrician or the patient. There have been a few case reports and excellent descriptions of this technique for cesarean section.[17–19] It is used much more frequently in third world countries but, on occasion, has a place in the management of the obstetric patient under various circumstances, including the obstetric patient with a difficult airway.

■ General Anesthesia

If general anesthesia is chosen for the obstetric patient with a possibly difficult airway, certain considerations must be kept in mind. As previously discussed, before the administration of general anesthetic, all patients should be thoroughly evaluated, receive aspiration chemoprophylaxis, and be positioned in the optimal position for intubation. Meticulous positioning can make the difference between success and failure at intubation and is extremely important for airway management in the obstetric patient.

Unrecognized Difficult Intubation

■ Calm, Detailed Plan of Action

Failed intubation usually occurs in situations in which the degree of possible difficulty in establishing an airway was not fully appreciated. Regardless of all safeguards, there will always be patients who undergo rapid sequence induction and in whom difficulty with intubation is encountered. It cannot be overemphasized that a plan of action should be detailed beforehand and followed once the situation occurs. As soon as serious difficulty is recognized, help should be requested. Desaturation in the obstetric patient occurs much faster than in a nonpregnant patient, and another pair of trained hands may make a difference in the welfare of both the mother and the fetus. If difficulty arises, the patient's position may be altered, a different laryngoscope handle or blade may be used, or a more experienced or different anesthesia practitioner may become involved. The key is to not keep trying the same thing over and over and to not panic. A maximum of three attempts at oral laryngoscopy and intubation should be allowed. After multiple attempts, edema formation, particularly hazardous in the obstetric patient with edema intrinsically present, makes the airway completely unmanageable. Continued laryngoscopy may also increase the likelihood of aspiration. After three reasonable attempts at oral laryngoscopy and intubation using different maneuvers, the likelihood of success is much lower than the probability of losing the airway completely due to edema and trauma. One should stop and reassess the situation.

■ Mask Ventilation

Failure to intubate the obstetric patient is often followed by difficulty with mask ventilation and possibly by pulmonary aspiration. Either of these conditions rapidly leads to hypoxemia for both the mother and the fetus. The adequacy of mask ventilation and the presence or absence of fetal distress are extremely important factors that must be taken into account in these situations. Although fetal distress is *not* the deciding factor in the algorithm, it is an important factor if mask ventilation is adequate.

Adequate Mask Ventilation, No Fetal Distress

In situations in which there is no fetal distress, it would be foolish to place the mother at risk of further airway complications by continuing with a surgical procedure. Even if mask ventilation is easy and steps were taken to minimize the chance and severity of possible aspiration, the patient should be awakened. Cricoid pressure should be maintained until the obstetric patient is fully able to protect her airway. Once the patient is awake, a decision needs to be made whether to proceed with regional anesthesia, perform awake intubation, or use straight local anesthesia. Again, the obstetric patient is at too high a risk of aspiration to continue with general anesthesia administered by face mask in the absence of other strong contributing factors such as significant fetal distress.

Adequate Mask Ventilation, Fetal Distress

This situation poses a somewhat different scenario in which there is concern for both the mother's and the child's welfare, and these concerns must achieve a delicate balance. Again, the first step is to evaluate the adequacy of mask ventilation. Ventilation and oxygenation should be easy to maintain, rather than marginal or tenuous. If the airway is truly manageable, the case may be continued by mask, maintaining a level of anesthesia deep enough to prevent laryngospasm. Other options include the use of an LMA,[20, 21] an esophageal tracheal Combitube (ETC), a lightwand, or other specialized laryngoscopes.[22] All anesthesia practitioners should become facile with at least one alternative method of securing the airway. In the original failed intubation drill proposed by Tunstall,[23] recommendations included turning the patients to their side, passing an orogastric tube to empty the stomach, and providing inhalational anesthesia by mask. Regardless of the method chosen, cricoid pressure should be applied and continued unless it interferes with the maintenance of a clear airway.

The LMA has gained wide acceptance, and in fact many anesthesia practitioners today are probably more likely to use the LMA than hold a face mask for an entire surgical procedure. There have been many case reports of the successful use of the LMA for cesarean section when the airway could not be intubated by routine measures.[24] It is important to remember that although the use of this airway device may allow adequate ventilation, it does not protect against aspiration. An adequate depth of anesthesia must be maintained, not only before insertion of the LMA, but throughout the surgical procedure in order to prevent gagging and laryngospasm. Anesthesia may be maintained with either inhalational or intravenous agents with appropriate provisions for the possibility of neonatal depression.

Cricoid pressure should be applied but not if it interferes with airway management (Fig. 13–2). Initial attempts to place the LMA should be made while maintaining cricoid pressure. If LMA placement is unsuccessful, cricoid pressure may be released with the next insertion attempt. Once inserted, cricoid pressure should be continued. If cricoid pressure with the LMA in place does not hinder the ease of airway maintenance, then it should be continued. If not, cricoid pressure should be discontinued and the patient allowed to resume spontaneous ventilation, if possible, in order to lessen the likelihood of regurgitation (see Chapter 2).[25] Another option is to secure the airway with a cuffed endotracheal tube using the LMA as a conduit.[26–29] Blind intubation techniques by way of an LMA have been successfully accomplished[30, 31] yet risk failure. The most effective and safest approach may be using fiberoptic endoscopic-guided intubation.

The ETC is a relatively new device that may gain more widespread acceptance and use in this situation. It is easily placed and may offer better airway protection against aspiration than the LMA. Studies are currently in progress at our institution to assess this matter.

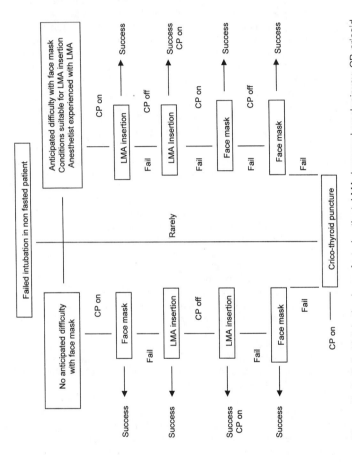

Figure 13–2 Failed intubation in nonfasted patient. LMA, laryngeal mask airway; CP, cricoid pressure. (From Brimacombe J, Berry A: The laryngeal mask airway for obstetric anesthesia and neonatal resuscitation. Int J Obstet Anesth 3:211, 1994.)

Inadequate Mask Ventilation

If mask ventilation is inadequate, maternal considerations come before all others. As discussed earlier, the obstetric patient desaturates much faster than the average nonobstetric patient, and the consequences of failure to oxygenate will be devastating if corrective steps toward adequate oxygenation are not taken *immediately.* Remember, there are simple physical maneuvers that may help open the airway, including a head tilt, a two-handed jaw thrust,[32] and bag ventilation by a third party. These maneuvers may open the airway and allow adequate oxygenation.

If the basic maneuvers do not immediately remedy the situation, time is of the essence and decisions must quickly be made to take actions toward establishing a patent airway and restoring oxygenation. Either the LMA or the ETC may be useful in this situation in order to resecure the airway. If the necessary equipment is available, retrograde intubation may also be considered. However, it is a technique that the practitioner should be facile with when used in this type of situation. In untrained hands, it may be too time-consuming and thus inappropriate.

Transtracheal jet ventilation via a catheter placed through the cricothyroid membrane is probably the fastest route to oxygenation in a patient who is desaturating. When performing jet ventilation, it is extremely important to ensure adequate exhalation in order to prevent excessive barotrauma. Again, equipment must be readily available, and this is a large part of what is meant by preparation of the operating area for the possibility of failed intubation at *any* time. Many centers maintain a jet ventilator in all anesthesiology locations. If this is not feasible, a jet ventilator should be immediately available in a nearby containment area. Oxygenation via transtracheal jet ventilation is usually a temporary measure of airway establishment and used for resuscitative purposes. It must be maintained by someone dedicated solely to holding the catheter at the patient's neck and is not to be considered a secure airway. After a cannot intubate, cannot ventilate situation, the patient should be allowed to awaken and the operative procedure postponed until a more secure airway is achieved. Also, one must remember that when a difficult airway situation arises, surgical consultation, if immediately available, should be summoned in the event that a tracheostomy is required. If surgical intervention is not available, then a surgical percutaneous cricothyrotomy may be performed. If oxygenation is not restored in an expedient manner and cardiac arrest ensues, resuscitation of the obstetric patient is much more effective when left uterine displacement is maintained.

■ Emergency Airway Cart

The emergency airway cart should be an integral part of every obstetric unit. A regimen should be instituted to ensure that equipment is secured and checked on a regular basis. Nursing staff, as well as anesthesia personnel, should know its location and have at least a rudimentary idea of what maneuvers may be necessary should a difficult intubation present after the induction of general anesthesia.

STAYING OUT OF TROUBLE: PREGNANT

P **Preoperative** evaluation of patients who may need surgical or anesthetic intervention, or both (i.e., *all* patients should be evaluated for medical or physical factors that would complicate their management). It has been suggested that as many as 87% of urgent or emergent cesarean sections may be predicted by the relevant medical history and by regularly observing the patient, labor pattern, and fetal heart tones.

R **Regional** anesthesia (spinal or epidural) is a viable option for many patients. It often allows the safest anesthetic and avoids manipulation of the airway. It is not fail-safe and must not be undertaken without a backup plan if complications occur.

E **Expectation.** Expect the worst-case scenario and have predetermined plans of action.

G **Get** the patient and all equipment ready and in order.

N **No,** I do not rush and make hasty decisions; the mother's safety is the first priority. No matter how urgent the situation, position properly and calmly proceed with a rational plan. There is no situation for mother or fetus that will be improved by maternal hypoxemia.

A **Assess** changes (e.g., fetal distress, prolonged second stage, worsening PIH, and the adequacy of regional block). These are all situations that may occur and change quickly, mandating a change in medical management.

N **kNow** your obstetrician and maintain good communication. Potential difficulties should be discussed *before* the crisis. Agree on patient management in advance.

T **Tracheal** intubation options are numerous with the airway gadgets now available. Familiarize yourself with a variety of intubation tools and techniques.

DIFFICULT AIRWAY CART

Topicalization and Preparation
Cotton-tipped applicators
Gauze (4 × 4s)
Tongue blades
Atomizer
Lidocaine (Xylocaine: 2% jelly, 2% injectable, 4% liquid, 10% spray)
Phenylephrine (Neo-Synephrine) nose drops (1% solution)
Syringes and needles of assorted sizes, including a 25-gauge 3.5-inch spinal needle
Medicine cups or similar containers suitable to contain 20 mL or more
Lubrication jelly

Intubation Equipment

Oropharyngeal and nasopharyngeal airways of assorted sizes
Ovassapian airways (two)
Laryngoscope handles and blades
> Two handles and backup battery supply
> Assortment of sizes and styles of blades

Magill forceps
Endotracheal tubes
> Regular orotracheal and Endotrol tubes if available
> 3.0 mm to 6.0 mm uncuffed, including half sizes (two of each)
> 6.0 mm to 8.0 mm cuffed (two of each)

Stylets for endotracheal tubes in appropriate sizes

Ancillary Equipment

Yankauer suction tubes (two)
Suction catheters of assorted sizes
Face masks of assorted sizes
Ambu bag
Tape and adhesive spray

Emergency Equipment

Endotracheal guides
> Gum elastic bougie (Eschmann catheter)
> Airway exchange catheters (rigid and hollow core allowing ventilation)
> Lightwand (Trachlight)

Fiberoptic intubation equipment and light source
LMAs (sizes 3, 4, and 5)
Esophageal tracheal Combitubes (small adult and regular adult)
Retrograde intubation equipment
Emergency cricothyrotomy kit
Emergency tracheostomy kit
Shiley tracheostomy tubes (sizes 6 and 8)
Angiocatheters of assorted sizes (three each)
Stethoscope
End-tidal CO_2 monitor
Oxygen source
Transtracheal jet ventilator setup

REFERENCES

1. Glassenberg R: General anesthesia and maternal mortality. Semin Perinatol 15:386–396, 1991.
2. Lyons G: Failed intubation: Six years' experience in a teaching maternity unit. Anaesthesia 40:759–762, 1985.
3. Mascia MF, Matjasko MJ: Emergency airway management by anesthesiologists. Anesthesiology 79:A1054, 1993. As stated by Deem S, Bishop M: Evaluation and management of the difficult airway. Crit Care Clin 11:1–27, 1995.
4. Atrash HK, Koonin LM, Lawson HW, et al: Maternal mortality in the United States, 1979–1986. Obstet Gynecol 76:1055–1060, 1990.
5. Department of Health: Reports on confidential enquiries into maternal deaths in England and Wales 1967–1969, 1970–1972, 1973–1975, 1976–1978, 1979–1981, 1982–1984, London.

6. Farcon EL, Kim MH, Marx GF: Changing Mallampati score during labour. Can J Anaesth 41(1):50–51, 1994.
7. Cheek TG, Gutsche BB: Maternal physiologic alterations during pregnancy. *In* Shnider SM, Levinson G (eds): Anesthesia for Obstetrics, 3rd ed. Baltimore, Williams & Wilkins, 1993, p 3.
8. Bogod DG: The postpartum stomach—When is it safe? Anesthesia 49:1, 1994.
9. MacLennan FM: Maternal mortality from Mendelson's syndrome: An explanation? Lancet 1:587, 1986.
10. Samsoon GLT, Young JRB: Difficult tracheal intubation: A retrospective study. Anaesthesia 42:487–490, 1987.
11. Rocke DA, Scoones GP: Rapidly progressive laryngeal oedema associated with pregnancy—Aggravated hypertension. Anesthesia 47:141–143, 1992.
12. Hood DD, Dewan DM: Anesthetic and obstetric outcome in morbidly obese parturients. Anesthesiology 79:1210–1218, 1993.
13. Barton S, Williams JD: Glossopharyngeal nerve block. Arch Otolaryingol 93:186–188, 1971.
14. D'Alessio JG, Ramanathan J: Fiberoptic intubation using intra oral glossopharyngeal nerve block in a patient with severe pre-eclampsia and HELP syndrome. Int J Obstet Anesth 4:168–171, 1995.
15. Woods AM, Lander CJ: Abolition of gagging and the hemodynamic response to awake laryngoscopy. Anesthesiology 67:A220, 1987.
16. Godley M, Reddy AR: Use of LMA for awake intubation for caesarean section. Can J Anesth 43:299–302, 1996.
17. Busby T: Local anesthesia for cesarean section. Am J Obstet Gynecol 87:399, 1963.
18. Cooper MG, Feeney EM, Joseph M, et al: Local anesthesia infiltration for cesarean section. Anaesth Intensive Care 17:198–212, 1989.
19. Ranney B, Stanage WF: Advantages of local anesthesia for cesarean section. Obstet Gynecol 45:163, 1975.
20. Gataure PS, Hughes JA: The laryngeal mask airway in obstetrical anaesthesia. Can J Anaesth 42(2):130–133, 1995.
21. Priscu V, Priscu L, Soroker D: Laryngeal mask for failed intubation in emergency cesarean section. Can J Anaesth 39:893, 1992.
22. Cohn AI, Hart RT, McGraw SR, Blass NH: The Bullard laryngoscope for emergency airway management in a morbidly obese parturient. Anesth Analg 81:872–873, 1995.
23. Tunstall ME: Failed intubation in the parturient. Can J Anaesth 36:611–613, 1989.
24. Brimacombe J, Berry A: The laryngeal mask airway for obstetric anesthesia and neonatal resuscitation. Int J Obstet Anesth 3:211, 1994.
25. Brimacombe J, Berry A, White A: An algorithm for use of the laryngeal mask airway during failed intubation in the patient with a full stomach. Anesth Analg 77:398–399, 1993.
26. Hagberg C, Abramson D, Chelly J: A comparison of fiberoptic orotracheal intubation using two different intubating conduits. Anesthesiology 83:A1220, 1996.
27. Hasham F, Kumar CM, Lawler PGP: The use of the laryngeal mask airway to assist fiberoptic orotracheal intubation [letter]. Anaesthesia 46:891, 1991.
28. Heath JL, Allagain J: Intubation through the laryngeal mask: A technique for unexpected difficult intubation. Anaesthesia 46:545, 1991.
29. Benumof JL: The laryngeal mask airway and the ASA difficult airway algorithm. Anesthesiology 84:686–699, 1996.
30. Chadd GD, Ackers JWL, Bailey PM: Difficult intubation aided by the laryngeal mask airway [letter]. Anaesthesia 44:1015, 1989.
31. Allison A, McCrory J: Tracheal placement of a gum elastic bougie using the laryngeal mask airway [letter]. Anaesthesia 45:419–420, 1990.
32. Benumof JL: The ASA Management of the Difficult Airway algorithm and explanation-analysis of the algorithm. *In* Benumof JL (ed): Airway Management Principles and Practice. St Louis, Mosby–Year Book, 1996, p 153.

Chapter 14

Management of the

Traumatized Airway

Michelle Bowman-Howard

Patients with a compromised or traumatized airway present multiple problems for the anesthesia practitioner throughout the perioperative period. These patients require a detailed history and physical examination in order to prepare for the difficulties of airway management. It is helpful to acknowledge factors that make airway management difficult or impossible even before sedative or paralytic medications are administered. This chapter reviews the evaluation of the traumatized airway, types of trauma to the airway, associated injuries that affect airway management, airway management techniques, and use of pharmacologic agents in patients with airway trauma.

EVALUATION OF THE AIRWAY

Airway trauma may include injuries of the nasopharynx all the way to the bronchi. Associated injuries of importance to the airway include those that limit or influence airway management, such as cervical spine instability and closed head injury. Additional factors that contribute to difficult intubation in the trauma patient may include a "full stomach," with the associated increased risk of vomiting and aspiration, blood or secretions, or both, in the airway, and neurologic injury with confusion or coma.[1-3] Airway trauma or damage should be suspected in patients with external tracheal or laryngeal damage, hoarseness, stridor, subcutaneous emphysema, dysphagia, dyspnea, or a "rocking boat" pattern of respiration.[1, 2, 4-10] In particular, the patient may require the sitting position in order to maintain the airway, thus allowing gravity to relieve obstruction due to oropharyngeal edema, blood or secretions in the oropharynx, or the tongue itself. Thus, the airway should be inspected for foreign material, and blood and secretions should be suctioned. Immediate airway assessment and management are critical in these patients, as unrelieved hypoxia will cause death within 3 to 5 minutes.[1]

TYPES OF TRAUMA TO THE AIRWAY

Airway trauma includes both blunt and penetrating injury. Either may lead to significant facial fractures that are not readily apparent yet may develop into an unstable airway. In particular, penetrating injuries (i.e., gunshot wounds) may cause much greater internal than external damage, with blood, bone, and tissue forced into the mouth and pharynx.[1] Blood and edema may compromise the integrity of the airway. Blunt injury may be more dangerous than penetrating injury as it offers less indication of the underlying structural damage.[6] Although these patients may be stable on arrival, up to 35% subsequently deteriorate over the next few hours, mandating emergency airway management.[7] These patients may have a high incidence of associated hypoxia as a common cause of death, making airway management critical.[11, 13, 14] In discussing trauma to the airway, it is necessary to include the structures from the face to the trachea. The following sections discuss the relevant structures, proceeding externally to internally in an anatomic progression.

Maxillofacial Injury

The most common causes of blunt maxillofacial trauma include motor vehicle accidents, direct facial blows during physical disputes, and sports injuries. The type of maxillofacial damage may indicate the amount of force involved in the injury.[6] Low-impact injuries, such as most sports and physical dispute injuries, usually cause self-limiting facial fractures of the midface and mandible.[6] These fractures rarely impact the airway itself, unless excessive bleeding compromises the airway, which might also increase the risk of aspiration. Fractures involving the mandible may compromise mandibular opening and limit laryngoscopy.[6] Those that involve the temporal bone may cause temporomandibular joint (TMJ) dysfunction, locking the jaw closed and consequently impairing orotracheal intubation. High-force injuries are typically caused by motor vehicle accidents, gunshots, and assault with heavy weapons. These injuries may have an associated mortality rate of up to 12%.[10, 11] Death is commonly due to the associated injuries, such as neurologic damage, rather than to the maxillofacial trauma itself.[6, 10, 11] Neurologic injury may occur in 36% of cases of maxillofacial trauma, and cervical spine injury in 5%.[12, 13] Neurologic consequences may include meningitis, subarachnoid hemorrhage, ocular nerve palsies, and blindness.[14] Most of the literature regarding maxillofacial trauma minimizes the grave risks associated with this type of damage, as the data indicate low mortality in patients with such isolated injuries. However, it should be noted that maxillofacial injury may be associated with airway compromise or unsuspected massive blood loss, ultimately leading to death.[11]

Facial Fractures

■ Mandibular Fractures

Mandibular fractures occur at points consistent with the cause of injury. High-velocity and high-impact injuries usually produce fractures of the angle and ramus, whereas low-velocity and low-impact injuries tend to cause fractures of the body and symphysis.[1] Mandibular fractures may make airway evaluation difficult, as mouth opening may be limited by either pain, trismus (masseter muscle spasm), or functional obstruction of the TMJ by a condylar fracture.[15, 16] Limitation of mouth opening due to pain and acute trismus does not usually limit laryngoscopy, as it responds to the administration of an anesthetic and a muscle relaxant.[16, 17] Limitation of mouth opening from TMJ injury may require subluxation of the joint by jaw thrust to provide an adequate airway opening[6, 18, 19] or fiberoptic intubation.[16] If trismus persists for 2 weeks or more, fibrosis of the masseter muscles may prevent relaxation of the muscles in response to the administration of muscle relaxants.[17] An jaw that is immobile because of masseter muscle fibrosis may therefore necessitate an awake intubation. High-impact injuries of the mandible or maxilla, or both, may traumatically remove the tissues normally obstructing visualization of the vocal cords. Therefore, it may be quite easy to place an endotracheal tube (ET) using simple laryngoscopy or direct digital visualization, without having to resort to an emergent surgical airway procedure.[16] Fifty percent of mandibular injuries involve more than one fracture site.[6, 17] Bimandibular fractures usually occur at the most vulnerable points of the mandible at the level of the first and second molars[20] and may be caused by hitting the chin from below by either falling or striking the steering wheel in a motor vehicle accident.[1] The anterior portion of the fracture may be forced posteroinferiorly by the muscles in the floor of the mouth,[21, 22] compromising ventilation and requiring manual fracture reduction and anterior tongue displacement to reopen the airway.[1, 16, 21, 23] Hematoma formation in the floor of the mouth may also cause airway obstruction by pushing the tongue against the palate, which can oftentimes be relieved by artificial airway insertion.[6, 24] When one is preparing for intubation, TMJ dysfunction must always be considered with mandibular fractures.[1, 20] Parasymphyseal and bilateral anterior mandibular fractures are the types most likely to cause airway obstruction.[1] The anesthetic care provider should ascertain the success of mask ventilation before the administration of sedatives or muscle relaxants.[16] It is prudent to also have equipment immediately available for cricothyrotomy or transtracheal jet ventilation.[16]

■ Maxillary Fractures

Midface (maxillary) fractures were originally described in 1901 by Le Fort, who tried to determine the relationship between the presence of facial fractures and the external signs of facial trauma.[1, 25] He concluded that a reliable inference cannot be made solely on the basis of external tissue damage: severe external facial injury can be present with no facial fractures, and conversely, minimal external facial injury may hide severe facial fractures.[1, 25] During his studies he also denoted the common lines of facial fractures: Le Fort I, Le Fort II, and Le Fort III (Fig. 14–1). The Le Fort I injury, or *floating palate*, is a transverse fracture that separates the lower maxilla, hard palate, and pterygoid process from the rest of the maxilla. The Le Fort II, also referred to as the *floating maxilla*, is a pyramidal fracture of the midface that separates along the nasofrontal suture laterally to the floor of the orbit, zygomaticomaxillary sutures, and pterygoid process. The Le Fort III is *craniofacial separation* that divides the midface from the cranium by extending the Le Fort II fracture parallel with the base of the skull.[1, 23, 26] Le Fort I and II fractures rarely affect airway integrity, although Le Fort II fractures may be associated with basilar skull fractures. Instrumentation of the nasopharynx is relatively contraindicated in these types of injuries.[17] Devices (an ET or nasogastric tube) inserted into the nasopharynx may project through the fracture line in the cribriform plate and into the subarachnoid space, which may directly damage the intracranial contents or may cause development of subsequent meningitis (Fig. 14–2).[17, 27] The typical facial appearance of the patient with a Le Fort III fracture includes a triad of raccoon facies (circumorbital ecchymosis), severe midfacial edema, and marked lengthening of the face. These fractures may complicate the management of the patient, causing air-

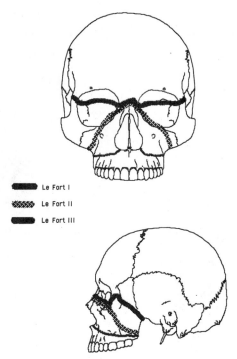

Figure 14–1 Le Fort fractures. (From Cicala RS: The traumatized airway. *In* Benumof JL [ed]: Airway Management Principles and Practice. St Louis, Mosby–Year Book, 1996, pp 736–759.)

way obstruction and bleeding.[6, 28] Airway obstruction may be caused by soft tissue obstruction due to either loss of the skeletal integrity of the face or negative pressure generated during inspiration.[6, 28] Aspiration of blood and tissue may also cause hypoxia in both conscious and unconscious patients.[6, 29] The Le Fort IV fracture is a maxillofacial fracture that extends farther, into the frontal bones, and has clinical symptoms similar to those found with a Le Fort III fracture.[16] Treatment of any of the Le Fort fractures oftentimes requires intramaxillary fixation and open reduction and fixation of the fractures, usually with plating or wiring.[1, 23, 26] Also, good medical management is necessary since multiple organ system involvement is common in those patients who sustain Le Fort III or IV fractures. As maxillary fractures are more commonly associated with airway compromise, the decision to secure the airway should be made early before decompensation occurs.[16] Mask ventilation may be extremely difficult owing to instability and airway debris. Significant injury may mandate immediate ET placement, whereas the stable patient may require only changing from a supine to a lateral position to allow the drainage of blood and secretions.[16]

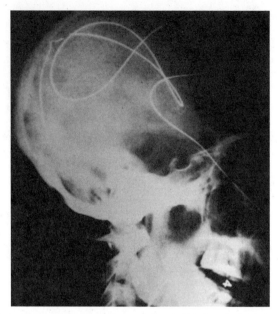

Figure 14–2   Nasogastric tube in the cranial vault. This is one of the dangers of inserting catheters through the nasal passage in head injury patients. (From Aileen P, Temple RN, Katz J: Management of acute head injury. AORN J 46:1068, 1987.)

Laryngotracheal Trauma

Laryngeal damage may also be caused by either blunt or penetrating trauma. Blunt trauma usually leads to one or more of the following: (1) laryngeal compression against the fixed, solid cervical spine, (2) fracture of the cartilage, or (3) bruising or laceration of the airways.[5] Life-threatening injury may occur in spite of insignificant or little external evidence of damage.[16] Since patients with laryngeal injury may rapidly deteriorate,[1, 23] they must be evaluated carefully with a thorough physical examination and possibly fiberoptic endoscopy to ascertain the degree of injury. Computed tomography may also be helpful in the evaluation. Penetrating injuries are usually visually apparent, but high tracheal injury may be masked by immediate intubation in the field by emergency personnel.[26] Preparation should be made for emergent tracheostomy as bleeding and tissue edema may rapidly compromise the airway[1, 26] and tissue distortion may make endotracheal intubation difficult or impossible.[1] Even initially patent airways may become acutely compromised while the patient is undergoing further diagnostic evaluation. Therefore, elective intubation should be considered to protect the airway from later deterioration, especially in patients with a gunshot wound to the face.[6]

Laryngeal injuries can be separated into supraglottic, tracheal, and infraglottic injuries.[5] Glottic damage is commonly associated with either supraglottic or infraglottic lesions.[5] Supraglottic injuries usually produce early obstruction with wheezing and dyspnea.[5] Infraglottic injuries are associated with late-onset increasing breathing difficulties such as paroxysmal coughing, hemoptysis, and progressive cervical emphysema.[5] Blunt trauma (direct blows) to the airway most commonly damages the larynx or cricoid cartilage, whereas blows to the larynx could fracture the thyroid cartilage.[6, 8] Such injuries may damage the thyroarytenoid ligaments, cause false cord–true cord separation, and create false passages that are seen on laryngoscopy.[6, 8, 9] Rarely, severe flexion-extension injuries such as "whiplash" injuries sustained in restrained motor vehicle accident victims cause laryngotracheal separation.[6, 7] Cricoid injury is much less common than thyroid cartilage damage but much more compromising to airway integrity.[6, 30] This may cause unanticipated obstruction or difficulty with intubation when cricoid pressure is applied.[6, 30, 31]

Clinical symptoms of tracheal damage may include pneumothorax, subcutaneous emphysema, hoarseness, and respiratory distress. However, signs of airway obstruction may not be present even with complete laryngotracheal disruption.[5, 26] Patients with laryngotracheal disruption or dislocation are able to maintain a patent airway until intubation, which may cause dislodgment of the two severed ends of the larynx, leading to obstruction and hypoxia.[6, 32] For this reason, many clinicians recommend fiberoptic intubation with direct visualization of the passage of the tube past the damaged area.[16] The ET should be inserted distal to the damaged area to minimize further damage, emphysema, or airway distortion.[16] If fiberoptic endoscopy and intubation are impossible, then many authorities advocate performing tracheostomy under local anesthesia.[16] Cervical tracheal injuries are often associated with cervical esophageal injuries,[5] more frequently in patients with cervical spine injury.[33] The thoracic trachea is fairly well protected by the thoracic cage and lungs.[1] Blunt or penetrating damage to the trachea often involves nearby structures including the heart, lungs, nerves, and vasculature. Therefore, these injuries are oftentimes fatal.[1, 5] Accompanying cervical spinal cord injury also correlates with a poor prognosis.[6] As tracheobronchial injuries are frequently associated with esophageal damage, many clinicians advocate laryngoscopy, bronchoscopy, and esophagoscopy in all patients with suspected laryngotracheal injury.[8, 16]

Neck Injury

Blunt or penetrating injury to the neck may cause damage to the veins, arteries, larynx and trachea, pharynx and esophagus, brachial plexus, cranial nerves, and spinal cord.[2] Forty percent of patients with penetrating neck injury ultimately require intubation.[6, 34] The neck is conventionally divided into three zones (Fig. 14–3). Zone I includes the base of the neck, from the clavicles and the thoracic inlet up to the cricoid cartilage. Penetrating injuries to zone I occur less frequently than those to the other two zones[6, 34] but are often associated with life-threatening vascular or pulmonary injures necessitating emergency airway management.[6, 35] Zone II represents the midbody of the neck from the level of

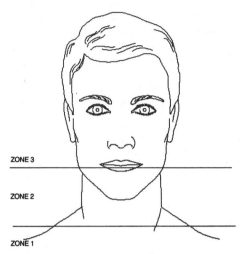

ZONE 3

ZONE 2

ZONE 1

Figure 14–3 Zones of penetrating injury to the neck. (From Cicala RS: The traumatized airway. *In* Benumof JL [ed]: Airway Management Principles and Practice. St Louis, Mosby–Year Book. 1996, pp 736–759.)

the cricoid cartilage to the angle of the mandible. The greatest number of injuries to the neck are contained in zone II, which typically is associated with the lowest mortality, as these injuries are easy to expose surgically. Penetrating injuries to zone II may cause airway obstruction from laryngeal damage, hematoma, and subcutaneous emphysema.[6] These complications may necessitate emergency airway management. Zone III includes the portion of the neck above the angle of the mandible to the base of the skull. Penetrating injuries to zone III are most commonly associated with vascular and pharyngeal injuries.[6] However, injuries at this zone are least likely to require airway management.[6] Injuries to the neck in zones I and III require angiography to assess vascular damage. Injuries in zone II are usually managed by surgical exploration.[26] Airway management is of primary importance in the assessment of neck injury, especially as extensive injury may be masked by minimal external evidence of damage.

ASSOCIATED INJURIES AND FACTORS AFFECTING AIRWAY MANAGEMENT

Associated injuries such as thermal damage, cervical spine injury, and thoracic injury are discussed in relation to their impact on airway management in the trauma patient. Additionally, the implications and risk of aspiration are addressed.

Thermal and Inhalational Injury

Thermal and inhalation injury can affect the airway in mainly four ways: carbon monoxide (CO) poisoning, upper airway edema resulting in obstruction, subglottic thermal and chemical burns, and chemical injury to lung tissue that impairs gas exchange.[6, 36]

CO is a colorless, odorless gas present in all forms of smoke. It readily binds with 200 times more affinity to hemoglobin than does oxygen, which may lead to hypoxia, asphyxia, and even death–depending on the degree of exposure. Carboxyhemoglobin cannot be differentiated from oxyhemoglobin on the infrared absorption spectrum of the pulse oximeter. Therefore, immediate serum carboxyhemoglobin levels must be obtained on arrival at the hospital.[6, 37] CO poisoning should be suspected in all fire victims, especially those from fires occurring in closed spaces. It should be treated with the administration of 100% oxygen, and intubation for patients with a decreased level of consciousness.[36] Hyperbaric oxygen therapy is reserved for patients with severe CO poisoning, or any patient who has been unconscious at the scene of a fire. Better results are obtained when hyperbaric oxygen therapy is administered within 6 hours of poisoning.[38–41]

Other potentially toxic substances, such as cyanide, ammonia, and chlorine, may be present in smoke from burning synthetic materials (e.g., plastic and rubber). These substances can cause chemical burns of both the airway and the lungs, thus leading to tissue edema. Cyanide poisoning can also be managed with hyperbaric oxygen therapy if standard pharmacologic therapy is unsuccessful.[38, 42–46] Upper airway edema may affect not only the face and pharynx but all supraglottic structures as well. Maximal swelling and tissue distortion may not occur until 12 to 24 hours after the burn; however, marked swelling may be seen in as early as 2 hours, causing inspiratory obstruction.[6, 36] If there is carbonaceous material in the mouth, nares, or pharynx, or if the patient displays stridor, hoarseness, or dyspnea, intubation should be performed sooner rather than later, as edema may cause complete airway obstruction.[6, 36] Swelling usually subsides in 3 to 4 days.[36] Subglottic thermal and chemical burns are best evaluated with fiberoptic bronchoscopy.[6] Airway obstruction may occur from bronchospasm, mucosal edema, and sloughed epithelium.[36] Inspired heat is usually absorbed in the upper airway, so thermal injury is uncommon in the distal trachea and lungs.[6, 36]

Chemical injury to lung tissue commonly results in pulmonary edema and should be treated with intubation and mechanical ventilation, along with the addition of positive end-expiratory pressure.[36] The severity of the pulmonary injury, as well as small-airway damage, can also be assessed with pulmonary function tests and serial arterial blood gas determinations.[6] Corticosteroids and prophylactic antibiotics have not been shown to be of benefit in treatment.[36] Burn patients must also be evaluated for other injuries secondary to an explosion or fall, such as cervical spine or intracerebral damage.[6]

Cervical Spine Injuries

Cervical spine and neck injury should be suspected when the patient is flaccid (especially with decreased rectal sphincter tone), exhibits diaphragmatic breathing, or has hemodynamic instability, specifically hypotension with bradycardia.[2] Cervical spine injuries are often missed since 5% to 10% of these patients have no neurologic deficits on arrival to the hospital. However, permanent deficits may develop while evaluation and treatment are performed.[6, 47] It is prudent to routinely use proper cervical spine precautions, as early interpretation of cervical radiographs is often inaccurate.[6, 47–49] An algorithm for the airway management of the patients with cervical injuries has been developed by Capan and colleagues[50] (Fig. 14–4).

An unstable cervical spine injury involves damage to all the support-

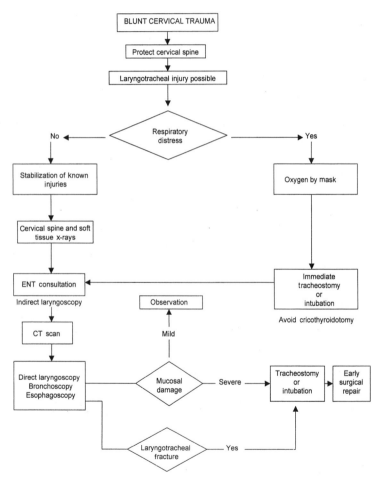

Figure 14–4 Algorithm for airway management in patients with cervical injuries to the airway. ENT, ear, nose, and throat; CT, computed tomography. (From Capan LM: Airway Management. *In* Capan LM, Miller SM, Turndorf H [eds]: Trauma Anesthesia and Intensive Care. Philadelphia[50], JB Lippincott, 1991.)

ing structures in either the anterior or the posterior portion of the vertebral column. Most trauma patients routinely have some type of neck immobilizer placed en route to the hospital to prevent excessive movement of the cervical spine. All or part of the immobilizer may need to be removed in order to proceed with intubation or to provide anterior neck access should a surgical airway be necessary. The head may be maintained in the neutral position with manual axial in-line traction (MAIT) by an assistant while the stabilizing devices are removed.

Although the risk of cervical spine injury must be considered, adequate oxygenation is of more importance in the trauma patient.[6]

Oral versus nasal intubation in the patient with suspected cervical spine injury remains controversial. Some argue that theoretically, orotracheal intubation with direct laryngoscopy may cause movement of unstable cervical elements, leading to spinal cord injury. MAIT has been radiologically demonstrated to distract and subluxate the spinal components during endotracheal intubation.[51, 52] Therefore, several authors advocate blind nasotracheal intubation for patients with cervical spine injuries; if this is unsuccessful, a cricothyrotomy should be performed.[3, 51, 52] Others believe that orotracheal intubation can safely be performed if MAIT or cervical immobilization is applied during laryngoscopy.[53] The traction must be continuously balanced against the forces applied by the intubator[53] and must be in the correct plane of the cervical injury. Flexion should be avoided in patients with posterior cervical spine injury, whereas extension should be avoided in those with anterior damage.[6] Nasotracheal intubation was once considered the safest method for intubating the cervical spine–injured patient. However, it is difficult to perform without cervical spine movement, especially in the combative trauma patient.[6, 53–57] Disadvantages of nasotracheal intubation include an increased risk of (1) aspiration (by stimulation of the gag reflex), (2) penetration of the brain (in skull or facial fractures), and (3) nasopharyngeal bleeding.[2] Nasotracheal intubation has been contraindicated in the presence of a coagulopathy, in basilar skull or complex facial fractures, and in patients with intranasal abnormalities.[2] Fiberoptic bronchoscopy may be an option in elective intubation of the cervical spine–injured patient, but rarely is it an option for emergent intubation, especially with the presence of intraoral bleeding.[6, 58, 59]

Closed Head Injury

Intracranial injury, due to either direct trauma or subsequent hypoxia, is still the most common cause of death and disability in trauma patients.[6] Associated closed head injury and the possibility of raised intracranial pressure (ICP) may mandate intubation with controlled ventilation and hyperventilation. Increased ICP may necessitate a smooth, well-controlled intubation, with management of associated hypertension.[60] Before induction, laryngoscopy, and intubation, the patient can spontaneously hyperventilate to decrease $PaCO_2$ and therefore ICP. A combative or comatose patient can also be hyperventilated with assistance before intubation by bag-mask, with cricoid pressure to prevent aspiration. Some believe that awake intubation is contraindicated in the patient with severe intracranial injury because of its associated hemodynamic changes.[6] However, it may be necessary in the unstable patient, with drugs available to treat hypertension and other associated responses.[6] Analgesics, induction agents, β-blockers, and lidocaine have all been used successfully to attenuate or treat the sympathetic response to laryngoscopy and intubation.[6] An algorithm for airway management in the head-injured patient is provided in Figure 14–5.

Some argue that increased ICP also precludes the use of nasal intubation (because of the sympathetic stimulation caused by nasal manipulation), whereas others believe that adequate topical anesthesia and sedation make nasal fiberoptic intubation the procedure of choice.[3, 49] Cricothyrotomy and retrograde intubation over a guide wire have also been used for the closed head–injured patient with associated cervical spine injury.[3, 49, 61–65] The combative patient usually requires sedation and muscle relaxation with a rapid sequence induction for intubation.[2, 3, 66] Care must be taken to maintain the cervical spine in the neutral position during intubation if there is a possibility of a cervical spine injury as well.[3, 66–69]

Thoracic Trauma

Thoracic trauma may also be either blunt or penetrating. Surprisingly, only 1% of cases of penetrating chest trauma lead to death, usually related to injury of the heart or great vessels.[6, 70] Approximately 5% of cases of blunt chest trauma are associated with major thoracic injuries; however, major blunt trauma has a higher mortality rate than penetrating chest trauma has.[6, 71] Blunt trauma may cause hemopneumothorax, interstitial emphysema, bronchial tears, rib fractures, chest wall contusions, flail chest, pulmonary contusion with delayed respiratory failure, or laceration of pulmonary vessels. Some of these patients may initially appear stable but quickly deteriorate, requiring emergency airway management, including intubation and ventilatory support.[6] Trauma patients with pulmonary vein laceration or open lung parenchymal injury may develop systemic air embolus, with a very poor prognosis. A high degree of clinical suspicion is necessary for this type of injury and complication, as the signs and symptoms are nonspecific (hemoptysis, hypotension, or seizures, or all of these).[6, 72]

Aspiration

The morbidity and mortality of aspiration are associated with an increased gastric volume (0.4 mL/kg of body weight), increased gastric acidity (pH less than 2.5), and the presence of particulate matter in the aspirate.[6, 73–75] Trauma patients are at increased risk of aspiration for several reasons: a full stomach from recent food ingestion, delayed gastric emptying (pain, shock), and altered consciousness (shock, head injury, substance abuse) with associated impaired airway reflexes.[6, 76–79] These factors may not subside with the passage of time, and thus

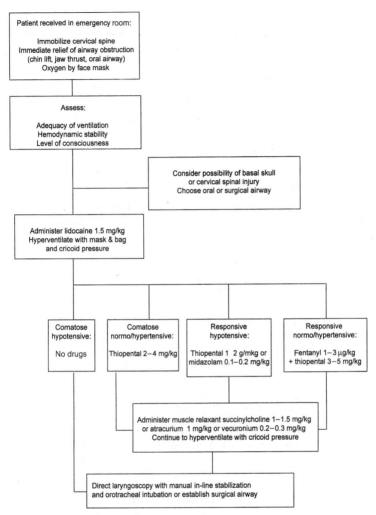

Figure 14–5 Algorithm for airway management in patients with head injury. (From Crosby ET: The difficult airway. II: Airway management in trauma patients. Anesthesiol Clin North Am 13:645, 1995.)

emergency surgery should not be postponed in efforts to decrease the risk of aspiration.[80, 81] Prevention may include endotracheal intubation with a cuffed ET to protect the airway, or gastric tube placement to decrease gastric distention and for aspiration of liquid matter present in the stomach. Pharmacologic intervention may include the use of nonparticulate antacids (may increase the pH within 15 minutes), metoclopramide (increases gastrointestinal motility as well as lowering esophageal sphincter tone), and histamine blockers (increase pH, but prolonged onset).[82] Signs and symptoms of aspiration include coughing, bronchospasm, wheezing, hypoxia, and visual identification of matter in the pharynx and trachea. If a patient is noted to aspirate, treatment should be instituted. The patient can be placed head down to prevent regurgitation of material in the trachea and then can be intubated.[6] Both suctioning and fiberoptic bronchoscopy may be performed to remove particulate matter via the ET. Positive-pressure ventilation with positive end-expiratory pressure may be required. Antibiotics should not be administered until a specific organism or specific organisms are identified. The use of steroids is controversial.

MANAGEMENT OF THE TRAUMATIZED AIRWAY

Indications for intubation include airway protection, pulmonary and tracheal toilet, positive-pressure ventilation, airway obstruction, coma, shock, and combativeness requiring sedation for diagnosis or treatment, or both.[2, 3, 60] There are a variety of methods by which the traumatized airway may be secured, depending on the nature of the injury, as well as the availability of and familiarity with specialized techniques and airway gadgets. A fully detailed algorithm for airway management in trauma patients, including those patients with suspected or diagnosed cervical spine trauma, is provided in Figure 14–6.

Airway Assessment

First, it is necessary to assess the patient and the patient's injuries. Patients can be divided into four groups depending on their need for airway management: those requiring immediate, emergent, urgent, and semi-elective airway management. Immediate airway management is mandated for patients in obvious respiratory distress. Emergent airway management is required by apneic patients. Care must be taken to find the cause of the apnea (foreign material, airway obstruction) and to consider associated injuries (cervical spine and intracerebral injuries).[6] Although the sequelae for cervical spine injury may be devastating, adequate oxygenation and ventilation may limit complications.[6, 49] Patients with impending respiratory distress, including patients with mandible and facial fractures, may require urgent or semielective airway management. These patients are usually stable with adequate ventilation but have the potential to develop respiratory distress. Thus, emergency medical personnel are able to coordinate airway management with the anesthesia practitioner and the surgeon. Patients with airway obstruction can be further divided into three groups. Those in the first group exhibit total or near-total airway obstruction that is often associated with hypoxia, hypercarbia, delirium, or unconsciousness. These patients must be intubated immediately.[83] Patients in the second group are able to maintain oxygenation but exhibit signs of obvious respiratory distress such as sternal retractions, labored respirations, stridor, and agitation. Fortunately, these patients are usually alert and cooperative, thus allowing the anesthesia practitioner and the surgeon

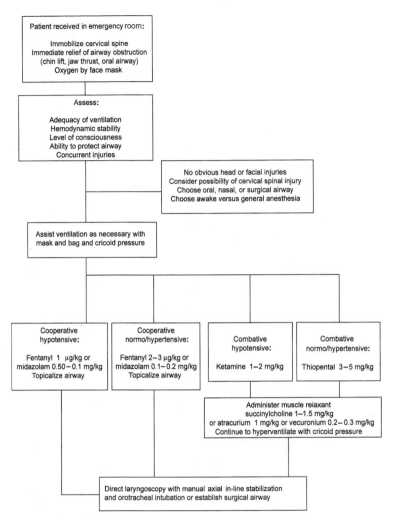

Figure 14–6 Algorithm for airway management in trauma patients, including those with suspected or diagnosed cervical spine trauma. (From Crosby ET: The difficult airway. II: Airway management in trauma patients. Anesthesiol Clin North Am 13:645, 1995.)

to formulate a treatment plan and approach to airway management.[83] The third group of patients includes those with impending respiratory distress. They do not have airway difficulties until they are sedated or manipulated.[83]

Trauma patients who require further assessment for airway management include those whose age, injuries, or medical condition places them at high risk for pulmonary problems.[6] This includes patients with confusion or obtundation on admission, burn injuries, hemodynamic instability requiring massive resuscitation, preexisting cardiopulmonary dysfunction, and thoracic or maxillofacial injury.[6, 83–87] Many of these patients may develop delayed respiratory insufficiency mandating emergency intubation and ventilatory support and therefore should be assessed and monitored closely in the resuscitative area.[6] Assessment may include physical examination, arterial blood gas analysis, chest radiography, computed tomography scanning, and bronchoscopy or laryngoscopy, or both. Physical examination may identify signs or symptoms of airway injury such as dyspnea, abrasions, ecchymosis, hoarseness, stridor, subcutaneous emphysema, or pneumothorax. Radiography is helpful in assessing the chest, ribs, and cervical spine.[6, 86] A computed tomographic scan may identify laryngeal injury and airway compromise.[6, 87–90] Laryngoscopy and bronchoscopy are considered procedures of choice to identify airway trauma, particularly vocal cord injury or laryngeal damage.[6, 86, 91]

Airway Management

The traumatized airway can be approached in a manner similar to that for the anticipated difficult airway. It is important to have proper head positioning as allowed by the associated injuries, and to have a variety of airway devices available. The approach to the airway is dictated by the airway and associated injuries from trauma. The initial procedure in airway management is to open the upper airway by either extending the neck and placing the patient in the sniffing position (not to be used in patients with potential cervical spine injuries), or to use the chin-lift and jaw-thrust maneuvers.[6, 18] Placement of nasopharyngeal or oropharyngeal airways may be necessary,[6] in addition to suction and removal of foreign material from the pharynx. Also it may be necessary to remove devices placed in the airway in the field by medical personnel, such as an esophageal-obturator airway.[6] Once a patent airway is established, different options to secure the airway may be considered. If the patient cannot be ventilated or intubated, immediate plans should be made to either perform transtracheal jet ventilation or create a surgical airway.[92] Nasotracheal intubation is contraindicated in the patient with a basilar skull fracture, intranasal deformities, or coagulopathy.[60, 62] During direct laryngoscopy, care must be taken to maintain the cervical spine in the neutral position to avoid theoretically exacerbating or causing a spinal cord injury.[3, 93] Rapid sequence induction should be employed for any patient with a full stomach to avoid aspiration, for even the obtunded patient may still have an intact gag reflex.[3] Fiberoptic intubation may be difficult in the trauma patient owing to decreased visibility by blood, secretions, or even injury. In addition, awake fiberoptic intubation may be impossible without either sedation of the patient or anesthetizing the airway. However, in the patient with a traumatized airway, the use of sedatives must be carefully weighed against the danger of causing respiratory embarrassment, loss of the airway, and aspiration.[3, 60, 94] Airway blocks are generally not indicated in the trauma patient owing to the risk of aspiration from obtunded airway reflexes.[95, 96] They have been used successfully in the trauma patient without associated aspiration or mishap;[97] however many anesthesia practitioners abstain from their use in this situation. Retrograde intubation with a guide wire may be particularly useful in those situations in which the view of the glottis is obscured by blood or heavy secretions. Cricothyrotomy or transtracheal jet ventilation may be indicated for severe trauma causing severe facial injury, upper airway obstruction, foreign body aspiration, or penetrating injury to the cervical area with hemorrhage.[3] It may also be used after unsuccessful oral or nasal intubation attempts.[3]

Airway devices that may be of assistance in managing the traumatized airway include the laryngeal mask airway, the esophageal-tracheal Combitube, the gum elastic bougie, and the Lightwand. The laryngeal mask airway has been used to blindly thread an ET into the trachea in the presence of excessive blood or secretions.[91, 98] Of course, there is no protection from aspiration with this technique. The esophageal-tracheal Combitube can also be used successfully in situations in which there is blood or vomitus, or both, in the oropharynx, as it does not require direct visualization for placement. It also does not require manipulation of the neck, thus avoiding the risk of cervical spine injury or exacerbation in the trauma patient. The role of the esophageal-tracheal Combitube has yet to be defined in managing the traumatized airway compared with traditional intubating techniques, especially in protecting against aspiration.

If the trachea is not visible on laryngoscopy, a gum elastic bougie, stylet, forceps, or Lightwand stylet may be used to assist with intubation.[60, 94, 99–103] Even in a bloodied pharynx, the aperture to the trachea may possibly be identified by bubbling, allowing an ET to be placed blindly. The gum elastic bougie may be particularly useful in the patient in whom laryngoscopy may be limited by a cervical collar or in-line traction, as it requires vision of only the epiglottis for placement.[104] Similarly, the Lightwand has also been used successfully in the trauma patient with limited neck movement and in children with an abnormal airway.[104, 105]

USE OF PHARMACOLOGIC AGENTS

Pharmacologic agents may be useful adjuncts to airway management even in traumatized patients. Medications commonly used in airway management include sedatives, opioids, lidocaine, induction agents, and neuromuscular blocking agents. Critically injured patients in shock need immediate resuscitation with the administration of 100% oxygen. Minimal anesthetic or sedative medications are needed in these unstable patients.[106] However, stable patients may require large doses of carefully titrated analgesics and sedatives to allow emergency room personnel to perform indicated procedures and to manipulate the airway.[106] Regional airway blocks may also be helpful in these patients, provided that the risk of aspiration is kept in mind. Hypertensive patients and those with elevated ICP may require medications to blunt the hemodynamic response to airway manipulation, such as hypertension, tachycardia, or increased ICP.[66, 106] Muscle relaxants may be used to maintain immobility and prevent coughing and bucking in response to laryngoscopy.[66] However, sedatives and muscle relaxants may also cause airway collapse or obstruction in a patient with a traumatized airway that is compromised by injury, blood, or secretions. The American Society of Anesthesiologists Difficult Airway Algorithm[92, 103] should still be applied in patients with traumatized airways, with awake intubation considered a conservative and effective means for securing the airway.[3, 66] The level of sedation may be slowly adjusted to maintain spontaneous ventilation, and topical anesthesia can be used to facilitate intubation.

Sedatives

The most commonly used sedatives for the trauma patient are midazolam and droperidol, although haloperidol has also been used successfully in the combative trauma patient.[3, 107–109] Midazolam is a short-acting, water-soluble benzodiazepine. It has sedative, amnestic, anxiolytic, and anticonvulsant properties. Incremental doses of midazolam (0.5 to 2 mg intravenously) may be titrated carefully to produce anxiolysis and retrograde amnesia within 1 to 2 minutes. Administered by itself, midazolam has minimal hemodynamic effects. If necessary, midazolam may be reversed by flumazenil, a benzodiazepine antagonist, in 0.5-mg increments. The half-life of flumazenil is shorter than that of midazolam, so the clinician must be prepared for possible resedation.[106, 109]

Droperidol is a butyrophenone that acts centrally to inhibit dopaminergic receptors. Hypotension may be caused by peripheral α-adrenergic blockade, although the blood pressure decrease is usually minimal.[106] Droperidol may be titrated carefully, with 2.5 to 5.0 mg usually causing reduced motor activity and anxiety, along with an indifference to the environment.[106] Droperidol has been used in combination with fentanyl to produce a cataleptic state with marked analgesia (neuroleptanalgesia). Side effects of droperidol include dysphoric reactions and extrapyramidal reactions (which should be treated with diphenhydramine), so its use should be avoided in patients with Parkinson's disease.

Haloperidol is also a butyrophenone that has been used to decrease anxiety accompanying psychoses. It has been advocated for use in the combative patient, to produce anxiolysis and cooperation without necessitating intubation.[3, 107, 109] Haloperidol is also titrated to effect in incremental 2.5- to 5.0-mg intravenous doses. Sedative drugs must be used with caution in trauma patients, particularly in elderly patients, to avoid side effects such as respiratory depression, dysphoria, or extrapyramidal reactions.

Opioid Agents and Lidocaine

Narcotics are frequently used to produce analgesia not only from the injuries but from the procedures performed during the patient's evaluation and care. Morphine is a naturally occurring opioid narcotic. Its synthetic analogues include fentanyl, alfentanil, and sufentanil. The newest synthetic opioid is the ultra-short-acting remifentanil, which is still undergoing clinical trials.[106]

Morphine has an onset of action of 15 to 30 minutes, with a peak effect within 45 to 90 minutes and a duration of action of 4 hours. It may cause hypotension from histamine release, among other side effects such as pruritus, urinary retention, somnolence, and nausea. It is usually reserved for hemodynamically stable patients requiring long-acting pain relief.

Fentanyl does not affect hemodynamic stability and has minimal side effects. It is usually titrated to effect in small doses of 0.5 to 1 μg/kg, up to 5 μg/kg. Larger doses produce a longer duration of action.[106] Alfentanil produces a transient peak effect with rapid redistribution and clearance. Sufentanil is approximately 10 times more potent than fentanyl and has a longer duration of action with cumulative doses. The synthetic narcotics are useful for analgesia and to help attenuate the hemodynamic response to intubation. Fentanyl (0.5 to 3 (μg/kg incrementally) and midazolam (0.5- to 1-mg increments) provide sedation, analgesia, and amnesia.[66] These must be administered cautiously in combination, as they can act synergistically and precipitate hypotension, especially in hypovolemic patients. The respiratory depressant effects may be enhanced in patients with central nervous system depression (i.e., from hypoxia, head injury, alcohol, or drugs). Opioid antagonists such as naloxone can be used to reverse the side effects of opioids such as respiratory depression, pruritus, urinary retention, vomiting, and biliary spasm.[106] Naloxone should be titrated slowly in 0.1-mg increments intravenously to produce the desired results without causing undesirable side effects such as cardiovascular stimulation (i.e., hypertension, tachycardia, pulmonary edema, and cardiac dysrhythmias).

Lidocaine (1.5 mg/kg) administered 2 to 3 minutes before intubation may also attenuate the hemodynamic response to intubation.[110, 111] Lidocaine can also be used as an adjunct to intubation topically or for airway blocks. It may blunt the increased responses of blood pressure, ICP, and intraocular pressure to intubation. It may also be used to attenuate or block the injection site pain of propofol and etomidate.[106]

Induction Agents

An uncooperative or combative patient may require a rapid sequence induction before intubation in order to allow medical intervention. The components of rapid sequence induction include preoxygenation, cricoid pressure (applied until proper ET placement is confirmed), and administration of a rapid-onset induction agent (hypnotic agent) and a muscle relaxant. Positive-pressure mask ventilation is avoided (unless the patient becomes hypoxic) to prevent gastric insufflation and aspiration. Other indications for rapid sequence induction include head trauma requiring hyperventilation, loss of consciousness, and uncontrolled seizure activity.

Induction agents include thiopental (Pentothal), propofol, etomidate, and ketamine. Also, midazolam may be used for induction. The doses and possible side effects are listed in Table 14–1.[106, 111] Note that the drug dosages should be decreased in the hypovolemic or unstable patient.

An alternative to the use of induction agents is to administer lidocaine (1.5 mg/kg) intravenously, followed 2 to 3 minutes later by propofol (1 to 2 mg/kg). The use of a muscle relaxant may be avoided as the propofol produces profound general anesthesia and blunts airway reflexes until it quickly redistributes. The patient's response to any of the induction agents depends on the injuries present and the associated volume of hemorrhage, severity of shock and of cardiopulmonary dysfunction, and degree of sympathetic stimulation. All these induction agents, with the exception of ketamine, increase ICP, cerebral metabolic oxygen consumption, and cerebral blood flow. However, they also decrease mean arterial blood pressure and potentially decrease cerebral perfusion pressure (Table 14–2).[106, 110–112] Thus, etomidate is often recommended as an induction agent for the hypovolemic head-injured patient, as it is the most cardiac stable of the induction agents.

Neuromuscular Blocking Agents

Muscle relaxants can facilitate laryngoscopy while preventing bucking and coughing. However, these medications may allow the oropharyngeal tissue to relax and distort the airway, making intubation either difficult or impossible, especially in an airway already compromised by trauma, blood, or secretions. The muscle relaxant most commonly used to facilitate laryngoscopy and intubation in traumatized patients is succinylcholine, because of its rapid onset (30 to 60 seconds) and short duration (8 to 10 minutes). However, it is contraindicated in patients with extrajunctional acetylcholine receptors (e.g., patients with neuromuscular disorders, a history of recent unhealed burns, or upper

Table 14–1 Comparison of Induction Agents

Agent	IV Dose* (mg/kg)	Side Effects
Thiopental	3–5	Sedation, nausea
Propofol	1–2	Pain on injection; antiemetic
Etomidate	0.3	Pain on injection, myoclonus, nausea, adrenal suppression
Ketamine	1–2	Tracheobronchial secretions, emergence delirium, sympathetic stimulation
Midazolam	0.1–0.2	Apnea, prolonged sedation, hypotension when given with opioids; retrograde amnesia

* In healthy patients.
Data from Smith CE: Pharmacologic adjuncts for emergency airway management in the adult trauma patient. Anesth News Oct:16, 1996; and Bedford RF, Persing JA, Pobereskin L, Butler A: Lidocaine or thiopental for rapid control of intracranial hypertension? Anesth Analg 59:435, 1980.

Table 14-2 Cardiovascular and Neurologic Effects of Induction Agents

Agent	HR	BP	Cardiac Contractility	ICP	CBF	CMRO$_2$
Thiopental	Increase	Decrease	No change or decrease	Decrease	Decrease	Decrease
Propofol	No change	Decrease	Decrease	Decrease	Decrease	Decrease
Etomidate	No change	No change	No change	Decrease	Decrease	Decrease
Ketamine	Increase	Increase	Decrease or increase	Increase	Increase	Increase
Midazolam	No change	Decrease	No change	Decrease	Decrease	Decrease

*Ketamine is a direct myocardial depressant but may increase BP via sympathetic stimulation, provided the patient is not already maximally sympathetically stimulated.

HR, heart rate; BP, blood pressure; ICP, intracranial pressure; CBF, cerebral blood flow; CMRO$_2$, cerebral metabolic oxygen consumption.

Data from Smith CE: Pharmacologic adjuncts for emergency airway management in the adult trauma patient. Anesth News Oct:16, 1996; Thomas H Jr, Schwartz E, Petrilli R: Droperidol versus haloperidol for chemical restraint of agitated and combative patients. Ann Emerg Med 21:407, 1992; Bedford RF, Persing JA, Pobereskin L, Butler A: Lidocaine or thiopental for rapid control of intracranial hypertension? Anesth Analg 59:435, 1980; Stoelting, RK: Pharmacology and Physiology in Anesthetic Practice, 2nd ed. Philadelphia, Lippincott-Raven, 1991.

Table 14-3 Nondepolarizing Muscle Relaxants

Agent	Normal Intubating Dose	Duration of Action (min)	Side Effects
Mivacurium	0.30 mg/kg in divided doses of 0.15 mg/kg each	20	Histamine release (hypotension) if given as single dose
Atracurium	0.5 mg/kg	20–30	Histamine release (hypotension), laudanosine metabolite (seizures)
Cisatracurium	0.2 mg/kg	30	
Vecuronium	0.1 mg/kg	30	
Rocuronium	0.6 mg/kg	30	Vagolysis with light anesthesia
Pancuronium	0.1 mg/kg	40–70	Tachycardia

Data from Smith CE: Pharmacologic adjuncts for emergency airway management in the adult trauma patient. Anesth News Oct:16, 1996; Bedford RF, Persing JA, Pobereskin L, Butler A: Lidocaine or thiopental for rapid control of intracranial hypertension? Anesth Analg 59:435, 1980; Fragen RJ, Avram MJ: Comparative pharmacology of drugs used for the induction of anesthesia. *In* Stoelting RK, Barash PG, Gallagher TJ (eds): Advances in Anesthesia, Chicago, Year Book Medical, 1986, p 103. Smith CE, Peerless JR: Rational use of neuromuscular blocking agents for emergency airway management in the trauma patient. Presented at the International Trauma Anesthesia and Critical Care Society Symposium, Baltimore, May 1995.

or lower motor neuron disease), as it may cause an acute hyperkalemic response and precipitation of life-threatening cardiac dysrhythmias. Other side effects include malignant hyperthermia, muscle fasciculations causing postoperative myalgias, and increased ICP, intraocular pressure, and intragastric pressure.[106, 112] The dose of succinylcholine in adults is 1 mg/kg, and in children 2 mg/kg.

Nondepolarizing muscle relaxants have also been used at twice the intubating dose, in order to speed their onset of action to facilitate rapid intubation. The selection of nondepolarizing agents should be based on clinical requirements (i.e., their duration of action; Table 14–3).[106, 111, 113–115] Although the newer agents such as rocuronium have minimal cardiovascular side effects, they may be more expensive.

Airway management is paramount in the trauma patient to avoid complications of brain damage, aspiration, and cardiopulmonary collapse. Pharmacologic agents should be administered carefully in light of airway compromise and cardiac instability.

REFERENCES

1. Gotta AW: Management of the Traumatized Airway. ASA Refresher Course 156:1–2, 1997.
2. Priano LL: Trauma and burns. In Barash P, Cullen BF, Stoelting RK (eds): Clinical Anesthesia, 3rd ed. Philadelphia, Lippincott-Raven, 1997, pp 1173–1204.
3. Walls RM: Airway management. Emerg Med Clin North Am 11:53, 1993.
4. Butler RM, Moser FH: The padded dash syndrome: Blunt trauma to the larynx and trachea. Laryngoscope 78:1172, 1968.
5. Green R, Stark P: Trauma of the larynx and trachea. Radiol Clin North Am 16:309, 1978.
6. Cicala RS: The traumatized airway. In Benumof J (ed): Airway Management Principles and Practice. St Louis, Mosby–Year Book, 1996, pp 736–759.
7. Dolin J, Scalea T, Mannor L, et al: The management of gunshot wounds to the face. J Trauma 33:508, 1992.
8. Mathison DJ, Grillo H: Laryngotracheal trauma. Ann Thorac Surg 43:254, 1987.
9. Trone TH, Schaefer SD, Carder HM: Blunt and penetrating laryngeal trauma: A 13 year review. Otolaryngol Head Neck Surg 88:257, 1980.
10. Luce EA, Tubb TD, Moore AM: Review of 1,000 major facial fractures and associated injuries. Plast Reconstr Surg 63:26, 1979.
11. Thaller SR, Beal SL: Maxillofacial trauma: A potentially fatal injury. Ann Plast Surg 27:281, 1991.
12. Hills MW, Deane SA: Head injury and facial injury: Is there an increased risk of cervical spine injury? J Trauma 34:549, 1993.
13. Conforti PJ, Haug RH, Likavec M: Management of closed head injury in the patient with maxillofacial trauma. J Oral Maxillofac Surg 51:298, 1993.
14. Haskell R: Applied surgical anatomy. In Rowe NL, Williams JL (eds): Maxillofacial Injuries. Edinburgh, Churchill Livingstone, 1994, pp 1–37.
15. Redick LF: The temporomandibular joint and tracheal intubation. Anesth Analg 66:675, 1987.
16. Murphy MT, Latham P: Anesthetic management of trauma to the airway. Anesth News Oct:43, 1996.
17. Shepard SM, Lippe MS: Maxillofacial trauma: Evaluation and management by the emergency physician. Emerg Med Clin North Am 5:371, 1987.
18. Guildner CW: Resuscitation–Opening the airway: A comparative study of techniques for opening an airway obstructed by the tongue. J Am Coll Emerg Physicians 5:588, 1976.
19. Sosis M, Lazar A: Jaw dislocation during general anesthesia. Can J Anesth 34:407, 1987.

20. Halazonetis JA: The weak regions of the mandible. Br J Oral Surg 6:37, 1968.
21. Seshul MB, Sinn DP, Gerlock AJ: The Andy Gump fracture of the mandible: A cause of respiratory obstruction or distress. J Trauma 18:611, 1978.
22. Capan LM, Miller SM, Glickman R: Management of facial injuries. In Capan LM, Miller SM, Turndorf (eds): Trauma Anesthesia and Intensive Care. New York, JB Lippincott, 1991, pp 385–408.
23. Stevenson TR, Jurkiewicz MJ: Plastic and reconstructive surgery. In Schwartz SI, Shires GT, Spencer FC (eds): Principles of Surgery. New York, McGraw-Hill, 1989, pp 2081–2132.
24. Cawood JI, Thind GS: Supraglottic obstruction. Injury 15:277, 1983.
25. Le Fort R: Etude experimentale sur les fractures de la machoire superieure. Rev Chir 23:208, 360, 479, 1901.
26. Jurkovich GJ, Carrico CJ: Trauma: Management of acute injuries. In Sabiston DC (ed): Textbook of Surgery. Philadelphia, WB Saunders, 1991, pp 286–289.
27. Muzzi DA, Losasso TJ, Cucchiara RF: Complication from a nasopharyngeal airway in a patient with a basilar skull fracture. Anesthesiology 74:366, 1991.
28. Bowegtz MS, Katz JA: Airway management of the trauma patient. Semin Anesth 4:114, 1985.
29. Arajarvi K, Lindquist C, Santavirta S, et al: Maxillofacial trauma in fatally injured victims of motor vehicle accidents. Br J Oral Maxillofac Surg 24:251, 1986.
30. Cicala RS, Kudsk K, Nguyen H: Airway injury in multiple trauma patients: A review of 48 cases. Clin J Anesth 3:91, 1991.
31. Reece GP, Shatney CH: Blunt injuries of the cervical trachea: Review of 51 patients. South Med J 81:1542, 1988.
32. Reese CA, Jenkins J, Nelson W, et al: Traumatic transection of the trachea anesthetic management: A case report. J Am Nurse Anesth 41:228, 1970.
33. Reddin A, Stuart ME, Diaconis JN: Rupture of the cervical esophagus and trachea associated with cervical spine fracture. J Thorac Cardiovasc Surg 42:218, 1961.
34. Shearer VE, Giesecke AH: Airway management for patients with penetrating neck trauma: A retrospective study. Anesth Analg 77:1135, 1993.
35. Eggen JT, Jorden RC: Airway management, penetrating neck trauma. J Emerg Med 11:381, 1993.
36. Furman WR: Burns. In Hoyt JR, Tonneson AS, Allen SJ (eds): Critical Care Practice. Philadelphia, WB Saunders, 1991, pp 392–399.
37. Barker SJ, Tremper KK: The effect of carbon monoxide inhalation on pulse oximetry and transcutaneous P_aO_2. Anesthesiology 66:667, 1987.
38. Haponik EF, Summer WR: Respiratory complications in burned patients: Diagnosis and management of injury. J Cont Care 2:121, 1987.
39. Moylan JA, Alexander LG: Diagnosis and treatment of inhalation injury. World J Surg 2:185, 1978.
40. Norkool DM, Kirkpatrick JN: Treatment of acute carbon monoxide poisoning with hyperbaric oxygen: A review of 115 cases. Ann Emerg Med 14:1168, 1985.
41. Monafo WW: Initial management of burns. N Engl J Med 335:1581–1586, 1996.
42. Ivanov KP: The effect of elevated oxygen pressure on animals poisoned with potassium cyanide. Pharmacol Toxicol 22:476, 1959.
43. Skene WG, Norman JN, Smith G: Effect of hyperbaric oxygen in cyanide poisoning. In Brown IW, Cox B (eds): Proceedings of the Third International Congress on Hyperbaric Medicine. Washington, DC, National Academy of Sciences, National Research Council, 1966, p 705.
44. Cope C: The importance of oxygen in the treatment of cyanide poisoning. JAMA 175:1061, 1968.
45. Trapp WG: Massive cyanide poisoning with recovery: A Boxing Day story. Can Med Assoc J 102:517, 1970.
46. Pruitt BA, Goodwin CW, Pruitt SK: Burns. In Sabiston DC (ed): Textbook of Surgery, 14th ed. Philadelphia, WB Saunders, 1991, pp 178–203.
47. Roon AJ, Christiansen N: Evaluation and treatment of penetrating cervical injuries. J Trauma 9:397, 1979.
48. Woodring JH, Lee C: Limitations of cervical radiography in the evaluation of acute cervical trauma. J Trauma 34:32, 1993.

49. Crosby ET, Liu A: The adult cervical spine: Implications for airway management. Can J Anaesth 37:77, 1990.
50. Capan LM: Airway management. *In* Capan LM, Miller SM, Turndorf H (eds): Trauma Anesthesia and Intensive Care. Philadelphia, JB Lippincott, 1991, pp 69–70.
51. Majernick TG, Bienek R, Houston JB, et al: Cervical spine movement during orotracheal intubation. Ann Emerg Med 15:417, 1986.
52. Bivens HG, Ford S, Bezmalinovic Z, et al: The effect of axial traction during orotracheal intubation of the trauma victim with an unstable cervical spine. Ann Emerg Med 17:53, 1988.
53. Grande CM, Barton CR, Stene JK: Emergency airway management in trauma patients with a suspected cervical spine injury in response. Anesth Analg 68:416, 1989.
54. Capan LM: Airway management. *In* Capan LM, Miller SM, Turndorf H (eds): Trauma Anesthesia and Intensive Care. Philadelphia, JP Lippincott, 1991, pp 43–81.
55. Layman PR: An alternative to blind nasal intubation. Anaesthesia 38:165, 1983.
56. Dronen SC, Merigian KS, Hedges JR, et al: Comparison of blind nasotracheal and succinylcholine assisted intubation in the poisoned patient. Ann Emerg Med 16:650, 1987.
57. Wright SW, Robinson GG, Wright MB: Cervical spine injuries in blunt trauma requiring emergency intubation. Am J Emerg Med 10:104, 1992.
58. Wang JF, Reves JG, Gutierrez FA: Awake fiberoptic laryngoscopic tracheal intubation for anterior cervical spinal fusion in patients with cervical cord trauma. Int Surg 64:69, 1979.
59. Messeter KH, Petterson KI: Endotracheal intubation with fibre-optic bronchoscope. Anaesthesia 35:294, 1980.
60. Mallanpati SR: Airway management. *In* Barash PG, Cullen BF, Stoelting RK (eds): Clinical Anesthesia, 3rd ed. Philadelphia, Lippincott-Raven, 1997, pp 573–594.
61. Shantha TR: Retrograde intubation using the subcricoid region. Br J Anaesth 68:109, 1992.
62. Morris IR: Fibre-optic intubation. Can J Anaesth 41:996, 1994.
63. McGill J, Clinton JE, Ruiz E: Cricothyroidotomy in the emergency department. Ann Emerg Med 11:361, 1982.
64. Walls RM: Cricothyroidotomy. Emerg Med Clin North Am 6:725, 1988.
65. King J, Huntington C, Wooten D: Translaryngeal guided intubation in an uncooperative patient with maxillofacial injury: Case report. J Trauma 36:885, 1994.
66. Crosby ET: The difficult airway. II: Airway management in trauma patients. Anesthesiol Clin North Am 13:645, 1995.
67. Redan JA, Livingston DH, et al: The value of intubating and paralyzing patients with suspected head injury in the emergency department. J Trauma 31:371, 1991.
68. Kuchinski J, Tinkoff G, Rhodes M, et al: Emergency intubation or paralysis of the uncooperative trauma patient. J Emerg Med 9:9, 1991.
69. Hickey D: Paralyzing a combative trauma patient before intubation. J Trauma 31:1455, 1991.
70. Guest JL, Anderson JN: Major airway injury in closed chest trauma. Chest 72:63, 1977.
71. Jackson J: Management of thoracoabdominal injuries. *In* Capan LM, Miller SM, Turndorf H (eds): Trauma Anesthesia and Intensive Care. Philadelphia, JB Lippincott, 1991, pp 481–510.
72. Trunkey D: Initial treatment of patients with extensive trauma. N Engl J Med 324:1259, 1991.
73. Bynum LJ, Pierce AK: Pulmonary aspiration of gastric contents. Am Rev Respir Dis 114:1129, 1979.
74. Greenfield J, Singleton RP, McCaffree DR: Pulonary effects of experimental graded aspiration of hydrochloric acid. Ann Surg 170:74, 1969.
75. Schwart DJ, Wynne JW, Gibbs CP: The pulmonary consequences of aspiration of gastric contents at pH values greater than 2.5. Am Rev Resp Dis 121:119, 1980.

76. Giesecke AH, Hodgson RM, Phulchand PR: Anesthesia for severely injured patients. Orthop Clin North Am 1:21, 1970.
77. Azricznyj B, Rockwood CA, O'Donaghue DH, et al: Relationship between trauma to the extremities and stomach motility. J Trauma 17:920, 1977.
78. Simpson KH, Stakes AF: Effect of anxiety on gastric emptying in preoperative patients. Br J Anaesth 45:1057, 1973.
79. Howard JM: Gastric and salivary secretion following injury: The systemic response to injury. Ann Surg 141:342, 1955.
80. Davies JAH, Howell TH: The management of anesthesia for the full stomach case in the casualty department. Postgrad Med J 49:58, 1973.
81. Scalea TM, Simon HW, Duncan AD, et al: Geriatric blunt multiple trauma: Improved survival with early invasive monitoring. J Trauma 30:129, 1990.
82. Mecca RS: Postoperative recovery. In Barash RG, Cullen BF, Stoelting RK (eds): Clinical Anesthesia. Philadelphia, Lippincott-Raven, 1997, pp 1279–1304.
83. Brown ACD, Sataloff RT: Special anesthetic techniques in head and neck surgery. Otolaryngol Clin North Am 14:587, 1981.
84. Jurkovitch GJ, Gussack GS, Luterman A: laryngotracheal trauma: A protocol approach to a rare injury. Laryngoscope 96:660, 1986.
85. Lambert GE, McMurry GT: Larygotracheal trauma: Recognition and management. J Am Coll Emerg Physicians 5:883, 1976.
86. Angood PB, Attia EL, Brown RA, et al: Extrinsic civilian trauma to the larynx and cervical trachea: Important predictors of long term morbidity. J Trauma 26:869,1986.
87. Mandal AK, Oparah SS: Unusually low mortality of penetrating wounds of the chest: Twelve years experience. J Thorac Cardiovasc Surg 97:119, 1989.
88. Mancuso AA, Hanafee WN: Computed tomography of the injured larynx. Radiology 133:139, 1979.
89. Schaefer SD, Brown OE: Selective application of CT in the management of laryngeal trauma. Laryngoscope 93:1473, 1983.
90. Urschell HC, Razzuk MA: Management of acute traumatic injuries of the tracheobronchial tree. Surg Gynecol Obstet 136:113, 1973.
91. Ecker RR, Libertini RV, Rea WJ, et al: Injuries of the trachea and bronchi. Ann Thorac Surg 11:289, 1971.
92. Benumof JL: Laryngeal mask airway and the ASA difficult airway algorithm. Anesthesiology 84:686, 1996.
93. Sinclair D, Schwartz M, Gruss J, et al: A retrospective review of the relationship between facial fractures, head injuries, and cervical spine injuries. J Emerg Med 6:109, 1988.
94. Rayburn RL: Lightwand intubation. Anaesthesia 34:677, 1979.
95. Stone DJ, Gal TJ: Airway management: In Miller RE (ed): Anesthesia, 4th ed. New York, Churchill Livingstone, 1994, pp 1403–1436.
96. Walts LF: Anesthesia of the larynx in the patient with a full stomach. JAMA 192:121, 1965.
97. Kopman AF, Wallman SB, Ross K, et al: Awake endotracheal intubation: A review of 267 cases. Anesth Analg 54:323, 1975.
98. Hagberg C, Abramson D, Chelly J: A comparison of fiberoptic orotracheal intubation using two different intubating conduits. Anesthesiology 83:3A 1995.
99. McIntyre JWR: The difficult tracheal intubation. Can J Anesth 34:2, 204, 1987.
100. Cobley M, Vaughan RS: Recognition and management of difficult airway problems. Br J Anaesth 68:90, 1992.
101. Cass NM, James NR, Lines V: Difficult direct laryngoscopy complicating intubation for anaesthesia. BMJ 1:488, 1956.
102. Samsoon GLT, Young JRB: Difficult tracheal intubation: A retrospective study. Anaesthesia 42:487, 1987.
103. ASA Task Force on Management of the Difficult Airway: Practice guidelines for management of the difficult airway. Anesthesiology 78:597, 1993.
104. Good ML: Airway Gadgets. ASA Refresher Course 531:1–6, 1994.
105. Holzman RS, Nargozian CD, Florence FB: Lightwand intubation in children with abnormal airways. Anesthesiology 69:784, 1988.

106. Smith CE: Pharmacologic adjuncts for emergency airway management in the adult trauma patient. Anesth News Oct:16, 1996.
107. Ovassapian A: Fiberoptic assisted management of the airway. ASA Refresher Course Lectures 254:1, 1990.
108. Clinton JE, Sterner S, Stelmachers Z, Ruiz E: Haloperidol for sedation of disruptive emergency patients. Ann Emerg Med 16:319, 1987.
109. Thomas H, Schwartz E, Petrilli R: Droperidol versus haloperidol for chemical restraint of agitated and combative patients. Ann Emerg Med 21:407, 1992.
110. Reves JG, Glass PSA, Lubarsky DA: Nonbarbiturate intravenous anesthetics. *In* Miller RD (ed): Anesthesia, 4th ed. New York, Churchill Livingstone, 1994, pp 247–292.
111. Bedford RF, Persing JA, Pobereskin L, Butler A: Lidocaine or thiopental for rapid control of intracranial hypertension? Anesth Analg 59:435, 1980.
112. Stoelting RK: Pharmacology and Physiology in Anesthetic Practice, 2nd ed. Philadelphia, Lippincott-Raven, 1991.
113. Hemelrijck JV, White PF: Nonopioid intravenous anesthesia. *In* Barash PG, Cullen BF, Stoelting RK (eds): Clinical Anesthesia, 3rd ed. Philadelphia, Lippincott-Raven, 1997, pp 311–328.
114. Smith CE, Peerless JR: Rational use of neuromuscular blocking agents for emergency airway management in the trauma patient. Presented at the International Trauma Anesthesia and Critical Care Society Symposium, Baltimore, May 1995.
115. Smith CE, Peerless JR: Use of neuromuscular blocking agents for trauma patients in the intensive care unit. Presented at the International Trauma Anesthesia and Critical Care Society Symposium, Baltimore, May 1995.

Chapter 15

Difficult Airway in the

Intensive Care Unit

C. Lee Parmley

CHALLENGES OF THE INTENSIVE CARE UNIT AIRWAY PRACTICE

Setting

Airway management in the intensive care unit (ICU) often presents unique challenges. Patients are admitted for intensive care because of numerous medical and surgical conditions that are considered sufficiently critical to require special levels of care. Occasionally ICU admission is based solely on airway factors, such as when progressive airway edema, obstruction, and respiratory embarrassment are anticipated. Extubation following intubation of a compromised airway or following a difficult intubation (see Chapter 16), may need to be delayed, necessitating an interval of ICU care.

Frequently, the need for airway control in the ICU is due to an emergent need to improve oxygenation or ventilation, or both, and by the time an anesthesia practitioner arrives on the scene, the situation has progressed to one of impending disaster.[1] Complications occur more frequently with emergency intubations than with routine intubations, approximating a 2% incidence in various locations. Complications from intubation depend on patient factors to some degree[2] but are also influenced by the equipment and process used. Intubations that are performed hurriedly in patients who are inadequately sedated, anesthetized, or relaxed and in patients in whom positioning is improper or visualization is poor often result in injury and complications.[3] One of the worst complications is cardiac arrest, which was reported in one study to occur in approximately 1% of emergency intubations.[4]

Although intubations in the ICU are in many respects similar to those routinely performed in the operating room, certain characteristics differ. In many ICUs, individuals performing intubations are less experienced in airway management than are individuals who perform intubation on a daily basis, such as anesthesia care providers and trained emergency medicine physicians. Likewise, ICU personnel are less familiar with the procedures and devices employed in airway management. They may not prioritize issues correctly, anticipate problems, or deal adequately with complications that occur.

Equipment needed for the management of a difficult airway, which may be readily available in the operating room, may be floors away from the ICU. Sending for the necessary or desired equipment is often time-consuming and difficult since the messengers are not familiar with the requested equipment. Many medications commonly used for anesthetic induction and intubation are not located in the ICU, and the acquisition of these medications may be difficult. Being properly prepared for a difficult airway in the ICU by having ready access to various airway devices and medications requires planning, education, and organization.

The management and administration of ICUs varies within and between institutions. Some hospitals have unit-based intensivists who may have been trained in a variety of specialties. Others rely on medical staff from other areas of the hospital to respond to emergencies. Any individual who may be called upon to respond to airway emergencies in a hospital may encounter a difficult airway in the ICU.

Modern airway practice has developed through the work of anesthesia practitioners who perform intubations as a routine part of anesthetic management. Assessment of the airway is an important part of a preanesthetic evaluation in which a patient's medical history and current conditions are reviewed and carefully considered when an anesthesia plan is developed. Most ICU patients could be classified as American Society of Anesthesiologists (ASA) Physical Status III or greater (i.e., those at increased risk for anesthesia-related complications). Compounding this is the fact that when intubation is required for an ICU patient, it is usually because the patient's medical status is deteriorating. These factors must be taken into consideration when planning which technique or medications should be used. Also, the fact that surgical stimulation does not follow an intubation, as it does in the operating room, must be taken into account. Any anesthetic or sedative agents that are administered may have significant consequences for the critically ill patient.

The multiple physician specialties and health care disciplines whose members practice in critical care units consult the anesthesia practitioners for guidance in airway practice. Although ICU intubations are frequently performed by nonanesthetists, if difficulties with intubation are anticipated or encountered, special expertise is often required. The ASA guidelines for management of the difficult airway are widely recognized and are also recommended for airway practice in the ICU.[5]

Patient

In general there are two categories of patients in whom intubation is required: those who will undergo general anesthesia and those with existing or impending respiratory failure. The general goals of intubation are the maintenance of upper airway patency, protection against gastric aspiration, the application of positive-pressure ventilation, and suctioning of the tracheobronchial tree. Although these goals may vary in importance, they are the same whether a patient requires intubation for anesthesia or because of impending respiratory failure.

Intubation may be necessary or desirable for a number of reasons in the ICU. Respiratory failure due to cardiac, neuromuscular, pulmonary, or metabolic illness may be associated with increased work of breathing and progressive fatigue to the point where intubation and mechanical assistance are needed. Obtundation from neurologic disease, medications, or metabolic conditions may progress, leading to the loss of protective airway reflexes and thus necessitating tracheal intubation for airway protection. Intubation may also be required when airway embarrassment or obstruction follows extubation, trauma, surgical procedures involving the head or neck, or allergic reactions. Finally, the need to establish an airway for cardiopulmonary resuscitation is widely recognized.

There are subjective and objective elements recognized as indicators that intubation is needed. Some variation in criteria may be based on the existence of chronic as opposed to acute respiratory failure, but both have thresholds based on the ability to oxygenate and ventilate. Mechanical ventilatory failure due to decreased lung volumes and a loss of motor function can be assessed by bedside measurement of the forced vital capacity and negative inspiratory force. A patient who is unable to generate a negative inspiratory force of 25 cm H_2O or whose forced vital capacity is less than 15 mL/kg (at least 1 liter) meets criteria for intubation based on mechanical criteria. Other objective indications for intubations are poor or inadequate oxygenation and ventilation. An arterial PO_2 less than 55 mm Hg on room air and less than 200 mm Hg on an FIO_2 of 1 indicate the need for intubation. Intubation is also indicated for a respiratory rate greater than 40 (30 recognized by many) or less than 6, or when PCO_2 acutely rises above 65 mm Hg.[6]

Contrasting the clear objective thresholds, subjective indicators for intubation may be subtle but must not be overlooked. ICU patients may have several reasons to be restless, anxious, tachycardic, and hypertensive, yet any of these symptoms may be indicators of impending respiratory failure. Dyspnea, cyanosis, the use of accessory respiratory muscles, and pursed-lip breathing are less subtle signs of respiratory distress. Any signs of existing or impending respiratory failure may necessitate intubation. Respiratory failure itself may be the result of pulmonary or nonpulmonary conditions that must appropriately influence decisions for proper airway management.

In addition to factors that constitute indications for intubation in the ICU patient, airway management must be performed with a clear recognition of physiologic changes produced by positive-pressure ventilation. Decreased venous return with resultant reduced cardiac output and hypotension may follow close behind tracheal intubation or become apparent soon after the stimulation of laryngoscopy has dissipated. This hypotension may be confused with or compounded by the effects of sedative or anesthetic agents employed for intubation. Positive-pressure ventilation also affects pulmonary vascular resistance and may impair right ventricular function. This effect may be worsened if bronchospasm and air trapping accompany airway manipulation.

EVALUATION OF THE INTENSIVE CARE UNIT PATIENT

Anatomic Characterization and Practice Rationale

Techniques and practice rationale for airway management have evolved largely through work with patients undergoing general anesthesia. In the operating room population of patients, approximately 4% of intubations are considered difficult.[7] Difficult intubation is traditionally based on anatomic features and exposure limitation rather than the potential for catastrophe with intubation. When a routine intubation from an anatomic perspective cannot be performed without significant physiologic consequences such as hypoxemia, cardiovascular compromise, or a risk of neurologic insult, it could be considered difficult. Although physiologic conditions have not been added to the ASA definition of a difficult airway, certainly characteristics common to ICU patients add degrees of difficulty to the management of an airway that may not be difficult from an anatomic standpoint.

Anatomic characteristics that may indicate the likelihood of difficulty with intubation can often be identified by careful assessment of the airway, which is discussed in detail in Chapter 2. A thorough airway assessment of an ICU patient may not be possible and will most likely not be ideal. Nevertheless, attention should be directed at the joint mobility for axis alignment, the mandibular space size, and the tongue size in relationship to the pharynx. With limitations of time and the participation of the patient, as much information as possible should be obtained by physical examination, a review of medical records, and discussion with staff, family, and the patient, if conversant.

Pathophysiology of Patient Groups

Separate from airway evaluation, there must be a consideration of underlying illnesses and associated pathophysiology. Traditionally, a preanesthetic evaluation identifies diseases and conditions that allow assignment of an ASA Physical Status for classification of anesthetic risk. Such an evaluation allows consideration of anesthetic options that are most appropriate for the particular patient. Much of the anesthetic plan focuses on how to conduct induction and intubation. The same issues must be weighed when dealing with intubations in the ICU setting. However, attention must be directed not only at conditions qualifying the patient for ICU admission in the first place, but also to recent developments in the patient's condition and the indications for intubation. Several conditions of particular concern require special focus.

■ Trauma

Reports from Level I Trauma Centers indicate that 93% of victims need emergency airway access. A surgical airway, such as a cricothyrotomy, is needed in one of eight patients.[8]

Trauma victims in critical care units may require intubation for a number of reasons. Bleeding, edema, distortion, and disruption of the airway may accompany head and neck trauma. Visualization of the anatomy may be impaired or impossible, presenting serious intubation difficulties that are discussed in Chapter 14. In most institutions, especially those designated as a Level I Trauma Center, anesthesia practitioners are responsible for airway management of trauma victims.[9] For all ICU trauma patients, the possibility of reduced circulating blood volume must be considered and the potential of cardiovascular instability weighed in selecting medications and airway management techniques.

Trauma to the thorax is often associated with injuries that complicate airway management. Pulmonary injuries often result in reduced lung volumes and hypoxemia, which may not respond well to preoxygenation. Positive-pressure ventilation can worsen ventilation-perfusion relationships and may even precipitate a tension pneumothorax. Cardiac dysrhythmias and impaired contractile function can accompany cardiac contusion and may manifest themselves during manipulation of the airway or the initiation of positive-pressure ventilation, or both. This can decrease cardiac filling and possibly impair right ventricular outflow. If chest injuries include bronchopleural fistulae, unilateral abnormality, or pulmonary hemorrhage, the use of a double-lumen tracheobronchial tube may be indicated.

Inhalational injuries and burns present significant challenges for airway management. Underlying hypoxemia from pulmonary injuries is often accompanied by impaired cardiac output and depletion of intravascular volume, which may be substantial. If the airway is not secured early in the management of the patient, edema may progress toward airway obstruction and the need for intubation. Recognition of airway structures at this time may be extremely difficult.

■ Cardiovascular

Patients with cardiovascular diseases are at increased risk of complications associated with airway management.[10] Direct laryngoscopy and intubation without pharmacologic interventions produce significant hemodynamic changes, particularly tachycardia and hypertension,[11] which can easily induce ischemia in patients with coronary artery disease. Medication to blunt these responses should be considered in this patient population regardless of the technique selected for intubation.

Impending respiratory failure is often seen in patients with congestive heart failure and critically ill patients with poor myocardial function or reserve. These patients may be extremely sensitive to anesthetic agents and can become hypotensive with very small doses of sedative agents. The stress of respiratory decompensation for these patients results in elevated levels of circulating catecholamines.[12] Intubation and relief of this respiratory stress cause a reduction in catecholamine levels that may lead to hypotension. Severe hypotension and possibly cardiovascular collapse can be precipitated in a patient with cardiac tamponade or a mediastinal mass by initiating positive-pressure ventilation.[13] Thus, spontaneous ventilation should be maintained in these patients, if possible.

■ Pulmonary

In critically ill patients, hypoxemia can exist for a variety of reasons, including ventilation-perfusion mismatching and increased intrapulmonary shunting, the latter being unresponsive to increased FiO_2. The existence of hypoxemia itself may necessitate intubation and present significant challenges in airway management. Arterial desaturation often occurs rapidly in patients with reduced functional residual capacity, even after proper attempts at preoxygenation. When dealing with a hypoxemic patient, it is best to anticipate a difficult intubation and prepare alternative airway management plans, especially if anesthetic induction for intubation is considered necessary.

Coughing and bucking on the endotracheal tube (ET) result from intact airway reflexes and can occur when intubation or airway instrumentation is performed in a responsive, unanesthetized patient. The movement from these reactions may have detrimental effects in patients with cervical spinal cord injuries and intracranial hypertension. The increased intrathoracic pressure these movements produce decreases venous drainage from the jugular system into the thorax and can significantly elevate intracranial pressure in patients with compromised intracranial compliance. Bronchospasm may also develop as a reaction to the presence of foreign objects in the airway and is more likely to occur in lightly anesthetized patients and in those who are prone to bronchospasm, such as smokers and asthmatics. Special considerations should be made for patients with reactive airway disease if awake intubation is necessary.

Pulmonary hemorrhage may be an indication for ICU admission, or it may develop in ICU patients. Trauma, infection, neoplasm, vascular abnormalities, interstitial lung disease, and airway diseases are among the causes of pulmonary hemorrhage, as are iatrogenic causes such as bronchoscopy and pulmonary artery catheterization. Mortality is related to the rate of hemorrhage and is greater than 70% with a 600-mL blood loss occurring in less than 4 hours. Death is due to asphyxiation and can occur within the first 30 minutes.[14] Control of the bloody airway with a large-bore ET may be lifesaving. The use of a double-lumen tube may also be helpful in separating the lungs to maintain adequate gas exchange.

■ Neurologic

Like the respiratory responses to intubation, the cardiovascular responses to airway manipulation must be carefully considered and managed when dealing with patients with central nervous system (CNS) abnormality. When autoregulation is intact, the cerebral blood flow remains constant over a wide range of mean arterial pressures. By contrast, when autoregulation is disrupted by any of a number of intracranial abnormalities, fluctuations in the mean arterial pressure are associated with similar fluctuations in cerebral blood flow. In situations in which intracranial compliance is compromised, an increase in cerebral blood flow produces an elevation of intracranial pressure, which can have devastating consequences.[15]

Patients with traumatic brain injury, CNS tumors, and edema from surgery or infarct are at increased risk of intracranial hypertension, which may be critically affected with airway management. These patient may require intubation for airway protection due to a deteriorating neurologic status, to provide mechanical ventilatory support, or even to safely accomplish diagnostic studies. Aspiration, hypercapnia, hypoxemia, and hypertension are risks to be anticipated in selecting medications and techniques for airway management in these patients. Stable hemodynamics with a low-normal blood pressure are desirable.

The hemodynamic effects of intubation and positive-pressure ventilation are also important factors to consider in dealing with patients with cerebrovascular lesions. Patients with unclipped cerebral aneurysms, arteriovenous malformations, and hemorrhagic infarcts are at risk of hemorrhage with increases in blood pressure and cardiac output. Declines in blood pressure, on the other hand, increase the potential for ischemic insults in patients with long-standing hypertension who have recently suffered an ischemic infarct or who have developed cerebral vasospasm after a subarachnoid hemorrhage. Airway manipulation in any of these patient populations may involve significant cerebrovascular risks.

Cervical spine injuries represent a recognized difficult airway; the cervical spine must remain immobile to avoid spinal cord injury or prevent worsening of an existing insult. Depending on the level and severity of cervical cord injuries, different degrees of respiratory failure can be anticipated. Loss of intercostal muscle function may be tolerated if diaphragmatic function remains intact. High cervical cord injuries, such as those above C5, can be expected to involve diaphragmatic function. Serial evaluations of the inspiratory force and vital capacity provide data indicating the stability and adequacy of respiratory mechanics. A patient whose vital capacity falls below 1 liter, or 15 mL/kg, or who is unable to generate 25 cm of inspiratory force, meets mechanical criteria for intubation.[6] These parameters can also be applied for respiratory failure due to neuromuscular disease.[16, 17]

■ Metabolic

Critically ill diabetic patients may require intubation. Life-threatening diabetic ketoacidosis accounts for approximately 10% of diabetic deaths in the United States, usually from coexisting cardiovascular or renal disease.[18] Many of the deaths in patients younger than 45 years are due to potentially reversible metabolic complications.[19] Diabetic ketoacidosis, usually precipitated by infection,[20] presents with abdominal pain, nausea, vomiting, and ileus induced by electrolyte disturbances. Osmotic diuresis due to hyperglycemia leads to dehydration and hypovolemia as well as hypotension. Hypotension may be exacerbated by peripheral vasodilatation caused by acidosis. Diabetic gastroparesis and the risk of aspiration must be considered, as must cardiovascular responses to sedation, airway manipulation, and positive-pressure ventilation when airway management is required for this patient population.[21]

Acute pancreatitis presents with abdominal pain, nausea, and vomiting, mimicking the acute surgical abdomen. Although severe pancreatitis is relatively uncommon, it carries mortality and serious morbidity that may exceed 50%. Hypovolemia may result from extensive fluid losses, which are accompanied by the release of pancreatic enzymes and vasoactive agents into the systemic circulation. Systemic complications appear during the early stages of an acute attack, including renal failure, respiratory failure, disseminated intravascular coagulopathy, gastrointestinal bleeding, and cardiovascular collapse.[22] Hypoxemia is often severe enough to require intubation. An inability to effectively preoxygenate the patient, as well as an increased possibility of gastric aspiration and cardiovascular instability, must be considered when planning airway management and mechanical ventilation in these patients.

Decompensated hepatic cirrhosis is often complicated by gastrointestinal bleeding, aspiration, adult respiratory distress syndrome, renal failure, and encephalopathy. Intubation of such patients is frequently required and often challenging. Although the blood volume is increased, the effective circulating volume seems to be decreased, and these patients present with a hyperdynamic cardiovascular system.[23] Mild to moderate hypoxemia and hypocapnia is often seen in arterial blood gas measurements.[24] Ascites and increased intraabdominal pressure elevate the diaphragm, resulting in basal lung unit closure[25] and reduction in the functional residual capacity. Changes in the pulmonary blood flow and vascular dilatation have been described and are believed to be responsible for inadequate hypoxic pulmonary vasoconstriction.[26, 27] Preoxygenation may be suboptimal in these patients, and intubation is often complicated by brisk gastrointestinal bleeding, making visualization difficult.

Intoxication and overdoses from ethanol, opiates, sedatives, stimulants, and other substances are frequently seen in patients admitted with CNS injury[28] and in trauma victims.[29] Substance abuse itself also accounts for numerous admissions to critical care units.[30] With progressive CNS depression, airway protection and cardiopulmonary support are often required. The risk of aspiration must always be considered, and circulatory instability must be anticipated for a number of reasons, including intravascular depletion and alterations in physiologic responses brought about by depletion of neurotransmitters and chronic intoxication.[31]

RISK OF GASTRIC ASPIRATION

The risk of gastric aspiration must always be considered in the ICU patient population when airway management is planned. Gastric aspiration is known to occur more frequently in older patients, in those in whom intubation is performed under nonelective conditions, and in those with significant systemic illness (i.e., those with ASA Physical Statuses IV and V).[32] A combination of these factors is common in ICU patients and should be taken into consideration whenever considering any airway manipulation. The risk of gastric aspiration is increased by numerous factors, including opioid administration, hypotension, increased gastric volume, decreased lower esophageal sphincter pressure, incompetent laryngeal reflexes, age, disability, and CNS and neuromuscular disease (Table 15–1).[33–35]

Consequences of Aspiration

The clinical consequences of aspiration range from benign to fatal.[36] A significant portion of patients who aspirate perioperatively require

Table 15–1 Risk Factors in Gastric Aspiration

PERIOPERATIVE
> Parturition
> Emergency
> Obesity
> Outpatient status
> Gastrointestinal dysfunction
> Hiatal hernia
> Scleroderma
> Intestinal obstruction
> Esophageal diverticulae
> Gastroesophageal reflux

DEPRESSED CONSCIOUSNESS
> Head injury
> Drug overdose
> Metabolic coma
> Infection of central nervous system
> Seizure
> Hypothermia
> Sepsis

LARYNGEAL INCOMPETENCE
> Central nervous system disease causing bulbar dysfunction
> Guillain-Barré syndrome
> Multiple sclerosis
> Brain stem cerebrovascular accident
> Posterior fossa tumor
> Muscular dystrophy
> Myasthenia gravis
> Amyotrophic lateral sclerosis
> Traumatic vocal cord paralysis
> Extensive surgery of pharynx and hypopharynx

NASOGASTRIC FEEDING

ARTIFICIAL AIRWAYS
> Tracheotomy tube
> Endotracheal tube

GASTROINTESTINAL HEMORRHAGE

From Goodwin S: Aspiration syndromes. *In* Civetta JM, Taylor RW, Kirby RR (eds): Critical Care, 2nd ed. Philadelphia, JB Lippincott, 1992, p 1262.

mechanical ventilatory support. Aspiration has been implicated as the cause of approximately 40% of cases of adult respiratory distress syndrome [37] Although the overall mortality from aspiration is relatively low, patients who die as a result of perioperative aspiration are those with poor physical status, who often constitute the population of patients cared for in the ICU setting.

Risk of Aspiration

It is important to remember that just because an ICU patient has had nothing by mouth for several days or has been on nasogastric suctioning, the risk of aspiration is not eliminated. In fact, gastroesophageal reflux is known to occur even when a nasogastric tube is in place[38] since it does not ensure gastric emptying.[39, 40] Also, gastric emptying is delayed by numerous factors found during critical illness, including pharmacologic agents such as opioids or anticholinergics, endogenous or exogenous sympathetic stimulation, sepsis, and abdominal abnormality.[41, 42] Thus most, if not all, ICU patients should be considered as "full stomachs" and managed accordingly.

Considering the relatively high risk of gastric aspiration in ICU patients in conjunction with the significant consequences for this patient population, practices intended to reduce the potential for gastric aspiration might best be employed for intubation of virtually all ICU patients. Pharmacologic aspiration prophylaxis may be possible if time permits, although concurrent medical therapy and conditions may limit its effectiveness. Nonetheless, efforts at decreasing the gastric volume and increasing the gastric pH should be considered.

Aspiration Prophylaxis

In the absence of intestinal obstruction, intravenous metoclopramide may be effective in increasing gastric emptying within 10 to 20 minutes of administration,[43] although this effect appears inconsistent with the coadministration of opioids.[44] The gastric pH may be increased by the oral administration of nonparticulate antacid solutions, such as sodium citrate.[45] The administration of 15- to 30-mL volumes of 0.3 M sodium citrate have been studied in regard to the effect on gastric pH in a variety of surgical patients with inconsistent findings.[46] The neutralization of gastric acid requires adequate mixing of the antacid with gastric fluid, which is influenced by the gastric volume, the time, and the movement of the patient.

The gastric pH may also be increased by the timely administration of H_2 antagonists such as cimetidine,[47] ranitidine,[48] and famotidine.[49] Ideally, such agents should be administered 8 to 12 hours before the scheduled intubation, as well as 1 to 2 hours before the time of actual intubation. An increase in gastric pH (above 2.5) may be seen as early as 30 to 60 minutes after an intravenous dose, but the maximal effect requires 60 to 90 minutes,[50] and the desired effect is not always obtained.[51] Rapid intravenous administration of cimetidine has been associated with hypotension[52] and cardiac dysrhythmias,[53] which are not well tolerated by ICU patients. Concurrent administration of metoclopramide and either cimetidine[54] or ranitidine[55] has been shown to be effective in decreasing the gastric acidity and volume. However, no combination of antacid, metoclopramide, and H_2 antagonists can guarantee both a low gastric fluid volume and an increased gastric fluid pH.

Gastric emptying can be accomplished, at least in part, by suction applied to an orogastric or nasogastric tube. Many ICU patients already have such a tube in place, and if not, it may be prudent to insert a gastric tube for decompression while protective reflexes are still intact. The presence of such a tube in the pharynx may interfere with laryngoscopy and intubation, and if this is the case the tube may need to be removed to allow an optimal intubation attempt. Some believe that an orogastric or nasogastric tube promotes silent regurgitation by rendering the gastroesophageal sphincter incompetent.[56, 57] Although this has not been proved, the application of appropriate cricoid pressure should effectively prevent any regurgitation.

Cricoid Pressure

Cricoid pressure can and should be applied if the induction of anesthesia is necessary or heavy sedation is used to accomplish intubation. Even in the presence of a gastric tube, cricoid pressure can protect against gastric reflux with intraesophageal pressures up to 100 cm H_2O.[58] The key to success with the use of cricoid pressure is proper application until the airway is protected (i.e., the ET with an inflated cuff is positioned within the trachea).

Many individuals who are very skilled at caring for ICU patients are unfamiliar with these critical aspects of airway management. Cricoid pressure is best applied by a skilled hand, which carefully identifies the cricoid cartilage and firmly applies pressure, compressing and occluding the esophagus between the cricoid cartilage and the cervical vertebra.[59] Although the pressure may have to be adjusted while laryngoscopy is performed, it is not released until the correct placement of the ET is confirmed. A careful explanation of the significance of this maneuver must be given to any unskilled assistants who provide cricoid pressure.

TECHNIQUES

Once a reasonable assessment of the patient's condition and airway has been completed, decisions regarding the technique of intubation can be made. Although the decision-making process may require the consideration of many factors, the intubation choices are fairly simple. The following questions should be addressed before any manipulation of the patient's airway: Is it better to secure the airway with the patient awake, or is it safe or even necessary to induce anesthesia for intubation? Should the approach be oral or nasal, or is this a case in which a surgical airway should be the first choice?

If the patient has a known history of difficult intubation, or if evaluation of the airway has identified the likelihood of a difficult airway, awake intubation should be the first choice. Awake intubation is recommended for postsurgical patients who have undergone certain facial, oral, or cervical procedures, as well as those with trauma to the face, upper airway, or cervical spine. Awake intubation is also indicated for patients at high risk of aspiration, in respiratory failure, or experiencing hemodynamic instability, patients commonly cared for in the ICU setting. For these patients, awake intubation is desirable because it preserves spontaneous breathing, airway patency, and protective reflexes, as well as the ability to monitor neurologic status. Contraindications to awake intubation are few and include the patient's refusal, combativeness, an inability to cooperate, and true allergies to local anesthetics.

Awake Versus Anesthetized

When anatomic or historic findings make a difficult intubation seem likely, awake intubation is an appropriate choice, but it is not required for all ICU intubations. In fact, if the operator lacks experience, skill, and practice, efforts at awake intubation may be extremely stressful for a patient with compromised physiologic reserves. Airway preparation and topical anesthesia may be less than optimal, and sedation may be problematic. Also, spontaneous breathing, airway patency, and protective reflexes may be lost at any time; thus the operator must be adequately prepared for several plans of airway management.

Whether intubation should be performed awake or with anesthetic induction, the principles applicable to airway practice in the operating room apply to ICU intubations as well. Ascertaining the availability of functional airway equipment, including suction and oxygen dedicated solely to the airway, is crucial. The oxygen tubing and flow must be checked, as must the bag-valve mask device, which may be different from the ones ordinarily used in the operative setting. Space at the head of the ICU bed is often crowded with tubing and monitoring lines. Access may be further complicated by the presence of a headboard, and positioning may be less than optimal because of a soft mattress or a patient's inability tolerate the supine position. All necessary efforts must be directed at providing an optimal attempt at intubation.

Oral Endotracheal Intubation Under Direct Laryngoscopy

Oral endotracheal intubation under direct laryngoscopy is the technique commonly chosen for ICU intubations. This technique is quick and reliable and can be performed in awake or anesthetized patients. At times, a metal stylet, bougie (Eschmann catheter), or other devices may help facilitate intubation. The risk of gastric aspiration should always be recognized and precautions taken accordingly. Cricoid pressure should be applied routinely and held until endotracheal intubation is accomplished.

If the initial intubation attempt is unsuccessful, mask ventilation with cricoid pressure should be performed and subsequent attempts at intubation should be made under more optimal conditions. If after an anesthetic induction has been performed, mask ventilation is impossible or inadequate, the ASA Difficult Airway Algorithm should be followed. If difficulty in establishing an airway is encountered in this sick patient population, the luxury of awakening the patient to perform an awake intubation may not be available. A quick attempt at airway control with a laryngeal mask airway (LMA) or Combitube may be appropriate, but there must be no reluctance or delay in establishing an airway; one must provide transtracheal jet ventilation or perform cricothyrotomy if necessary.

Blind Nasal Intubation

Blind nasal intubation is often desirable for ICU intubations. With adequate topical anesthesia and vasoconstrictors applied to the nasal mucosa, intubation can frequently be accomplished with minimal discomfort and little sedation in an awake patient. Nasal intubation should be avoided in patients with coagulopathy, basal skull fractures, and nasal deformities. As blind nasal intubation often requires movement of the neck, it should be avoided in patients with cervical spine instability if adequate precautions are not taken.

Fiberoptic Intubation

Fiberoptic intubation has become a popular technique in ICU airway practice. Described in Chapter 5, this technique can be employed for nasal or oral intubation in awake patients. With proper patient preparation, it can be less stimulating than intubation performed under direct laryngoscopy. The timely administration of an antisialagogue, the application of topical anesthesia, or the administration of nerve blocks, or all of these, as well as light sedation, greatly facilitate the procedure. Since all the necessary equipment to perform fiberoptic intubation may not be readily available in the ICU setting, proper preparation for the circumstances is necessary.

Retrograde Intubation

Retrograde intubation, as described in Chapter 6, is a technique useful in a variety of settings such as maxillofacial trauma,[60] jaw ankylosis, and upper airway masses.[61] The usefulness of this technique in the critical care setting is limited because of the time required for the procedure. In addition, airway anesthesia needed for successful retrograde intubation eliminates protective airway reflexes, further limiting its application in patients at risk for gastric aspiration.

Laryngeal Mask Airway

Applications and use of the LMA are described in Chapter 8 and elsewhere.[62] The availability of an LMA for use in critical situations where attempts at intubation and mask ventilation have failed is crucial for airway management. Cricoid pressure may prevent proper insertion of the LMA,[63] and the device itself does not protect against gastric aspiration. This limitation, in addition to an inability to provide high inflation pressure, limits the use of the LMA for airway management in the critical care setting.

Esophageal Tracheal Double-Lumen Airway, or Combitube

The esophageal tracheal double-lumen airway, or Combitube, is discussed in Chapter 8. Compared with the endotracheal airway for cardiopulmonary resuscitation, the Combitube has been found to have a shorter intubation time and is associated with comparable blood gas results.[64] When the distal cuff is positioned in the esophagus, as is the usual case, the Combitube affords some protection against gastric aspiration; however, in this position, suctioning of the tracheobronchial tree is not possible. The Combitube is contraindicated in patients with intact gag reflexes, irrespective of their level of consciousness; thus it is not commonly used in the critical care setting but may prove beneficial in the cardiopulmonary arrest situation.

Transtracheal Jet Ventilation

Transtracheal jet ventilation, described in Chapter 9, is a technique that may prove lifesaving in operating room practice, as well as in the critical care setting. Both the availability of equipment and familiarity with its use are crucial for success. In our ICU practice, jet ventilation equipment is set up and tested before tube changes and intubations for which difficulty is anticipated. Jet ventilation can be provided by attaching the device to the suction port of a fiberoptic bronchoscope, through a cannula placed in the cricothyroid membrane or through a jet stylet.

Surgical Airways

Surgical airways are commonly needed for the management of critically ill patients. Fortunately, this most frequently involves elective tracheostomy for ongoing respiratory support. When a surgical airway is required emergently, as when the upper airway is obstructed or when intubation attempts fail and the patient cannot be ventilated adequately, a cricothyrotomy is the technique of choice. Compared with emergency tracheostomy, cricothyrotomy has fewer immediate complications.[65-68] The cricothyroid membrane is relatively superficial, with no important structure lying between it and the skin. The procedure can be performed quickly, with few instruments, and by properly trained anesthesia practitioners. By contrast, the cervical trachea lies behind muscles and vascular structures, making tracheostomy a more complex technique that should be performed by surgeons, optimally under nonemergent circumstances.

Tracheostomy, although seldom the surgical airway of choice in emergency situations, is frequently needed for airway management in the critical care setting. The presence of an ET leads to irritation, edema, and injury to mucosa and underlying structures.[69] Laryngotracheal tubes characteristically tend to damage the medial arytenoid and posterior half of the vocal cords, the cricoid surface, and the anterior tracheal wall. Tracheostomy affords protection against further laryngeal injury, but trauma may still occur at the site of the inflated cuff, or at the tip of the tracheostomy tube. Erosion into the esophagus and brachiocephalic artery can occur with prolonged laryngotracheal intubation but is more commonly seen after tracheostomy. Erosion of the tracheal cartilages can result in tracheomalacia and potentially in tracheal collapse. After tissue erosion, healing may result in granuloma formation and fibrosis.[70, 71] Consequences of this nature may not become apparent until months after extubation when hoarseness persists and when scarring restricts the tracheal diameter.

Elective tracheostomy may be needed in patients who are unable to protect their airway or who require chronic or prolonged ventilatory support. Others include patients with obstructive sleep apnea, facial trauma, and lesions partially obstructing the airway. Although it limits laryngeal damage, long-term complications of intubation are not entirely eliminated by tracheostomy, which brings with it additional risks related to surgery such as hemorrhage, infection, injury to other structures, and even death. These risks considered, laryngotracheal intubation is commonly accepted for 3 weeks or longer.[72]

Elective tracheostomies are performed in the operating room setting in some institutions, whereas others have found that this procedure can be satisfactorily performed within the critical care unit. In our institution, many routine tracheostomies are performed in the ICU setting by a procedure team consisting of a surgeon and assistant, a technician, and an anesthesia practitioner. A percutaneous technique, using a guide wire and sequential dilators, significantly limits surgical trauma and instrumentation. The procedure is facilitated by the use of fiberoptic visualization via the translaryngeal tube, confirming proper placement of the guide wire within the trachea and below the end of the existing ET, which must be withdrawn somewhat, early in the procedure.

EQUIPMENT

Equipment readily available for intubations in an ICU is usually limited to basic devices needed for routine airway management. Some units have prepared intubation cases or trays with an assortment of ETs, stylets, and laryngoscope blades. Other ICUs rely on others to bring the needed equipment with them, usually in a "code" box that is taken to the scene of emergency resuscitation when they are called for a cardiac or respiratory arrest.

For most intubations, this basic equipment is sufficient. When a difficult airway is encountered, however, other devices are necessary. At times, the need for more sophisticated devices develops quickly, and the time required to locate and employ them becomes critical. The ASA practice guidelines for management of the difficult airway list equipment that should be located in a portable cabinet or cart, readily available for a response when a difficult airway is encountered[73] (Fig. 15–1). Many anesthesia departments have set up such portable equipment carts. It may be necessary to develop a similar airway cart devoted to the ICU if operating room equipment cannot be made immediately available or supplies are limited.

In our ICUs, where anesthesia practitioners act as primary intensivists, we have found dedicated airway carts to be most useful. As set forth by the ASA, these carts contain a selection of laryngoscope blades and ETs, Combitubes, LMAs, a retrograde intubation kit, a broncho-scope and light source, a cricothyrotomy kit, tube exchangers, a jet stylet and jet ventilation equipment, lightwand, suctioning equipment,

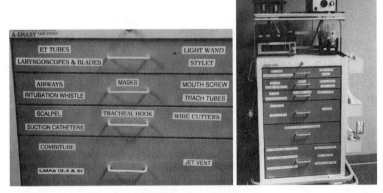

Figure 15–1 Well-stocked, clearly labeled, dedicated airway cart proves useful for airway practice in critical care units.

tracheostomy tubes, and a means for CO_2 detection. The layout is simple and uncluttered with each drawer clearly labeled, indicating its content (see Fig. 15–1).

If the ICU airway cart is used for all intubations, staff can become familiar with its contents and feel more comfortable in using these devices. The cart must be restocked after every use and inventoried on a regular basis. Maintaining the cart under lock and key (with the keys in the custody of the charge nurse and respiratory therapist) may be helpful to ensure that it remains stocked.

Anticipating medications that may be needed for intubation can help avoid delays. The desired medications are often not as available in the ICU as in the operating room. ICU stock medications often do not include a large selection of muscle relaxants, and narcotics or sedatives are routinely locked in a cabinet. Anesthetic induction agents often have to be ordered from another area of the hospital. For individuals who frequently work in the ICU, it may be prudent to put in place a mechanism by which desired medication can be made readily available. It may be easier for anesthesia practitioners to be responsible for the provision of the necessary medications when they are called to go to the ICU to provide airway management.

CHANGING ENDOTRACHEAL TUBES IN CRITICALLY ILL PATIENTS

"Electively changing an indwelling ET is one of the most hazardous airway interventions undertaken in a critically ill patient."[74] Unfortunately, there are a number of reasons for which this may be necessary. Malfunction of the pilot tube valve or a cuff leak may render an ET inadequate to maintain necessary airway pressure. A different-sized tube may be required for bronchoscopy to be performed, or a different type of tube may be necessary, such as a double-lumen tube when independent lung ventilation is needed for the management of pulmonary hemorrhage or unilateral pulmonary abnormality. Likewise, it may be necessary to convert from a double-lumen to a single-lumen tube, or to replace an ET that has become partially obstructed. Exchanging a nasal for an oral tube to treat or avoid sinusitis, or exchanging an oral for a nasal tube in order to improve the patient's comfort, is often needed in ICU practice.

An initial determination of the urgency and desired route of tube replacement, oral versus nasal, is necessary. Available techniques include direct laryngoscopy, the use of a tube exchanger, and fiberoptic techniques. If the new tube can be placed by the same route as the existing tube, a tube exchanger can be used. The tube exchanger is passed beyond the tip of the existing tube and held firmly in place as the existing tube is removed over it. The replacement tube is then advanced over the tube exchanger and into the trachea. The tube exchanger is then removed, ET placement confirmed, and ventilation resumed.

Direct laryngoscopy and fiberoptic bronchoscopy can be used when it is necessary to place the new tube by an alternative route. Both these techniques require the aid of an assistant in handling the existing tube while the operator controls the replacement tube.

In many situations, tube exchange under laryngoscopic direct visualization can be accomplished. After preoxygenation, administration of sedation and a neuromuscular blocking agent may be considered, if appropriate. The airway should be suctioned and cleared and cricoid pressure applied, followed by direct laryngoscopy. When the existing tube and glottis are well exposed, the tip of the replacement tube is positioned such that as the assistant deflates the cuff and withdraws the old tube, the replacement ET can immediately be passed into the trachea.

In 1981, Rosenbaum[75] and others[76] described a technique for changing ETs in critically ill patients utilizing fiberoptic bronchoscopy. The technique, which involves passing the tube-loaded bronchoscope alongside the existing ET, has been described as cumbersome but is considered to offer the least likelihood of failure to reintubate.[77] Variations on this technique have proved useful in a number of settings, particularly when changing routes (oral versus nasal). The early administration of an antisialagogue and appropriate sedation often facilitate the procedure. The fiberoptic bronchoscope is used as a guide for placing the new tube, which is loaded on the scope before beginning the oral procedure, or passed through the nasopharynx before scope insertion for a nasal procedure. Attaching a bronchoscopy (Bodai) adapter on the new tube (Fig. 15–2) before inserting the scope often proves helpful. Initial visualization of laryngeal structures is often challenging. The use of special airways designed for oral fiberoptic procedures may also facilitate initial visualization of the larynx.[78–80]

The flexible fiberoptic bronchoscope is passed by way of the naris or the oropharynx into the larynx anterior to the existing tube, which occupies the posterior portion of the glottic opening. The cuff is deflated and the scope maneuvered beyond it to a depth just above the tracheal

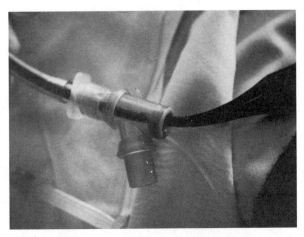

Figure 15–2 Incorporation of a bronchoscopy (Bodai) adapter on the replacement tube before insertion of the fiberoptic scope may prove helpful.

carina (Figs. 15–3 through 15–5). This scope position is maintained by the operator while an assistant withdraws the preexisting ET. The replacement ET is threaded over the bronchoscope into the trachea as soon as the old ET is above the larynx. Once the replacement tube is in place, ventilation can begin by way of the Bodai adapter. Without a Bodai adapter, the bronchoscope must be withdrawn and ventilation can be reestablished.

For additional security, a ventilating stylet (airway exchange catheter) can be passed through a Bodai adapter on the existing tube before beginning the procedure (Fig. 15–6). In the event of difficulty with the

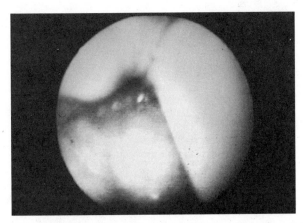

Figure 15–3 Flexible fiberoptic bronchoscope is passed via the naris or the oropharynx.

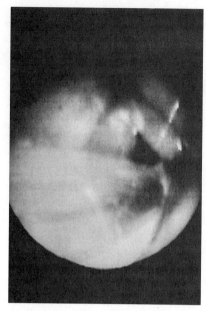

Figure 15–4 Flexible fiberoptic bronchoscope in the larynx anterior to the existing tube.

tube exchange (e.g., the replacement tube does not readily pass into the airway after the preexisting tube is removed), jet ventilation can be accomplished through the ventilating stylet.[81] Alternatively, jet ventilation can be performed by way of the suction port on the fiberoptic bronchoscope (Fig. 15–7).[82]

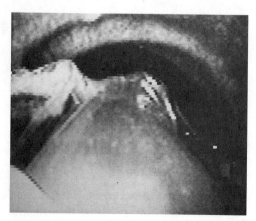

Figure 15–5 Cuff is deflated and the scope maneuvered beyond it.

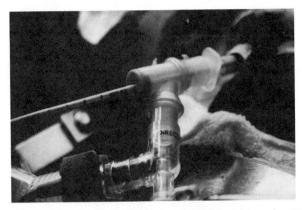

Figure 15–6   Before the procedure is begun, a ventilating stylet can be passed into the existing tube through a Bodai adaptor for jet ventilation.

SUMMARY

Although modern airway practice was developed in the intubation of patients for surgical anesthesia in the operating room, tracheal intubation is often required on locations outside the operating room. Among those locations is the ICU setting.[83–86]

Airway management in the critical care setting may be complex for a number of reasons. Physiologic factors increase the likelihood of hypoxemia and an undesirable cardiovascular response with intubation, even when the airway is not difficult to intubate anatomically. Airway assessment may be suboptimal. Medications, equipment, and capable assistance are often not readily available. The high risk of gastric aspiration must always be considered.

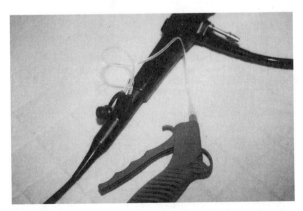

Figure 15–7   Jet ventilation can also be performed using the suction channel of the fiberoptic scope.

Alternative plans to establish an airway are necessary in the ICU just as in the operating room. Airway management in compliance with the ASA Difficult Airway Algorithm is appropriate, although awakening the patient and returning on a different day is usually not an option. Anticipation of problems, both anatomic and physiologic, and careful planning and preparation for intubation difficulties are essential for successful airway practice in the ICU setting.

REFERENCES

1. Mascia MF, Matajsko MJ: Emergency airway management by anesthesia practitioners. Anesthesiology 79:A1054, 1993.
2. Applebaum EL, Bruce DL: Tracheal intubation. Philadelphia, WB Saunders, 1976, p 77.
3. Stauffer JL, Olson DE, Petty TL: Complications and consequences of endotracheal intubation and tracheotomy. Am J Med 70:65, 1981.
4. Mort TC: Incidence and risks leading to cardiac arrest following emergency intubation. Crit Care Med 22:A137, 1994.
5. Castello DA, Smith HS, Lumb PD: Conventional airway access. *In* Shoemaker WC, Ayres SM, Grenvik A, et al (eds): Textbook of Critical Care, 3rd ed. Philadelphia, WB Saunders, 1995, p 701.
6. Ponpoppidan H, Geffin B, Lowenstein E: Acute respiratory failure in the adult (second of three parts). N Engl J Med 287:743, 1972.
7. Samsoon GLT, Young JRB: Difficult tracheal intubation. A retrospective study. Anaesthesia 42:487, 1987.
8. Hawkins ML, Shapiro MB, Cué JI, Wiggins SS. Emergency cricothyrotomy: A reassessment. Am Surg 6:52, 1995.
9. Committee on Trauma, American College of Surgeons: Resources for Optimal Care of the Injured Patient. Chicago, American College of Surgeons, 1993.
10. Prys-Roberts C, Greene, LT, Meloche R, et al: Studies of anaesthesia in relation to hypertension. II: Haemodynamic consequences of induction and endotracheal intubation. Br J Anaesth 43:531, 1971.
11. Bedford RF: Circulatory responses to tracheal intubation. Probl Anesth 2:201, 1988.
12. Parmley WW: Pathophysiology and concurrent therapy of congestive heart failure. J Am Coll Cardiol 13:771, 1989.
13. Ferguson DW: Sympathetic mechanisms in heart failure: Pathophysiologic and pharmacologic implications. Circulation 87:7, 1993.
14. Neuman GG, Weingarten AE, Abramowitz RM, et al: The anesthetic management of the patient with an anterior mediastinal mass. Anesthesiology 60:144, 1984.
15. Conlar AA, Hurwitz SS, Kriege L, et al: Massive hemoptysis. Review of 123 cases. J Thorac Cardiovasc Surg 85:120, 1983.
16. Shapiro HM, Wyte SR, Harris AB, Galindo A: Acute intraoperative intracranial hypertension in neurosurgical patients; mechanical and pharmacological factors. Anesthesiology 37:399, 1972.
17. Ropper AH, Kehne SM; Guillain-Barré syndrome: Management of respiratory Failure. Neurology 35:1662, 1985.
18. Gracy DR, Divertie MB, Howard FM: Mechanical ventilation for respiratory failure in myasthenia gravis. Mayo Clin Proc 58:597, 1983.
19. Faich GA, Fishbein HA, Ellis SE: The epidemiology of diabetic acidosis: A population-based study. Am J Epidemiol 117:441, 1983.
20. Connell FA, Louden JM: Diabetes mortality in persons under 45 years of age. Am J Public Health 73:1174, 1983.
21. Faich GA, Fishbein HA, Ellis SE: The epidemiology of diabetic acidosis: A population-based study. Am J Epidemiol 117:441, 1983.
22. Favin LA: Perioperative management of the diabetic patient. Endocrinol Metab Clin North Am 21:457, 1991.
23. Steer ML: Etiology and pathophysiology of acute pancreatitis. *In* Go VLW, Di-

Magno EP, Gardner JD, et al (eds): The Exocrine Pancreas: Biology, Pathobiology, and Diseases. New York, Raven, 1993, pp 581–592.

24. Glauser F: Systemic hemodynamic and cardiac function changes in patients undergoing orthotopic liver transplantation. Chest 98:1210, 1990.

25. Agustí AG, Roca J, Bosch J, Rodriguez-Roisin R: The lung in patients with cirrhosis. J Hepatol 10:251, 1990.

26. Hanson C, Ritter A, Duran W, et al: Ascites: Its effect upon static inflation of the respiratory system. Am Rev Respir Dis 142:39, 1990.

27. Krowka M, Cortese D: Hepatopulmonary syndrome: An evolving perspective in the era of liver transplantation. Chest 98:1053, 1990.

28. Hedenstierna G, Soederman C, Eriksson LS, et al: Ventilation-perfusion inequality in patients with non-alcoholic liver cirrhosis. Eur Respir J 4:711, 1991.

29. Heinemann AW, Mamott BD, Schnoll SH: Substance use by persons with recent spinal cord injuries. Rehabil Psychol 35:4, 1990.

30. Clark RF, Harchelroad F: Toxicology screening of the trauma patient: A changing profile. Ann Emerg Med 20:151, 1991.

31. Baldwin WA, Rosenfeld BA, Breslow MJ, et al: Substance abuse–related admissions to adult intensive care. Chest 103:21, 1993.

32. Lowinson JH, Ruiz P, Millman RB (eds): Substance Abuse, a Comprehensive Textbook, 2nd ed. Baltimore, Williams & Wilkins, 1985.

33. Warner MA, Warner ME, Weber JG: Clinical significance of pulmonary aspiration during the perioperative period. Anesthesiology 78:56, 1993.

34. Arms RA, Dines DE, Tintsman TC: Aspiration pneumonia. Chest 65:136, 1974.

35. Bynum LJ, Pierce AK: Pulmonary aspiration of gastric contents. Am Rev Respir Dis 114:1129, 1976.

36. Goodwin S: Aspiration syndromes. In Civetta JM, Taylor RW, Kirby RR (eds): Critical Care, 2nd ed. Philadelphia, JB Lippincott, 1992, p 1262.

37. Olsson GL, Hallen B, Hambraeus-Jonzon K: Aspiration during anaesthesia: A computer-aided study of 185,358 anaesthetics. Acta Anaesthesiol Scand 30:84, 1986.

38. Fowler AA, Hamman RF, Good JT, et al: Adult respiratory distress syndrome: Risk with common predispositions. Ann Intern Med 98:593, 1983.

39. Satiani B, Bonner JT, Stone HH: Factors influencing intraoperative gastric regurgitation. Arch Surg 113:721, 1978.

40. Taylor WJ, Champion MC, Barry AW, et al: Measuring gastric contents during general anaesthesia: Evaluation of blind gastric aspiration. Can J Anaesth 36:51, 1989.

41. Ong BY, Palahniuk RJ, Cumming M: Gastric volume and pH in out-patients. Can Anaesth Soc J 25:36, 1978.

42. Nimmo WS: Drugs, diseases and altered gastric emptying. Clin Pharmacokinet 1:189, 1976.

43. Mamel JJ: Gastric emptying disorders. In Nord HJ, Brady PG (eds): Critical Care Gastroenterology. New York, Churchill Livingstone, 1982, p 113.

44. Ciresi SA: Gastrointestinal pharmacology review and anesthetic application to the combat casualty. Mil Med 154:555, 1989.

45. McCammon RL: Prophylaxis for aspiration pneumonitis. Can Anaesth Soc J 33:S47, 1986.

46. Gibbs CP, Spohr L, Schmidt D: The effectiveness of sodium citrate as an antacid. Anesthesiology 57:44, 1982.

47. Manchikanti L, Grow JB, Colliver JA, et al: Bictra (sodium citrate) and metoclopramide in outpatient anesthesia for prophylaxis against aspiration pneumonitis. Anesthesiology 63:378, 1985.

48. Toung T, Cameron JL: Cimetidine as a preoperative medication to reduce the complications of aspiration of gastric contents. Surgery 87:205, 1980.

49. Andrews AD, Brock-Utne JG, Downing JW: Protection against pulmonary acid aspiration with ranitidine. Anaesthesia 37:22, 1982.

50. Dubin SA, Silverstein PI, Wakefield ML, et al: Comparison of the effects of oral famotidine and ranitidine on gastric volume and pH. Anesth Analg 69:680, 1989.

51. Stoelting RK: Gastric fluid pH in patients receiving cimetidine. Anesth Analg 57:675, 1978.
52. Toung T, Cameron JL: Cimetidine as a preoperative medication to reduce the complications of aspiration of gastric contents. Surgery 87:205, 1980.
53. Mahon WA, Kolton M: Hypotension after intravenous cimetidine. Lancet 1:828, 1978.
54. Cohen J, Weetman AP, Dargie HJ, et al: Life-threatening arrhythmias and intravenous cimetidine. Br Med J 2:768, 1979.
55. Solanki DR, Suresh M, Ethridge HC: The effects of intravenous cimetidine and metoclopramide on gastric volume and pH. Anesth Analg 63:599, 1984.
56. Manchikanti L, Colliver JA, Marrero TC, et al: Ranitidine and metoclopramide for prophylaxis of aspiration pneumonitis in elective surgery. Anesth Analg 64:903, 1984.
57. Stone SB: [letter]. J Trauma 21:996, 1981.
58. James, CF: Pulmonary aspiration of gastric contents. In Gravenstein N, Kirby RR (eds): Complications in Anesthesiology, 2nd ed. New York, Lippincott-Raven, 1996, p 176.
59. Salem MR, Joseph NJ, Heyman HJ, et al: Cricoid compression is effective in obliterating the esophageal lumen in the presence of a nasogastric tube. Anesthesiology 63:443, 1985.
60. Sellick BA: Cricoid pressure to control regurgitation of stomach contents during induction of anaesthesia. Lancet 2:404, 1961.
61. Barriot P, Riou B: Retrograde technique for tracheal intubation in trauma patients. Crit Care Med 16:712, 1988.
62. Waters DJ: Guided blind endotracheal intubation: For patients with deformities of the upper airway. Anaesthesia 18:158, 1963.
63. Pennant JH, White PF: The laryngeal mask airway: Its use in anesthesiology. Anesthesiology 79:144, 1993.
64. Ansermino JM, Blogg CE: Cricoid pressure may prevent insertion of the laryngeal mask airway. Br J Anaesth 69:465, 1992.
65. Staudinger T, Brugger S, Watschinger B, et al: Emergency intubation with the Combitube: Comparison with the endotracheal airway. Ann Emerg Med 22:1573, 1993.
66. Silva WE, Hughes J: Tracheotomy. In Rippe JM, Irwin RS, Alpert JS, Fink MP (eds): Intensive Care Medicine, 2nd ed. Boston, Little, Brown, 1991, pp 169–182.
67. Jorden RC, Rosen P: Airway management in the acutely injured. In Moore EE, Eiseman B, VanWay CW (eds): Critical Decisions in Trauma. St Louis, CV Mosby, 1984, pp 30–35.
68. Miklus RM, Elliott C, Snow N: Surgical cricothyrotomy in the field: Experience of a helicopter transport team. J Trauma 29:506, 1989.
69. Mulder DS, Marelli D. The 1991 Fraser Furd lecture: Evolution of airway control in the management of injured patients. J Trauma 33:856, 1992.
70. Blanc VF, Tremblay NAG: The complications of tracheal intubation: A new classification with a review of the literature. Anesth Analg 53:202, 1974.
71. Klainer AS, Turndorf H, Wu W, et al: Surface alterations due to endotracheal intubation. Am J Med 58:674, 1975.
72. Snow JC, Harnao M, Balough K: Post-intubation granuloma of the larynx. Anesth Analg 45:425, 1966.
73. Srauffer JL, Olson DE, Petty TL: Complications and consequences of endotracheal intubation and tracheotomy. Am J Med 70:65, 1981.
74. American Society of Anesthesia practitioners Task Force on Management of the Difficult Airway: Practice guidelines for management of the difficult airway. Anesthesiology 78:597, 1993.
75. Rosenbaum SH, Rosenbaum LM, Cole RP, et al: Use of the flexible fiberoptic bronchoscope to change endotracheal tube in critically ill patients, Anesthesiology 54:169, 1981.
76. Mecca RS: Management of the difficult airway. In Kirby RR, Gravenstein N (eds): Clinical Anesthesia Practice. Philadelphia, WB Saunders, 1994, p 176.

77. Watson CB: Use of a fiberoptic bronchoscope to change endotracheal tube endorsed. Anesthesiology 54:476, 1981.
78. Dellinger RP: Fiberoptic bronchoscopy in adult airway management. Crit Care Med 18:882, 1990.
79. Berman RA: A method for blind oral intubation of the trachea or esophagus. Anesth Analg 56:866, 1977.
80. Patil V, Stebling LC, Hauder HL, et al: Mechanical aids for fiberoptic endoscopy. Anesthesiology 57:69, 1982.
81. Ovassapian A: A new fiberoptic intubating airway. Anesth Analg 66:S132, 1987.
82. Bedger RC, Chang JL: A jet stylet endotracheal catheter for difficult airway management. Anesthesiology 66:221, 1987.
83. Tonnesen AS: Initial stabilization. *In* Hoyt JW, Tonnesen AS, Allen SJ (eds): Critical Care Practice. Philadelphia, WB Saunders, 1991, p 35.
84. Emergency Cardiac Care Committee and Subcommittees, American Heart Association: Advanced cardiac life support guidelines for cardio-pulmonary resuscitation and emergency cardiac care. JAMA 268:2199, 1992.
85. Committee on Trauma, American College of Surgeons: Advanced Trauma Life Support Protocol. Chicago, American College of Surgeons, 1993.
86. Bogdonoff DL, Stone DJ. Emergency management of the airway outside the operating room. Can J Anaesth 39:1069, 1992.

Chapter 16

Extubation of the

Difficult Airway

Carin A. Hagberg and Tyce Regan

Management of the difficult airway does not end with the placement of an endotracheal tube (ET). Much has been written about intubation, but equal emphasis should be placed on strategies that lead to safe and successful extubation. The anesthesia practitioner is faced daily with the extubation of patients in the operating room, the postanesthesia care unit, or the intensive care unit (ICU). Most of these extubations are uncomplicated and considered routine, but on occasion one is faced with extubation of a difficult airway. Although extubation usually takes place without incident, adverse outcomes related to extubation accounted for 7% of the respiratory related claims in the American Society of Anesthesiologists (ASA) Closed Claims Project.[1] The ASA Task Force on Management of the Difficult Airway has developed practice guidelines for managing the difficult airway that includes strategies for extubation of the difficult airway (Fig. 16–1).[2] They state that the strategy will depend in part on the surgery, the condition of the patient, and the skills and preferences of the anesthesia practitioner. They further recommend

1. Consideration of the risk-to-benefit ratio of awake extubation versus extubation in the deeply anesthetized state

2. Careful evaluation of factors that could impair ventilation after extubation

3. The formation of a plan to immediately regain control of the airway in the event that adequate ventilation is not achieved after extubation

4. Consideration of the short-term use of a stylet to act as a bridge to aid in reintubation or ventilation, or both, if extubation is not successful

Because of the anesthesia practitioner's frequent involvement in airway management of patients in various settings, it is important to be armed with techniques that successfully address extubation of the difficult airway and appreciate the potential complications associated with extubation.

THE DIFFICULT AIRWAY

The first question to ask when dealing with any airway is: *Does the patient have a difficult airway?* A difficult airway, as defined by the ASA Task Force, is the clinical situation in which a conventionally trained anesthesia practitioner experiences difficulty with mask ventilation, difficulty with tracheal intubation, or both.[2] Obviously, if one had difficulty with ventilation or initial endotracheal intubation, particular caution should be exercised at the time of extubation. Usually this scenario is seen after multiple attempts at securing the airway have resulted in airway trauma. The patient is extubated and obstruction is encountered because of edema from the initial intubation attempts. On the other hand, one may have had no problem with the initial airway management, but because of direct surgical procedures on or around the airway, positioning (e.g., prone or sitting with extreme neck flexion), inhalation injuries, or aggressive fluid management, the airway has progressed intraoperatively from an easy to a difficult one. More than one anesthesia practitioner has been placed in the unenviable position of trying to control a difficult airway after an extubation when the airway was easily managed after induction. One must remember that not all airways that are easy at the start of an anesthetic procedure are easy after the completion of surgery. Thyroidectomy, carotid endarterectomy, anterior cervical spine procedures, and maxillofacial surgery are only a few examples of surgical procedures that may result in difficult airways after extubation. Most extubation problems associated with

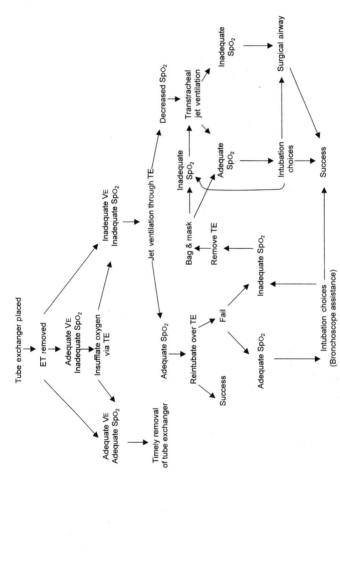

Figure 16–1 Algorithm for extubation of the difficult airway that is suggested as one of several stepwise approaches to difficult airway management after extubation. The patient's condition and the clinical skills of the practitioner dictate specific management. ET, endotracheal tube; TE, tube exchanger. (From Miller KA, Harkin CP, Bailey PL: Postoperative tracheal extubation. Anesth Analg 80:149–172, 1995.)

surgical procedures involve postoperative bleeding, nerve damage, or direct tissue trauma. Certain coexisting medical conditions may also cause problems at the time of extubation; these include rheumatoid arthritis, obstructive sleep apnea, hypoventilation disorders, neuromuscular conditions, and depressed levels of consciousness. The anesthesia practitioner should also be careful of devices placed near the airway around the time of extubation (e.g., a cervical collar, maxillomandibular fixation equipment, a large dressing on the head or neck). These devices may make it difficult to reestablish an airway. The answer to this initial question determines what equipment and personnel are needed at the time of extubation.

Once it has been determined that the patient has a difficult airway, the next question is: *Can I extubate the patient?* This question is not always easy to answer, especially if one had a great deal of difficulty in originally securing the airway. The main goal of extubating the difficult airway, as with any airway, is to avoid reintubation if at all possible. This goal is extremely important when faced with a difficult airway because reintubation is almost always more hazardous. At the time of reintubation, one may be faced with emergent situations such as poor oxygenation or ventilation, or both, an uncooperative patient, a compromised airway, and inadequate expert help if reintubation takes place outside the operating room. If not properly addressed, these factors combined with a difficult airway may lead to a less than desirable outcome.

Another important question is: *Where should I extubate the patient?* Patients are usually extubated immediately after surgery in the operating room, postanesthesia care unit, or ICU. There appears to be a higher percentage of reintubations in the ICU compared with the postanesthesia care unit (4% versus 0.19%, respectively).[3, 4] The higher percentage of reintubations in the ICU may be due to the patients' overall debilitated state, neurologic status, impaired mucociliary clearance, extreme age, or inability to control the underlying disease state, or all of these, that put these patients in the intensive care setting originally.[5] When and where a patient is extubated depend on both airway and nonairway issues. The usual criteria should be met, for example, hemodynamic stability, a satisfactory oxygen-carrying capacity, normothermia, an adequate respiratory rate and tidal volume, good oxygen saturation, and a conscious alert patient who is able to clear secretions and protect the airway. Issues specific to the airway should revolve around the possibility of airway obstruction, ventilatory problems, and aspiration. Patients at high risk for failed extubation are those with any potential for hypoventilation, a ventilation-perfusion mismatch, a failure of the pulmonary toilet, or airway obstruction. One should also take into consideration the patient's future operative schedule. It makes no sense to extubate a patient with a difficult airway and later find out that the patient will be returning the next morning for follow-up surgery!

Two maneuvers common to anesthetic practice are often performed when determining the feasibility of extubation. The first is the performance of direct laryngoscopy before extubation. This practice, frequently taught as a way to evaluate edema around the airway, is of limited value. The ET blocks the operator's view of the laryngeal inlet, and anatomy is deformed by the ET in situ, leading to an underestimation of the difficulty of reintubation. No studies have shown that direct laryngoscopy before extubation decreases the incidence of reintubation. The second maneuver commonly performed is testing for a cuff leak.[6] This is accomplished in a spontaneously ventilating patient by removing the patient from the ventilation circuit and occluding the end of the ET with a finger while simultaneously deflating the cuff. If no significant edema is present, the patient will be able to breathe around the ET. A cuff leak test should be performed on any patient who it is felt may demonstrate obstruction after extubation. The incidence of reintubation and the need for tracheostomy is greater in the absence of a cuff leak. Should a possibly difficult airway be extubated in the absence of a cuff leak? In our opinion, three options exist:

1. One can wait until a cuff leak develops.
2. If the patient has been ventilated for a "reasonable" time, a tracheostomy may be in order.
3. One can perform controlled extubation over a jet stylet (described later).

Once the decision has been made that the patient can be extubated, strategies for a safe extubation can be formulated.

STRATEGIES FOR EXTUBATION

The anesthesia practitioner must understand the various options for extubation and formulate a plan of action to regain control of the airway if extubation fails. Benumof considers a controlled, gradual, step-by-step, reversible withdrawal of airway support as the optimal approach to the difficult airway extubation,[7] and we are in agreement. There are basically three approaches to extubation of the difficult airway:

1. Extubate with the patient in a deep plane of anesthesia (deep extubation).
2. Extubate conventionally with the patient awake and hope for the best.
3. Extubate with the patient awake, with a "bridge" to full extubation.

We support the last option because it agrees with the concept of a controlled withdrawal of airway support.

The ASA Task Force on Management of the Difficult Airway recommends that the risk-to-benefit ratio of an awake extubation versus an extubation with the patient in the deeply anesthetized state should be considered.[2] The so-called deep extubation or modified deep extubation, in which a laryngeal mask airway is placed after the patient is extubated in a deep plane of anesthesia, has been described in patients with difficult airways. Extubation while the patient is in a deep plane of anesthesia has been widely taught as a means to decrease the risk of laryngospasm or bronchospasm, or both, but there are no adequate studies indicating any real benefit from this approach. Although the performance of deep extubation is elegant, the risk of obstruction is ever present, and therefore we feel that this practice should generally be discouraged in the face of a difficult airway. Awake extubation is the most appropriate method of removing the ET in most patients with a difficult airway.

Some practitioners choose to extubate a difficult airway in a conventional manner (i.e., removing the ET as in the uncompromised airway). Those who elect this method state that if reintubation is needed, the likelihood of reintubation is enhanced by prior knowledge of the initial intubation. We discourage this "sink or swim" approach for two reasons: First, the assumption that what worked originally will work again is wrong. The airway is not static but dynamic, and a completely different airway may be seen the second time around. Second, alternative methods allow more control in the advent that reintubation is needed. Most of these options revolve around placing a stylet-type device through the ET and removing the ET over the stylet.

Many devices have been used in the extubation of the difficult airway. Most of these devices were first described for ET exchange, and many are still used for that purpose. Bronchoscopes,[8] nasogastric tubes,[9] gum elastic bougies,[10] and endotracheal ventilation catheters[11] are just some of the devices that have been used in the extubation and reintubation of patients. The jet stylet catheter is a product specifically designed for extubation of the difficult airway. The commercial tube changers make ideal jet stylets. There are numerous manufacturers for these types of catheters (Table 16–1), but all basically work on the same principle: a long hollow tube device is inserted into the in situ ET to a predetermined depth; the ET is removed over the catheter; and the catheter remains in place to insufflate oxygen, act as a guide to intubation if reintubation is necessary, or intermittently measure end-tidal carbon dioxide ($P_{ET}CO_2$) from the trachea. These products come in a variety of sizes and have different features depending on the manufacturer. The jet stylet that we most frequently use is the Cook airway exchange catheter produced by Cook Critical Care (Fig. 16–2).[12] The

Table 16–1   Endotracheal Ventilation Catheters

Bedger jet stylet
Metro (Cook)
Airway exchange catheter (Cook)*
Patil two-part intubation catheter (Cook)*
TTX (Sheridan)
ETX (Sheridan)*
JETTX (Sheridan)
Endotracheal ventilation catheter (CardioMed)

*Capable of double-lumen endotracheal tube exchange.

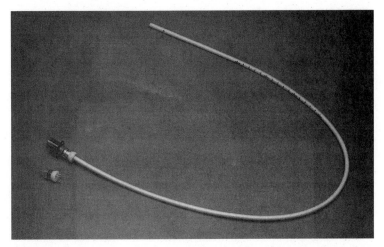

Figure 16–2 Cook airway exchange catheters. Proximally, a 15-mm endotracheal tube connector is attached, although a second Rapi-Fit adapter for jet ventilation is available. Distally, note the side holes and single end hole. (Courtesy of Cook Critical Care.)

device comes with a Rapi-Fit 15-mm connector for connection to the anesthesia machine or Ambu bag and a Luer-Lok connector for jet ventilation (Table 16–2). The catheters have distance markings to allow proper depth determination. In order to minimize barotrauma, these catheters should not be inserted to a depth greater than 26 to 27 cm when used for orotracheal intubation. The Patil two-part intubation catheter is also manufactured by Cook Critical Care (Fig. 16–3). It is 63 cm long with an outer and inner diameter of 6 and 3.4 mm, respectively. It is suitable for endotracheal tubes with a 7 mm or greater inner diameter and has a total of eight side ports in addition to an end hole. A malleable stylet inserted through the "first part" may be used to facilitate intubation when the "second part" is connected to the first. It can be used as a tube exchanger or to perform reversible extubation.

Sheridan tracheal exchange catheters (Fig. 16–4), on the other hand,

Table 16–2   Characteristics of Cook Airway Exchange Catheters

Semirigid radiopaque polyurethane catheters
Available in six sizes (2.7–6.33 mm OD, 1.6–3.4 mm ID)
Single distal end hole and two distal side holes (with one exception)
Rapi-Fit adapters for both routine and jet ventilation
Distance markings every centimeter until 30 cm
Length (cm)
  Pediatric 45
  Adult   83

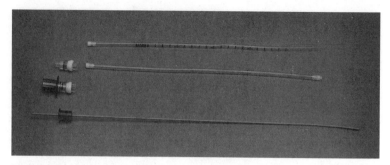

Figure 16–3 Patil two-part intubation catheter, showing the disassembled two-part intubation catheter, along with a malleable stylet and two Rapi-Fit connectors. (Courtesy of Cook Critical Care.)

do not come equipped with ready-made adaptations for ventilation (Table 16–3). On ET removal, the catheter is left in place, with the proximal end taped to the patient's shoulder and labeled appropriately. Adult patients usually tolerate the catheter well with minimal, if any, coughing if proper analgesics are given before extubation. The catheter is usually left in place for 30 to 60 minutes since obstruction usually occurs within this amount of time, although additional time may be necessary. A variety of techniques may increase the utility of these catheters, including insufflation of humidified oxygen through the central lumen; the use of a face mask to supplement the fraction of inspired oxygen (FIO_2); nebulization of racemic epinephrine (to decrease mucosal edema); and administration of helium-oxygen (heliox).[13] Although these catheters are good for acting as a guide for reintubation, their use as ventilation catheters for any length of time is questionable. The possibil-

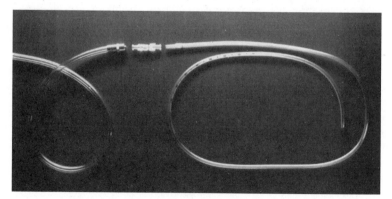

Figure 16–4 Sheridan tracheal tube exchanger, which is available in four sizes. The exchanger has one distal end hole and no side holes. Although many adaptations may be used for connection to a jet ventilation device, a plastic Luer-Lok adapter is pictured here. (Courtesy of Sheridan.)

Table 16–3   Characteristics of Sheridan Jet Stylet Catheters

Available in four sizes (2.0–5.8 mm OD)
Single distal end hole (ends are identical)
Relatively soft but firm
No ready-made attachments for ventilation
Distance markings every 2 cm until 28 cm
Length (cm)
Pediatric	56
Adult	81.25
ETX	100

ities of catheter whip and barotrauma are ever present.[14] Therefore, we recommend that the catheter be used in conjunction with an oxygen source for insufflation as opposed to jet ventilation, if at all possible. Also, patients should be kept fasted for the duration of catheter use, and any respiratory care therapies should continue to be administered.

If ventilation is necessary, several considerations should be kept in mind in order to minimize the incidence of barotrauma, including

1. Assurance of a maximally patent upper airway by placing the patient in the optimal "sniffing" position.
2. Delivery of an appropriate oxygen supply through the use of an in-line regulator initially using 15 psi. (Even experienced users of airway exchange catheters can have an 11% incidence of barotrauma when they are used for 50-psi jet ventilation.)[15, 16]
3. Using the appropriate inspiratory time. According to Gaughan and colleagues, a 1-second inspiratory time at 25 psi with an FIO_2 near 1 will provide at least *partial* life-sustaining ventilatory support with even the smallest sized commercially available catheters, whereas a 0.5-second inspiratory time will provide *total* ventilatory support with either the medium- or larger-sized catheters.[17, 18]

By maintaining a maximally patent airway and delivering an appropriate tidal volume taking into consideration both the pressure and the inspiratory time, the incidence of barotrauma should be minimized.

RECOMMENDED TECHNIQUE FOR EXTUBATION OF THE DIFFICULT AIRWAY

Following is the technique recommended by the ASA for extubation of the difficult airway:

1. Administer 100% oxygen.
2. Suction the oropharynx.
3. Deflate the ET cuff (check for cuff leakage).
4. Insert an airway exchange catheter through the ET to a predetermined depth.

5. Extubate the patient over a jet ventilation catheter.
6. Apply oxygen by face mask or insufflation through a jet ventilation catheter.
7. Tape the proximal end to the patient's shoulder to stabilize it.
8. Remove the jet ventilation catheter after 30 to 60 minutes if no obstruction appears.

PROBLEMS ASSOCIATED WITH EXTUBATION

The potentially difficult airway is not the only situation that the anesthesia practitioner may encounter at the time of extubation. Complications common to extubation can and do occur. Even routine extubations can present the practitioner with a variety of problems. Some problems are mild and transient, requiring no treatment, whereas others can be life threatening and necessitate quick diagnosis and rapid therapy.

Hemodynamic Changes

Hemodynamic changes, which usually include an increase in heart rate and blood pressure of approximately 20%, occur in most patients at the time of extubation.[19, 20] These changes are usually transient and rarely require treatment. Catecholamine release due to ET stimulation is thought to be responsible for the change in hemodynamics. Although these hemodynamic responses are well tolerated in most individuals, patients with cardiac disease, pregnancy-induced hypertension,[12] and increased intracranial pressure[21] may be at particular risk for adverse consequences. Patients with cardiac disease have shown decreased ejection fractions at the time of extubation.[22] Management is focused on deep extubation or pharmacologic therapy, or both. Deep extubation may be appropriate for some patients but is inappropriate for those with a difficult airway, those at high risk for aspiration, and those in whom airway access is reduced. Pharmacologic strategies emphasize the importance of decreasing the heart rate, which is more likely to cause myocardial ischemia than increased blood pressure. β-Blockers appear to have the most consistent success with blunting the hemodynamic response to extubation. Esmolol, 1.5 mg/kg, given 2 to 4 minutes before extubation, has been shown to prevent rapid increases in heart rate and blood pressure during extubation.[23] Labetalol, 0.25 to 2.5 mg/kg, has also been used with success.[21] Although the calcium channel blocker diltiazem, in doses of 0.1 to 0.2 mg/kg, has shown promise, [24] inconsistent results have been obtained with lidocaine and high-dose narcotics.[25]

Laryngospasm

Laryngospasm is a common cause of airway obstruction and is a protective reflex mediated by the vagus nerve. This reflex is an attempt to prevent the aspiration of foreign bodies into the trachea. Various techniques have been used to attempt to decrease the incidence of this event, but none have proved superior to the others. Laryngospasm may be provoked by movement of the cervical spine, pain, vocal cord irritation by secretions, or sudden stimulation while in a light plane of anesthesia.[26] Management consists of suctioning the oropharynx before extubation and administering 100% oxygen with sustained positive pressure at the time of extubation. Severe cases may require a small dose of succinylcholine (20 mg for an adult) to "break" the spasm along with reintubation.[27]

Vocal Cord Malfunction

Injury to the vagus nerve or one of its branches can cause vocal cord paralysis. This rare complication is most often seen with thyroid, thoracic, and various neck surgeries.[12] Vocal cord malfunction can also be caused by cuff pressure from the ET near the anterior division of the recurrent laryngeal nerve.[28] Although the anesthesia practitioner has little control over the surgical causes of vocal cord injury, the incidence of anesthetic causes may be decreased by avoiding overinflation of the cuff of the ET and placement of the ET at least 15 mm below the vocal cords.[29] Unilateral vocal cord paralysis produces little more than hoarseness, and recovery usually occurs in weeks. Bilateral vocal cord paralysis can cause airway obstruction requiring immediate reintubation. Recovery is often delayed and a tracheostomy may be required. Diagnosis can be confirmed by fiberoptic evaluation.

Laryngeal Edema

Laryngeal edema is an important cause of postextubation obstruction. This condition has various causes and can be classified as being supraglottic, retroarytenoidal, or subglottic.[30] Supraglottic edema is most commonly seen as a result of surgical manipulation, positioning, hematoma formation, aggressive fluid management, decreased venous drainage, or coexisting conditions (e.g., preeclampsia, angioneurotic edema). Subglottic edema is more often seen in children, particularly neonates and infants. Factors associated with the development of subglottic edema in the young include trauma during tracheal intubation, intubation for greater than 1 hour, "bucking" on the ET, a change in head position, and a tight-fitting ET. Usually laryngeal edema presents as stridor within 30 to 60 minutes after extubation, but it may occur up to 6 hours after extubation. The cause of retroarytenoidal edema is less well described but may be local trauma or irritation. No matter what the cause, management depends on the severity of the condition and includes humidified oxygen, racemic epinephrine, positioning the patient head-up, and occasionally reintubation with a smaller ET. The practice of giving systemic steroids in the hopes of reducing edema is controversial, and studies are divided on their efficacy.[31]

Negative-Pressure Pulmonary Edema

Negative-pressure pulmonary edema may develop in spontaneously breathing patients after extubation when airway obstruction occurs. As a result of the obstruction, these patients generate significant negative intrapleural pressure leading to pulmonary edema from engorgement of the pulmonary vasculature and increased pulmonary capillary hydrostatic pressure.[32] This condition is seen within minutes after extubation and usually presents with pink frothy sputum and a decrease in oxygen saturation (SpO_2). Management involves removing the obstruction, oxygen support, close monitoring, and afterload reduction with furosemide or morphine, or both. Reintubation is rarely needed, and most cases resolve without complication.

Airway Trauma

Unlike trauma during intubation, airway trauma at the time of extubation has not been well described. Arytenoid cartilage dislocation has been reported after difficult as well as uncomplicated intubations.[33, 34] The symptoms become apparent soon after extubation and may be mild, consisting of difficulty swallowing and voice changes, or major, involving airway obstruction. Management depends on the severity of the condition but can involve reintubation, reduction of the arytenoids, or even tracheostomy. If this condition is suspected an otolaryngology consultation is warranted.

Airway Compression

External compression of the airway after extubation may lead to obstruction. An excessively tight postsurgical neck dressing is one cause of external compression that can be easily resolved. A more ominous situation is a rapidly expanding hematoma in proximity to the airway. This situation may be seen after certain surgeries (e.g., carotid endarterectomy, thyroidectomy) and must be quickly diagnosed and properly treated before total airway obstruction occurs.[12, 35] Immediate surgical reexploration is in order, but one should approach airway issues in these patients with extreme caution. Most anesthesia texts suggest that one should avoid general anesthesia until the wound is evacuated under local anesthesia, thus decreasing airway distortion. We agree with this approach, but airway obstruction may still occur because of edema caused by venous and lymphatic congestion. Therefore, routine induction techniques (especially involving the use of muscle relaxants) could still result in total airway obstruction at the time of induction, even after local evacuation of a neck hematoma. Management of the airway with an awake fiberoptic technique or inhalation induction without the use of muscle relaxants until the airway is secured are more conservative options. Another cause of external compression of the airway is tracheomalacia, which may occur for a number of reasons including prolonged compression from a goiter.[36] This condition is usually seen after the removal of the goiter, but tracheal collapse on induction after muscle relaxants were administered has been reported.[37] Airway obstruction becomes apparent soon after extubation and management includes reintubation, surgical tracheal support, or tracheostomy below the obstruction.

Aspiration

The problems associated with aspiration have long been recognized.[38] Burgess and colleagues have shown that laryngeal function is altered for at least 4 hours after extubation.[39] This alteration in laryngeal function, along with residual anesthesia, may make the patient more vulnerable to aspiration at the time of extubation. Aspiration is probably more widespread than we would like to admit. Why is aspiration not recognized more frequently? More than likely, most cases of aspiration are either minor and do not cause any change in the patient's postoperative course or the development of postoperative problems are attributed to other factors. Management consists of supportive measures and depending on the extent of aspiration may include reintubation and ventilation with positive end-expiratory pressure.

CONCLUSION

Extubation of the trachea is not without risk. The anesthesia practitioner needs to consider many factors, including the ease of the initial intubation, the patient's medical status, the setting in which extubation is going to occur, and finally, the practitioner's skills and preferences. The potential for reintubation after any extubation is always present. The strategy should carry low risk, cause minimal patient discomfort, and optimize the objectives of airway access, oxygenation, and ventilation. Several complications common to extubation can and do occur and may or may not require treatment. Tracheal reintubation over tube changers is neither without complications nor 100% successful; therefore, those who use these devices should be familiar with the equipment and techniques, their potential complications, and alternatives in case of reintubation failure. The anesthesia practitioner should be familiar with the extubation strategy developed by the ASA Task Force on Management of the Difficult Airway. Finally, high-risk patients should be identified if at all possible.

REFERENCES

1. Caplan RA, Posner KL, Ward RJ, Cheny FW: Adverse respiratory events in anesthesia: A closed claims analysis. Anesthesiology 72:828, 1990.
2. Caplan RA, Benumof JL, Berry FA, et al: Practice guidelines for management of the difficult airway, a report by the American Society of Anesthesiologists Task Force on Management of the Difficult Airway. Anesthesiology 78:597, 1993.
3. Rose DK, Cohen MM, Wigglesworth DR, DeBoer DP: Critical respiratory events in the postanesthesia care unit. Anesthesiology 81:410, 1994.
4. Demling RH, Read T, Lind LJ, Flanagan HL: Incidence and morbidity of extubation failure in surgical intensive care patients. Crit Care Med 16:573, 1988.
5. Mathew JP, Rosenbaum SH, O'Conner T, Barash PG: Emergency tracheal intubation in the postanesthesia care unit: Physician error or patient disease? Anesth Analg 71:691, 1990.
6. Fisher MM, Raper RF: The "cuff-leak" test for extubation. Anaesthesia 47:10, 1992.
7. Benumof JL: Management of the difficult adult airway. Anesthesiology 75:1087, 1991.
8. Dellinger RP: Fiberoptic bronchoscopy in adult airway management. Crit Care Med 18:882, 1990.

9. Steinberg MJ, Chmiel RA: Use of a nasogastric tube as a guide for endotracheal reintubation. J Oral Maxillofac Surg 47:1232, 1989.
10. Robles B, Hester J, Brock-Utne JG: Remember the gum-elastic bougie at extubation. J Clin Anesth 5:329, 1993.
11. Cooper RM, Levytam S: Use of an endotracheal catheter for difficult airway management. Anesthesiology 77:A1110, 1992.
12. Cooper RM: Extubation and changing endotracheal tubes. In Benumof JL (ed): Airway Management Principles and Practice. St Louis, Mosby–Year Book, 1996, p 864.
13. Loudermilk EP, Hartmannsgruber M, Stoltzfus DP, Langevin PB: A prospective study of the safety of tracheal extubation using a pediatric airway exchange catheter for patients with a known difficult airway. Chest 111:1660, 1997.
14. Benumof JL, Gaughan SD: Concerns regarding barotrauma during jet ventilation. Anesthesiology 76:1072, 1992.
15. Cooper RM: Extubation and changing endotracheal tubes. In Benumof JL (ed): Airway Management Principles and Practice. St Louis, Mosby–Year Book, pp 864–885, 1996.
16. Cooper RM, Cohen DR: The use of an endotracheal ventilation catheter for jet ventilation during a difficult intubation. Can J Anaesth 41:1196, 1994.
17. Gaughan SD, Benumof JL, Ozaki G: Quantification of the jet function of a jet stylet. Anesth Analg 74:582, 1992.
18. Gaughan SD, Benumof JL, Oaki G: Can an anesthesia machine provide for effective jet ventilation? Anesth Analg 76:800, 1993.
19. Bidwai AV, Bidwai VA, Rogers CR, Stanley TH: Blood pressure and pulse rate responses to endotracheal extubation with and without prior injection of lidocaine. Anesthesiology 51:171, 1979.
20. Wohlner EC, Usubiaga LJ, Jacoby RM, Hill CE: Cardiovascular effects of extubation. Anesthesiology 51:S194, 1979.
21. Muzzi DA, Black S, Lasasso TJ, et al: Labetalol and esmolol in the control of hypertension after intracranial surgery. Anesth Analg 70:68, 1990.
22. Coriat P, Mundler O, Bousseau D, et al: Response of left ventricular ejection fraction to recovery from general anesthesia: Measurement by gated radionuclide angiography. Anesth Analg 65:593, 1986.
23. Dyson A, Isaac PA, Pennant JH et al: Esmolol attenuates cardiovascular responses to extubation. Anesth Analg 71:675, 1990.
24. Katsuya M, Kahru N, Nobuhiro M, Hidefumi O: Attenuation of cardiovascular responses to tracheal extubation: Verapamil versus diltiazem. Anesth Analg 82:1205, 1996.
25. Paulissian R, Salem MR, Joseph NJ, et al: Hemodynamic responses to endotracheal extubation after coronary artery bypass grafting. Anesth Analg 73:10, 1991.
26. Rex MAE: A review of the structural and functional basis of laryngospasm and a discussion of the nerve pathways involved in the reflex and its clinical significance in man and animals. Br J Anaesth 42:891, 1970.
27. Chung DC, Rowbottom FJ: A very small dose of suxamethonium relieves laryngospasm. Anesthesia 48:229, 1993.
28. Ellis PDM, Pallister WK: Recurrent laryngeal nerve palsy and endotracheal intubation. J Laryngol Otol 89:823, 1975.
29. Cavo JW, Jr: True vocal cord paralysis following intubation. Laryngoscope 95:1352, 1985.
30. Hartley M, Vaughan RS: Problems associated with tracheal extubation. Br J Anaesth 71:561, 1993.
31. Darmon JY, Rauss A, Dreyfuss D, et al: Evaluation of risk factors for laryngeal edema after tracheal extubation in adults and its prevention by dexamethasone: A placebo-controlled, double-blind, multicenter study. Anesthesiology 77:245, 1992.
32. Kirby RR: Negative pressure pulmonary edema. ASCCA Interchange. March, 1994.
33. Frink EJ, Pattison BD: Posterior arytenoid dislocation following uneventful endotracheal intubation and anesthesia. Anesthesiology 70:358, 1989.

34. Tolley NS, Cheesman TD, Morgan D, et al: Dislocated arytenoid: An intubation-induced injury. Ann R Coll Surg Engl 72:353, 1990.
35. O'Sullivan JC, Wells DG, Wells GR: Difficult airway management with neck swelling after carotid endarterectomy. Anaesth Intensive Care 14:460, 1986.
36. Geelhoed GW: Tracheomalacia from compressing goiter: Management after thyroidectomy. Surgery 104:1100, 1988.
37. Wade H: Respiratory obstruction in thyroid surgery. Ann R Coll Surg Engl 62:15, 1980.
38. Mendelson CL: The aspiration of stomach contents into the lungs during obstetric anesthesia. Am J Obstet Gynecol 52:191, 1946.
39. Burgess GE, Cooper JR, Marino RJ, et al: Laryngeal competence after tracheal extubation. Anesthesiology 51:73, 1976.

Chapter 17

Effective Dissemination of

Critical Airway

Information

Tyce Regan and Michelle Bowman-Howard

Endotracheal intubation is a commonly performed procedure, and an unexpectedly difficult intubation may place the patient at serious risk for complications or even death. The American Society of Anesthesiologists (ASA) Task Force on Management of the Difficult Airway has defined a difficult airway as "the clinical situation in which a conventionally trained anesthesiologist experiences difficulty with mask ventilation, difficulty with tracheal intubation, or both."[1] Although unsuccessful or failed intubation occurs rarely, it continues to be associated with a high risk of catastrophic complications, including death. Adverse outcomes associated with respiratory events remain the largest class of injury in the ASA Closed Claims Project as reported by the ASA Committee on Professional Liability. The majority (89%) of adverse events in this class of claims relate to problems with airway management.[2]

The effective dissemination of airway information may be an overlooked part of difficult airway management. There seems to be no standard method of relaying information from one physician to another. Many anesthesiologists document their management of a difficult airway in the anesthesia record and discuss the problems encountered with the patient postoperatively, but this approach may not be enough. The MedicAlert Foundation offers a means by which critical information regarding the airway may be disseminated in an organized fashion.

WHAT IS MEDICALERT?

MedicAlert is a nonprofit, membership organization that provides a 24-hour emergency medical information service. Member benefits include a personalized MedicAlert emblem and a computerized medical file. MedicAlert was started by a physician in 1956 after his daughter had a severe reaction to tetanus antitoxin. MedicAlert relays information about medical conditions, allergies, medications, and special needs including difficult airway information. Other anesthesia-related medical problems such as malignant hyperthermia, pseudocholinesterase deficiency, latex allergy, prior laryngeal surgery, or tracheostomy information may be included in the MedicAlert database. There are 2.3 million Americans enrolled in MedicAlert. An additional 1.7 million are served by 17 MedicAlert affiliates all over the world. Currently, 3579 patients registered with MedicAlert have "difficult airway" as the main component in their database (D. Hunt, personal communication to C. Hagberg, March 3, 1999). MedicAlert was endorsed by the ASA in 1979.[3]

WHAT DOES THE PATIENT GET?

The components of MedicAlert are

1. A bracelet or necklace (Fig. 17–1) with the MedicAlert emblem on one side and the MedicAlert collect phone number, the patient's medical condition or main problem (e.g., difficult airway), and a unique patient ID number on the other side.
2. A record summary (Fig. 17–2) with the same information as the bracelet or necklace, as well as a more extensive database (75 lines) that may be helpful to the practitioner (e.g., clinical airway algorithm).
3. A 24-hour emergency response center that can fax a hard copy of the patient's past airway management database from the MedicAlert file.

WHAT DOES IT COST?

Basically, the membership fee covers the cost of the medical file and MedicAlert emblem. Designer emblem costs vary depending on the type of metal selected (silver, steel, or gold). Also, the patient may have a choice of ordering a bracelet or a necklace. By registering with MedicAlert, the patient receives a medical file, an ID number, and a

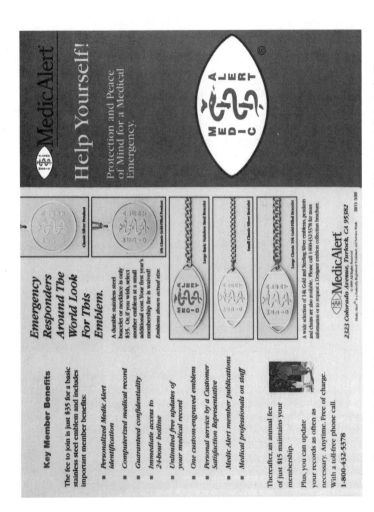

Figure 17–1 Bracelet and necklace selections. (Courtesy of MedicAlert, Turlock, Calif).

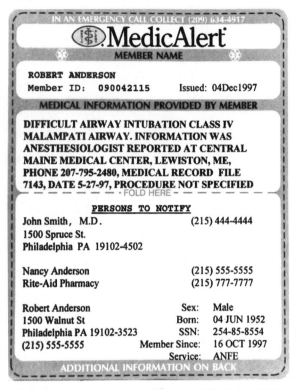

Figure 17–2 Sample record summary. (Courtesy of MedicAlert, Turlock, Calif).

record summary. The annual membership fee is $15, after an initial registration fee of $35 paid the first year. The membership fee includes 24-hour year-round emergency hotline service and unlimited free updating of the patient's computer record. The 24-hour response includes fax transmission of airway management records.

WHY BOTHER WITH MEDICALERT IDENTIFICATION?

Many anesthesiologists feel that detailed information regarding a difficult airway should be both documented on the anesthesia record and discussed with the patient, thus protecting against future airway complications. It must be remembered that patients often forget, and other events such as trauma or shock may prevent the patient from relaying this critical information. Also, an inability to retrieve old records or incomplete records may not allow a future practitioner to benefit from a past practitioner's experience. The greatest benefit of the MedicAlert system may be with the unanticipated difficult airway. Most physicians familiar with airway management develop a "feel" for a potentially

Your Vital Medical Facts
Available Worldwide, 24 Hours a Day

Allergies, medical conditions and medications can all have serious, even deadly, consequences in an emergency.

That's why nearly 2.3 million individuals nationwide have joined Medic Alert — and you should, too.

Medic Alert's logo is recognized by emergency responders around the world. When they see that emblem engraved with your personal ID number and essential medical condition, they call Medic Alert's 24-Hour Emergency Response Center.

We transmit your vital medical facts that help you receive the fast, accurate treatment that could save your life.

Call 1-800-432-5378
and Join Today!

Founded by a physician whose daughter nearly died from an allergic reaction, Medic Alert is a nonprofit membership organization. We are endorsed by leading medical and health organizations nationwide, and nearly 80,000 people across the country credit Medic Alert with helping them survive a medical emergency.

Medic Alert is for _everyone_ who understands the need for fast, accurate information in an emergency.

And it's easy to become a member. Simply call the toll-free number and you can join right over the phone. Or, if you prefer, mail in the attached application.

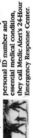

TO JOIN BY PHONE Call 1-800-432-5378 anytime. Please have the following information ready: 1 Credit card number and expiration date; 2 Medical information; 3 Name, telephone number and address of primary physician; name and phone number of emergency contacts; and 4 Bracelet size (when ordering bracelet).

TO JOIN BY MAIL Complete form and mail payment to Medic Alert, 2323 Colorado Ave., Turlock, CA 95382. *Please allow 4-6 weeks to process mail/fax orders, 7-10 working days for phone orders.*

1. **PREVIOUS/CURRENT Medic Alert MEMBER?** ☐ Yes ☐ No

2. **PERSONAL INFORMATION** *(please print or type clearly)*

   ☐ Mr. Last Name   First   Middle   Sex   If Mr., Enter Member Initial:
   ☐ Ms.
   ☐ Mrs.   M F   Social Security Number (optional)

   Mailing Address   Phone   Date of Birth
                                      Area Code (   )   Month Day Year

   City   State   ZIP

   EMERGENCY CONTACTS: As a member benefit, Medic Alert will advise your physician of your emergency events.

   Primary Physician's Phone   Phone   Person 1   Phone
                                               (   )   (   )
   Primary Physician's Address   Person 2   Phone
                                                                                        (   )

3. **TO BE ENGRAVED ON EMBLEM, your essential emergency medical information:** Medical conditions and allergies.
   Names, generic drugs, blood type, etc. Small bracelet: 6 spaces; large bracelet: 58 spaces; Necklace: 29 spaces. Allow one space between words. Do not abbreviate.
   For help, call 1-800-432-5378. Medical professionals are on staff.

4. **TO BE ADDED TO YOUR COMPUTERIZED MEDICAL FILE, these vital medical facts:**
   Additional medical conditions, allergies and medications. Dosage data not needed. Use additional paper if necessary.

   Health Number   Group Plan Number   Insurance Member Number

5. **ANNUAL MEMBER BENEFITS:**
   Membership is only $15 a year. Your first year's membership fee is subject. Your
   membership includes: establishing and maintaining your computerized medical file,
   record summary, and custom engraved emblem and chain. Annual Members also
   receive continued access to our 24-Hour Emergency Response Center, unlimited
   FREE updates to your medical file, member publications and special discounts on
   replacement emblems.

6. **EMBLEM SELECTION:**
   Check the box for your emblem selection, then transfer the cost to the form below:

	LARGE	SMALL	SMALL CHILD'S	COST
METAL/STYLE	NECKLACE	BRACELET	BRACELET	
Classic Stainless Steel	☐	☐	☐	$35.00
Classic Series				
Silver (Rhodium-Plated)	☐	☐	☐ (med only)	$50.00
10K Gold-Filled	☐	☐		$75.00

   "Bracelet Size: Measure your wrist snugly and add 1/2" to allow room for emergency
   personnel to turn the emblem over:
   ☐ 5-1/2" ☐ 5-3/4" ☐ 6-1/4" ☐ 7-1/4" ☐ 8-1/2" ☐ F
   Note: Designer collection sterling silver and 14k gold also available. Call for details.
   (Prices and terms are of SVR, subject to change without notice.)

7. **PAYMENT CALCULATION:**
   Emblem selection cost from above .... $ _____
   Complete Contribution: _____
   Medic Alert is a nonprofit organization that depends on free and
   contributions to support our Emergency Response Center) .... $ _____
   TOTAL AMOUNT ENCLOSED .... $ _____

8. **METHOD OF PAYMENT:**
   ☐ Check. ☐ MasterCard. ☐ VISA. ☐ Discover
   ☐ Money Order   Payment must accompany order.

   Sent to: Medic Alert, 2323 Colorado Ave., Turlock, CA 95382.
   NOTE: Annual Membership Fee after first year only $15.00
   ☐ Each year, please charge my credit card $15.00 to continue my Annual
     Member services.

   FAX it paying by credit card, you may fax this form to: 800-863-3429.
   Credit card number must be included.

   Card
   Number: _____ Exp. Date: _____

   X _____
   9. Signature of Member   Date

   IMPORTANT: When you receive your personalized Medic Alert
   emblem and the copy of your emergency medical file, please check both
   carefully for accuracy and call Medic Alert to report any errors. Also please
   be sure to notify Medic Alert 1-800-432-5378 whenever your physician,
   address, or family/physician information changes. Medic Alert believes that
   the information in your medical file is confidential and should only be
   released if printed or sent to a member's file. By accepting membership in
   Medic Alert, you do authorize Medic Alert to release information in emergencies or to healthcare personnel when you authorize. We welcome you as a
   new member and will do our very best to serve you well.

   3913
   SVR

Figure 17–3 Sample general application. (Courtesy of MedicAlert, Turlock, Calif.)

difficult airway based on standard criteria and experience, but it has been estimated that up to 3% of all patients undergoing anesthesia have unanticipated difficult airways.[4] Knowledge of a successful clinical algorithm in an unanticipated difficult airway may be lifesaving.

WHOM SHOULD I URGE TO JOIN MEDICALERT?

You should consider enrolling *any* patient who requires special techniques for airway management.

HOW DO I ENROLL A PATIENT?

First, get agreement from the patient to become a member of Medic-Alert. A general application form (Fig. 17–3) must be filled out, and information regarding how you managed the difficult airway should be included. The form is given to the patient to mail with the initial fee. Patients who cannot afford a membership can have the fee waived if appropriate documentation is supplied to MedicAlert.

SUMMARY

- Document carefully your airway management algorithm in the patient's chart and on the anesthesia record.
- Discuss with the patient in detail the importance of relaying airway management issues to future caregivers.
- If you used special techniques to secure the airway, consider taking the time to urge the patient to join MedicAlert.
- Follow up with the patient to make sure the patient sent all documentation to the MedicAlert Foundation, 2323 Colorado Avenue, Turlock, CA 95382.

REFERENCES

1. American Society of Anesthesiologists Task Force on Management of the Difficult Airway: Practice guidelines for management of the difficult airway. Anesthesiology 78:597, 1993.
2. Cheney F: American Society of Anesthesiologists, Committee on Professional Liability: Preliminary study of closed claims. ASA Refresher Course Lectures p. 156, October 15–19, 1994, San Francisco.
3. Temple WJ: MedicAlert Foundation International. ASA Newsletter 44:3, 1980.
4. Caplan RA, Posner K, Ward RJ, Cheney W: Adverse respiratory events in anesthesia: A closed claims analysis. Anesthesiology 72:828, 1990.

Index

....

Note: Page numbers in *italics* refer to illustrations;
page numbers followed by (t) refer to tables.